Prostitution and Victorian Social Reform

CROOM HELM SOCIAL HISTORY SERIES

General Editors

PROFESSOR J.F.C. HARRISON and STEPHEN YEO University of Sussex

Prostitution and Victorian Social Reform

Paul McHugh

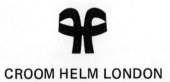

CROOM HELM LONDON

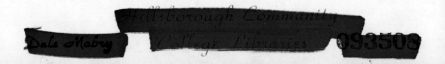

© 1980 Paul McHugh
Croom Helm Ltd, 2-10 St John's Road, London SW11

British Library Cataloguing in Publication Data

McHugh, Paul
    Prostitution and Victorian social reform. –
    (Croom Helm social history series).
    1. Prostitution – England – History –
    19th century 2. Social movements – England
    – History – 19th century
    1. Title
    345'.42'0253   KD8077

    ISBN 0-85664-938-4

Printed and bound in Great Britain by
Redwood Burn Limited
Trowbridge & Esher

CONTENTS

TABLES AND FIGURES

Tables

Figures

ABBREVIATIONS

Most repeal association titles ended with the suffix 'for the repeal of the Contagious Diseases Acts', some with 'for the Abolition of State Regulation of Vice'.

BCGF	British, Continental and General Federation
FA	Friends' Association
LNA	Ladies' National Association
MCEU	Midland Counties Electoral Union
NA	National Association
NCL	Northern Counties League
NMA	National Medical Association
SDL	Subjected Districts League
SNA	Scottish National Association
WMNL	Working Men's National League
EA	Association for Promoting the Extension of the Contagious Diseases Acts
NEL	National Education League
UKA	United Kingdom Alliance
VA	Vigilance Association (for the Defence of Personal Rights)
BL	British Library
EC	Executive Committee
FLB	Fawcett Library (Josephine Butler MSS)
FLW	Fawcett Library (H.J. Wilson MSS)
PP	Parliamentary Papers
PRO	Public Records Office

For Caroline

PREFACE

What makes the historian decide to work on a particular subject? In my case, I fear that I cannot claim that any elevated motive set me on the trail. In the Autumn of 1969, as a new postgraduate student in search of a suitable topic, I decided to read through the then standard work on the period of British history which most interested me — Sir Robert Ensor's *England, 1870–1914.* Upon reaching page 171, promisingly titled 'sex questions', I came across a two paragraph reference to the Contagious Diseases Acts which were then a mystery to me. As a summary of an agitation it aroused my interest, while the glowing tributes to Josephine Butler and James Stansfeld provoked a degree of irreverent scepticism. I was 'hooked'. I cannot remember whether or not I continued to plough on through Ensor, but certainly I have found no other subject which has exercised the same fascination for me as the resurrection of this apparently obscure and forgotten campaign.

Over the years, less opportunistic motives have come to the fore. I speedily abandoned any idea of a Lytton Strachey type demolition of Ensor's hero and heroine. His verdict stands up remarkably well even if he tended to exaggerate the deliberateness of Stansfeld's self sacrifice. Instead, I have tried to go beyond the biographical approach and to breathe some life into the campaign as a whole. I hope that the result is a study which sees the agitation not merely as a contribution to women's history, nor as simply one aspect of a changing moral climate, nor even as a part of the political history of the period, but as a campaign which needs to be assessed in its own right. My aim has been to reach a balanced assessment of the struggle for repeal, looking at Mrs Butler and Stansfeld not as 'makers' of the movement (with all the moral overtones thereby implied) but as pressure group leaders with strengths and weaknesses. In the process I hope that I have brought out the significance of humbler repeal activists more forcefully.

In the course of my research I have incurred numerous debts of gratitude to the staffs of many libraries and archives. To acknowledge all would fill too many pages, but if some may be singled out, I should say that the Bodleian Library was a most congenial place in which to read one's way into the repeal campaign, and that I received a kindly welcome and much assistance at the Library of the Society of Friends and at the Methodist Archives and Research Centre. My chief obligation, however, is to the Fawcett Library where I spent several summers working on repeal material. Its then Librarian, Miss M. Surry ALA, and the archivists were extremely kind in answering my requests. In particular, the library was good enough to grant me access to the Josephine Butler Papers while they were still being arranged. I am most grateful for this privilege, and I should like to extend my thanks to the cataloguer of these papers, Miss M. Burton, for much assistance on Mrs Butler, about whom her knowledge is surely unrivalled. As the arrangement of these papers and of the H.J. Wilson Papers at the Fawcett Library was not completed when I was working on them, some of my references are necessarily provisional, though I have tried to give the fullest possible details in all cases. It is a matter of relief and a cause for celebration that this splendid library, the future of which seemed unclear a few years ago, has now been rehoused intact at the City of London Polytechnic, where scholars receive the same warm welcome as in the old days at Westminster. Professor John Vincent of Bristol University was good enough to set me on the track of the Stansfeld Papers whose present owner, Mr W.J. Stansfeld, readily granted me access. I am indeed grateful to him for doing so, and I should also like to offer my thanks to his brother, Mr A. Stansfeld, for providing me with a copy of a letter from William Lloyd Garrison to James Stansfeld's sister-in-law, Madame Venturi.

This book is the revised version of a doctoral thesis originally submitted to Oxford University. Throughout the period in which I was working on this thesis, I received the greatest stimulus and encouragement from Brian Harrison, the most patient and scrupulous of supervisors. I am most grateful to him for all his kindnesses, which have not lessened since submission of the original thesis. My examiners, Mr M. Shock and Dr R.T. Shannon, in the course of a courteous and pleasant *viva* made a number of suggestions for improvement which I have tried to incorporate into the reworking of the book. I should also like to thank Dr Geoff Eley of Emmanuel College, Cambridge, who kindly agreed to read drafts of both thesis and book; I benefitted greatly from his criticisms. More recently, my colleagues at the Cambridgeshire College of Arts and Technology, Dr Piers Brendon, Mr Michael Murphy and Dr Michael Woodhouse, have been good enough to read and comment on revised chapters. While extremely grateful to all who have helped me in ironing this book into shape, responsibility for all errors and omissions remains mine alone.

Finally, I should like to thank my two expert and conscientious typists: Miss Rosemary Graham most cheerfully shouldered a burden at a difficult time; but to my wife, who typed the major part of the manuscript, my debt obviously extends very much further than words can say.

Paul McHugh
Cambridge

1 INTRODUCTION

One hundred years ago, 18 districts in England and Wales were still subjected to a system of regulated prostitution similar, in essence, to those systems of police-controlled and registered prostitution widely employed throughout continental Europe in the nineteenth century and still, in part, surviving in the twentieth. The United Kingdom's flirtation with regulation lasted only from 1864, when the first of the Contagious Diseases Acts was enacted, to 1886 when the system was abolished. The object had ostensibly been to protect members of the armed forces from the consequences of venereal disease, and the government from the resulting financial penalties and loss of manpower. The method employed was to identify prostitutes and submit them to examination by designated official doctors; if they were found to be diseased they were detained in hospitals for specified periods. To implement the Acts a specialised police force and purpose-built Lock wards were provided.[1]

In the nineteenth century, attitudes to the Acts ran deep. They were defended as examples of progressive sanitary enlightenment, berated as immoral abuses of the constitution. An agitation sprang up to campaign for repeal of the Acts which has recently been called 'one of the century's most notable protest movements'.[2] Certainly the repeal movement recruited an extraordinary variety of campaigners: moralists, feminists, individualists, opponents of medical pretensions and military arrogance were amongst those who found the Acts repugnant, and were prepared to work for their repeal in what were, at first, highly unfavourable circumstances.

However, consideration of the repeal movement has been excessively concerned with its place in the history of women's social and political emancipation.[3] This concentration on the Acts' relationship to women's rights has tended to obscure other equally interesting aspects of the campaign against them. This study will attempt to redress the balance by assessing the campaign's connections with non-feminist agitations, and with wider social and political questions. It will also analyse the movement's internal mechanisms in order to show how a Victorian pressure group operated, and why this particular one eventually succeeded where so many others failed.[4]

Yet this feminist bias is forgivable when one confronts the

assumptions which underpinned the Acts; assumptions memorably en-
capsulated in Keith Thomas's long-standing indictment of the Acts as
the high-water mark of the double standard of sexual morality.[5] The
Acts were based on the premisses that women but not men were responsible for the spread of venereal disease, and that while men would be
degraded if subjected to physical examination, the women who
satisfied male sexual urges were already so degraded that further
indignities scarcely mattered. Protection for males was supposed to be
assured by inspection of females.[6]

Why should these assumptions, grounded in sex discrimination still
to be found today, have borne fruit in the mid nineteenth century?
There are probably two reasons for the Acts' appearance at this
historical juncture.

Firstly, it seems likely that Victorian interest in prostitution, the
'social evil', was at its greatest in the 1850s and 1860s — in 1860, for
example, the *Saturday Review* noted its popularity as a subject for
discussion.[7] Furthermore the bulk of the discussion — in the medical
and weekly press — was in the direction of recognising the inevitability
of prostitution and reaching some accommodation with it. Dr William
Acton had published his *Prostitution* in 1857, an enormously
influential argument for humane treatment of prostitutes associated
with measures to keep them as free from disease as possible. As he
realised, most prostitutes eventually found their way back into the
community at large.[8] Upper-class males would be familiar with the
contemporary debate on the necessity for the prostitute if the pre-
marital virtue of upper-class females was to be preserved; a debate
clinched for many in Lecky's notorious phrase: 'Herself the supreme
type of vice, she is ultimately the most efficient guardian of virtue.'[9]
They would also be familiar with the sight of police-regulated
prostitution in European cities, which kept the streets decent and
apparently offered some protection from disease.[10] The whole discussion was, of course, couched in terms of society's needs being best
served by an authoritarian, albeit enlightened, provision of healthy
prostitutes. Humane concern for the prostitute herself may have
followed from this, but any concession to the notion of these women
as citizens with the right to lead independent lives was notably absent.

Secondly, the Acts can be seen as a response to the supposed
deterioration of health in the armed forces. In the aftermath of the
Crimean War and the invasion scare of the late 1850s, the army and
navy had, for a time, emerged from the neglect with which government
and public opinion alike usually treated them. Reform was in the air,

Royal Commissions exposed inadequacies, and serious fears were voiced about military ineffectiveness caused by the ravages of venereal disease.[11]

Living conditions were still appalling and marriage was restricted by regulation to about 6 per cent of enlisted men. Despite the efforts of philanthropic and religious workers, notably the Wesleyans from the early 1860s, this 'bachelor army' was accustomed to turn to prostitutes, hordes of whom were to be found in dockyard and garrison towns.[12] In 1865 the Inspector-General of Hospitals estimated the prostitute population of the eleven towns under the 1864 Act to be 7,339, of whom 929 were said to be diseased.[13]

Since the climate of upper middle class opinion was so strongly in favour of some form of regulation of prostitution, since the armed forces in particular seemed to be imperilled by venereal disease and since doctors were unable, in practice, to control it effectively given the then state of medical knowledge, some form of legislative onslaught on the 'carriers' of disease (however arbitrary that definition) was increasingly likely. Indeed it possessed almost a logic of its own in the early 1860s.

The reaction against this medico-military consensus was slow in manifesting itself. Not until 1870 did the movement against the Acts get off the ground, and even then amidst tensions and divisions which it will be a primary task of this study to analyse. One such tension was the contest between provincial radicalism, on its way towards the capture of the Liberal party, and the declining force of Metropolitan radicalism, The battle between these two groupings, so crucial to the future shape of British Liberalism, was fought out within the repeal movement. The provincials—Nonconformist, self-assured and convinced of the duplicity of all things metropolitan—eventually came to displace the secular, cosmopolitan, 'old radical' Londoners as prime movers of the agitation.[14]

To some extent, this contrast is reflected in the relationship between the leading personalities in the repeal movement: the charismatic Josephine Butler, the Liberal minister James Stansfeld and H.J. Wilson the Sheffield radical.

Josephine Butler (1828—1906) was first in the field and is normally regarded as the movement's leading light; so much so that brief references to it usually talk of 'Josephine Butler's crusade against the Contagious Diseases Acts'.[15] She came from a branch of the Grey family of Northumberland—her father, John Grey of Dilston, was a scientific farmer, a leading northern Liberal, a strong supporter of his kinsman Earl Grey at the time of the Reform Bill agitation and an anti-slavery

enthusiast. This Whiggish background was a splendid apprenticeship
for a lifetime of philanthropy — even though there was sometimes a
touch of wistful *noblesse oblige* about it, a feeling that she was the
last of her kind. Towards the end of her life she commiserated with
her son about 'the vulgarising influences of the present day, and the
decay of the best traditions through the advance of the money-making
class into all places of influence'.[16]

In 1852 she married George Butler, eldest son of Dr George Butler,
Dean of Peterborough and former headmaster of Harrow. The Butlers
were an academic family (one of George's younger brothers, Montague,
became Master of Trinity College, Cambridge) and George pursued a
predictable career of examining and schoolmastering.[17] After five
years of teaching at Oxford, he became vice-principal of Cheltenham
College where he remained from 1858 until 1866. While at Cheltenham,
the Butlers were struck by personal tragedy — the accidental death in
1864 of their youngest child Eva. Mrs Butler was understandably
prostrated by it, and throughout her life was haunted by the memory
of the child, having fallen down the stairs as she rushed to greet her
parents, dying in her father's arms.[18] The tragedy had two immediate
results: George Butler leapt at the offer of the principalship of
Liverpool College, and once they had moved there early in 1866,
Josephine Butler began to discover in philanthropy the solace for her
own grief — as she said, 'it was not difficult to find misery in
Liverpool'.[19] She began visiting the oakum sheds of the Brownlow
Hill Workhouse where she was confronted by the wretchedness of
destitute women. Moved by this, she founded first a house of rest, and
later an industrial home; she even took dying prostitutes into her own
home.[20] Subsequently she went on to champion women's education,
becoming president of the North of England Council for Promoting
the Higher Education of Women. She was also acutely aware of the
need to extend employment opportunities for women; and in correspondence with her friend Albert Rutson and with the positivist
Frederic Harrison, she angrily pointed out the connection between
unemployment and prostitution.[21] In 1869 she edited and introduced
a collection of essays, *Woman's Work and Woman's Culture*, which
served to emphasise the link between her two interests.[22]

Until 1869 Mrs Butler was thus a conventional advocate of women's
rights (though this is in itself remarkable enough), broader-minded than
most women of the day, more courageous in her personal espousal of
the cause of suffering women, but not yet offering any challenge to a
male-dominated society. That was to come when she took up repeal.
In all this, she was loyally supported by her husband, whose career
suffered as a result of his wife's activities. As a public school Head,

George Butler was initially a great success and his breadth of interests
make him one of the nineteenth century's more progressive headmasters,
but besides this, he also sustained Josephine in work which was from
that expected of a Head's wife.[23] The strain was great, and the last years
of his headmastership were unhappy; he was at odds with his directors
and his grip on the school faltered.[24] By 1877 the Butlers wanted to
retire, but were prevented by lack of alternative income; indeed
financial worries added to the strain. Mrs Butler's correspondence is
full of references to their grave problems: raising three boys on an
income which fluctuated with the College's roll, the need to maintain
an office on erratically provided funds from repeal bodies and the
temptation, which she was seldom able to resist, of plunging into her
own pocket to keep repeal work going — on occasions her bank
balance fell to 6d.[25]

All this had a crippling effect on her life. She sold her jewels to raise
funds, she begged money from wealthier repealers. Their response was
generous. Indeed two funds were raised to help the Butlers, the second
of which, in 1882, was originally designed to enable George to retire —
when he received a canonry at Winchester it was diverted to provide
Josephine with an annuity of £200 per annum.[26] Nevertheless,
shortage of money was always a difficulty, and she overworked herself in order to surmount it. The result, inevitably, was illness. Sometimes as in 1875, severe and prolonged illness made worse by the knowledge that convalescence was but an interlude 'and as soon as people
know I have got home, they call all day, and claims thicken and gather'.[27]
All this simply intensified her inner compulsion to identify through
shared suffering with the women she was helping. She told Rutson in 1868
that she was kept awake at night by visions of starving women: 'it is
difficult for friends to believe how my spirit can be darkened . . . until
it ends in an illness like this and my bodily sight is darkened too'. In
1876 she explained to a repealer that her breakdown in the previous
year had been partly caused by the outrages seen in Paris when visiting
hospitals for prostitutes.[28] This is some measure of the pain and sacrifice
which deep commitment to repeal involved for her and her family. Her
role in the movement will be discussed as part of the general analysis
of its progress and methods; but perhaps it is worth pausing here to
indicate those contributions which seem most significant.

First there is the insistence on a specifically female perspective;
Josephine Butler mobilised respectable middle-class women in the
defence of their working-class sisters, and her Ladies' National
Association (LNA) upheld the human rights of the prostitute, even

while disapproving of her occupation and knowing little of her
problems. However, Mrs Butler's philanthropic work meant that she
was better informed than her followers about prostitution, which
she saw as a social, not a sexual, problem:

> for the lessening of this enormous evil it needs only that men of
> education should apply themselves earnestly to the much neglected
> subject of social economy; for this is not a question of natural
> vice nearly so much as one of political and social economy.[29]

But while she demanded equality of treatment with men, she also
insisted that the struggle was one for higher moral standards. She was
horrified by the way the Acts deprived women of a sense of shame;
and found it abhorrent that prostitutes should be induced to welcome
the Acts because of slightly improved conditions.[30] Men, she declared,
could never really understand this argument, and so: 'it is to women
therefore that we must chiefly look for the initiative in fresh acts of
aggression against the conventional and accepted standard in society
concerning sexual morality.'[31] Moderate repealers stood little chance
against this sort of determination. She was amused to find that her
occasional appearances at meetings of the London-based National
Association for Repeal (NA) caused a storm;[32] but, unlike them, she
consistently urged an uncompromising attitude towards regulation,
which caused grave tactical problems, although it eventually became
the movement's orthodoxy. Women repealers saw their involvement in
militant terms, as 'a call to battle' and she called it 'a revolt against
and an aggressive opposition to a gross political and illegal tyranny'.[33]

The novelty of angry women made them all the more difficult to
deal with, and their strength of commitment proved a worthy counterweight to the other side's official support.[34] Here again, Josephine
Butler's personal contribution was crucial; her oratory attracted huge
crowds and she clearly possessed the power to move audiences. She
could inspire women to hold firm to a difficult cause: 'My one gift,
if I have one, is to breathe a little fire or courage into *individual*
workers.'[35] Nor were men untouched by her spell; the Regius
Professor of Divinity at Oxford commented that: 'Men could never
be the same again after they had seen and known Josephine Butler.
A new sense of what passionate pity could mean was brought home
to them.'[36] Reform movements usually prosper with charismatic
leaders and Mrs Butler was just this; her letters are dominated by
her belief in the superiority of voluntary action, she despised the

meddling state, and tirelessly invoked the deity to underline the excellence of individual endeavour. Strength of personality swept others along with her.

There remains the question of her judgement, and here opinions differ. She could be infuriatingly obtuse about political realities, and like most reformers she always affected to see her 'cause' as the most pressing matter in politics. What is one to make of this statement uttered in February 1879? — 'I hope there is no chance of this horrid Zulu War occupying all the evenings for debate and putting off this question and others.'[37] On occasions she permitted zeal and strength of conviction to carry her away, as with her notorious evidence to the Royal Commission in 1871. Yet her strategic judgement was, in general, very good — certainly far better than anything her followers displayed. She saw the need for a clear, undivided objective, and held to it whatever the tactical cost. She was an early advocate of working-class involvement in the campaign, she always stressed the need for work in the subjected districts themselves (although repeal strength was elsewhere) and towards the end of the campaign, she saw the need for the support of the Liberal party.

These are major contributions — sufficient in themselves to explain why her name has become synonymous with the repeal campaign. She had obvious failings: the darker side of inspiration was a tendency to hysteria; her determination to promote her agitation as vigorously as possible could be counter-productive, for instance, her hounding of Gladstone in the early 1870s; she admitted that she lacked organising ability (though in fact she did not do too badly); and in a way she lacked application — she tended to get agitations going and then move on to more thrilling projects. These are, however, minor objections when judged in the context of her overall significance for repeal.[38]

Josephine Butler was an incongruous leader for the repeal movement, as it eventually developed. She fitted comfortably into the 'intellectual aristocracy' with her Cambridge/public school/Anglican connections while her followers were characterised more by nonestablishment, nonconformist family ties. Similarly, James Stansfeld (1820—98) stood out from the mass of repealers — a Liberal frontbencher and private brewer in a movement of provincial temperance enthusiasts.[39] Stansfeld can also be cited as a metropolitan radical for most purposes. True, he was born into an old Unitarian family in Halifax, and represented the borough in parliament from 1859 until 1895; but after taking his degree at University College London

(debarred from Oxford and Cambridge by religious tests) he married one
of the daughters of the distinguished radical solicitor, William Ashurst.
In doing so, he married into London radicalism; the Ashursts were
friendly towards all Europe's subject peoples, and were particularly
devoted Mazzinians. Another Ashurst daughter, Emilie, married Major
Carlo Venturi, a Garibaldian adventurer. Through them, Stansfeld
came to know and value the friendship of Giuseppe Mazzini who
was often a visitor to his home in the 1850s and 1860s.[40]

Stansfeld was thus a representative of cosmopolitan, mid-century
Liberalism. He was interested in foreign affairs, and, like all staunch
radicals, wedded to the concept of a united Italy, with Mazzini and
Garibaldi as his heroes. The contrast with the narrow radicalism of
provincial England later in the century is only too plain. In parliament
he was a representative radical and an advocate of political economy —
for which reasons he was propelled into office by Palmerston in 1863.[41]
He was a capable administrator, fiercely interested in economy, and
further promotion would have been his without difficulty had he not
felt obliged to resign over the Greco affair in April 1864; he was in-
directly implicated in a scandal concerning an attempt on Napoleon
III's life via letters which had been addressed to Mazzini (using a
pseudonym) at Stansfeld's London home. This momentarily retarded
his progress, but he was back in office in 1866 and by 1871 had
entered the Cabinet as President of the Poor Law Board. His
reputation stood fairly high at that stage; he was one of the most
prominent radicals in parliament and one of the few who was clearly
front-bench material; the Mazzini episode had been forgotten except
in so far as it proved him to be, in Joseph Cowen's words, 'the man
who stands by his friends'. If not seen as a statesman, Stansfeld was at
least regarded as a serious politician.

Both Stansfeld and Mrs Butler had been successfully active in
public life before their involvement in the repeal campaign; neither
were 'created' by it, nor were they single-issue partisans. Mrs Butler
had been working for other women's rights issues and continued
doing so to a reduced extent; Stansfeld championed Italy, was a
Poor Law reformer and was also a firm supporter of suffrage and
medical education for women. Yet their historical reputations surely
rest on their work in this movement rather than any other. Repeal
rescues Stansfeld from being simply another forgotten Victorian
minister. It rescues Mrs Butler from being one more nineteenth-century
advocate of middle-class women's rights.

The conventional wisdom is that Mrs Butler provided the moral

leadership and Stansfeld the parliamentary ability. This is a fair judgement, in no great need of harsh revision — the verdict of contemporaries
will, broadly speaking, stand firm; but the picture needs to be sharpened,
and the claims of others deserve consideration.

Henry Wilson of Sheffield, the movement's workhorse, has clearly
been neglected in comparison with Mrs Butler and Stansfeld. This is
no more than a reflection of the fact that the history of the organisation
of repeal has been similarly neglected — for Wilson was above all the
'organisation man'.[42] His papers, well arranged and neatly docketed by
his private office, tell the story of the creation of a Victorian pressure
group; they also throw light on the nature of provincial radicalism of
which Wilson has been cited as the exemplar.[43] Indeed, it can be argued
that in the drive to convince the Liberal party of the necessity for
repeal, Wilson's devoted cultivation of contacts within the National
Liberal Federation was just as important as the contribution of the
better known leaders.[44] Of the leaders, it is he who came nearest to
catching the style of the rank and file repealer. Investigation of the
techniques and priorities of Wilson and his kind makes it possible to
delve beneath the great names and free the history of the campaign
from the biographical approach which has dominated it.[45] For while
the leaders of the agitation are of interest, so too are their followers,
their employees and their societies. Reformers and their organisations
as such need to be examined — all the more so given the nature of their
cause.

Indeed, it was a complex, and for that reason an exceptionally
interesting, cause; not only because of its relationship to the political
world of radicalism, but also for the very large number of associated
issues upon which it impinged. While these will be further discussed
at a later stage, they will be briefly considered now, in order to locate
the Acts in a more secure historical context.

One aspect of the Acts which the usual feminist-progressive treatment of them has tended to obscure is their place in the movement
towards preventive medicine. Excessive attention to them as a defeated
species of reactionary, libertinist, sexual politics has blinded many
historians to the fact that they can quite plausibly be seen in terms of
the interventionist public health legislation advocated by Chadwickian
officials and medical reformers.[46] Sir John Pakington, one of the
sponsors of the 1864 Bill and a leading defender of the Acts (he sat
on all the Commons committees which considered them up to his
electoral defeat in 1874, and was a member of the 1870—1 Royal
Commission) was a prominent Tory social reformer. He secured the

appointment of the Newcastle Commission on popular education in 1858, carried measures on beer houses and juvenile offenders in the 1840s, and compulsory vaccination in 1853.[47] He was no reactionary rake; nor were the leaders of the medical profession, nor the departmental civil servants who supported the Acts. Rather, here were pragmatic reformers confronted by an undeniable evil, testing an answer by temporary legislation (the 1864 Act), finding that it contained the seeds of a solution and therefore urging improvement and extension to the whole country much as they had pressed the advisability of setting up local Boards of Health.

The three enquiries into the Acts in the 1860s saw confident doctors pressing for extension, and working to create a climate of opinion which would make this possible. They believed, too confidently as it turned out, that they had the answer to venereal disease, and the growing respect for their profession almost brought them success. But not everybody was willing to go along with this growth of medical authority, nor were provincial doctors necessarily willing to follow the leaders of the profession in their enthusiasm for regulation. Repealers detected medical arrogance behind bland claims for the Acts and they mistrusted the influence over legislation which doctors were seeking. Josephine Butler talked about a 'superstitious reliance on medical opinion among the upper classes from the Queen down to MPs' and even questioned their integrity — it was a fight for women's bodies:

> If these doctors could be forced to keep their hateful hands off us, there would be *an end* to laws which protect vice, and to many other evils; for this indecent outrage is surrounded and connected on every side with fraud and lustful purpose.[48]

She was extreme in her dislike of male doctors, but repealers in general can be seen as part of a libertarian reaction against medical expertise; this, combined with their mistrust of intervention, makes them representative of a certain sort of late Victorian radicalism — seen also in the movements against vivisection and the Vaccination Acts.[49]

This leads us to those who opposed the Acts because they gave additional powers to the state; in parliament MPs such as the Tory, J.W. Henley, or the radical A.S. Ayrton, combatted the interventionism inherent in the Acts; outside parliament anti-state zealots championed repeal as a means of furthering their wider aims.[50] Josephine Butler consistently preached the superior merits of local voluntary action which government intervention could only sap; she took the view that moral behaviour was, in any case, not a proper area of government activity, and she warned about the perils of centralisation: 'you find no municipal spirit where the government have petted the people. They have grown unmanly, and they do not understand what municipal feeling is'.[51] Hostility to the state was one of the commonest repeal characteristics — as one of its leaders in parliament argued:

> the centralising, despotic, reforming state is not my idea of what a State ought to be, I like local influence and local good to be brought about by local people, and not either by the Home Secretary or the War Minister.[52]

Repealers could thus represent the Acts as offences against conscience and freedom—an argument vividly put to the Royal Commission on the Acts by John Stuart Mill — and as attacks on English liberty and the constitution.[53]

All of this could be set into a general attack on a corrupt governing class; dislike of 'lustful' and 'aristocratic' doctors led naturally to suspicion of the upper classes generally; *they* dominated parliament and the officer corps, *they* possessed the reputation for libertinism. Against them, repealers gratefully noted the sturdy morality of ordinary people. As a moderate repealer said:

> Our cause is never so safe as when it is in the hands of the working classes . . . a phalanx of very powerful officials are leagued together to thwart and defeat us . . . a host of specialists and of pseudo-scientists, and perhaps a majority of the officers of the army and navy, and we know not how many peers and potentates are amongst our foes.[54]

This is a classic exposition of the view that radical politics was a matter of waging war on a metropolitan elite; worldly, well represented in parliament and the professions and with advantageous aristocratic connections. Thus when Lord Charles Beresford gave notice of a motion on the Contagious Diseases Acts in 1875, the *Shield* commented: 'As there is nothing in the antecedents of his lordship to induce any hope that he intends to move a resolution in support of repeal, it will be wise to assume that the resolution will be hostile.'[55] The resolution came to nothing, but the *Shield*'s suspicions were later confirmed in the lobbies. This aristocratic coalition was well known to reformers.

Identified by the men of the anti-Corn Law League, it entered the
demonology of most subsequent agitations.

The impact which the Acts had on the armed forces has usually been
considered in a purely medical sense. But to consider thus is to endorse
the contemporary view that the ordinary soldier or sailor was a
depraved creature to be segregated from society, requiring special
discipline and 'social arrangements'.[56] Of all neglected aspects of the
agitation, this one will receive least attention in this study, but one
suggestion can surely be advanced.

It is possible to see the Acts as the end of a tradition which did seek
to cater for the needs of a mercenary soldiery. With Cardwell's
reforms, the growth of the volunteer movement, and the appearance of
a radical interest in the condition of the forces (exemplified not only
by the repeal campaign, but also by the struggle to abolish flogging),
the army and navy were, in a sense, becoming civilianised.[57] That is to
say, enlistment was no longer a disgrace, soldiers and sailors were
beginning to be seen as citizens in uniform rather than society's cast-
offs, and ferocious measures like the Contagious Diseases Acts,
appropriate to a half-wild and despised army, were no longer acceptable.
In short, just as conventional morality was changing, so too was the
expectation of military behaviour; the two combined to render the
Acts less publicly desirable. Research into attitudes to the Acts among
officers and men is needed to test this; the revival of interest in
regulation in wartime suggests that it is not unpopular among the
military. However, this study of the civilian campaign against the Acts
goes no further in plumbing the reaction of the Victorian armed
services to them.[58]

The basis of the repeal case was a deep belief in the immoral nature
of the Acts. Repealers approached the statistical side of the argument
with evident reluctance — Josephine Butler was indifferent to the
results of the Acts — but they felt obliged to challenge inflated claims
for the Acts' success, even while despising the whole business. Their
real triumph lay in forcing their choice of battlefield upon the enemy.
Where regulationists had once been satisfied with proofs that the Acts
diminished disease, they were eventually obliged to claim that
prostitutes were reclaimed by their agency. However, the brutalising
nature, the hardening effect of the Acts, above all, the open acceptance
and encouragement of vice, enabled repealers to dismiss this sort of
argument as belated cosmetic. They could easily dip into evidence
given to enquiries held before their agitation began, and come up with
innumerable rash statements demonstrating lack of concern for

prostitutes, even frank avowals of the need for legalisation of prostitution.[59] Repealers in contrast trumpeted their own consistency and ceaselessly preached their attachment to principle. Nor were they above attributing such obviously evil legislation to faults in the national character, Josephine Butler combined mistrust of the immoral French with topicality when in 1871 she warned:

> the attempt to regulate vice in this matter is so impious, that, if continued, I expect it will sooner or later draw down the judgements of heaven upon our country, as they have been drawn upon France.[60]

Moral decay was in the air which made fidelity to principle all the more important. It was no business of repealers to offer palliatives to vice: tidying up evil was what regulationists were aiming for — repeal's job was to defeat it.

Victorian agitations making moral claims, usually called in religion to legitimise their activities; so it was with repeal. Indeed religious support was crucial, given the murky nature of the subject matter.[61] Regulationists were denounced as hypocrites and reprobates, and repeal statements were inevitably couched in religiose terms; this was Mrs Butler's strength — she could be made physically ill 'to see those men [MPs] pleading for wickedness in such an exalted tone and in the name of Jesus', and she stressed the power of prayer as a means of rallying 'God's servants'.[62] Underpinned by this sort of spiritual decisiveness, repealers were helped to weather the first difficult years. But as a parade of public morality became more essential in politics, so the stridency and consistency with which they had proclaimed their monopoly of virtue over the years, stood them in good stead. By the 1880s, with strong nonconformist support, the repeal movement was freed from any earlier stigma and in the mainstream of radical politics. This remarkable shift illustrates the importance, in a period when society's attitude was changing, of building one's strategy around an immovably high moral standard and enlisting the support of religion to emphasise the validity of this stance.[63]

Yet if the repeal movement was an important part of this effort to raise moral standards, it also found itself eclipsed in the 1880s by a vigorous social purity movement which abandoned appeals to conscience and libertarian beliefs in favour of a coercive philosophy. While the National Vigilance Association (NVA) may well have inherited much of the support which had earlier gone to repeal, it jettisoned sympathy for the victim and concern for individual rights in favour of a wild and often undiscriminating repressive policy which has had enormous influence in shaping our view of attitudes towards morality and sexuality in the late nineteenth century.[64] It is important to be clear that the repeal campaign may have helped to contribute to the creation of such attitudes, may indeed be seen as the initiator of the social purity 'wave' of the 1880s, but also contained elements of humane concern and prickly individualism which differentiate it from the excesses of W.A. Coote and Mrs Ormiston Chant.[65]

Thus the repeal movement spans a crucial period and, in doing so, almost turns full circle. From combatting officially sanctioned prostitution in the 1860s, to seeing its heirs attempting to drive prostitutes from their traditional haunts in the 1890s; from resistance to 'aristocratic' legislation to the promotion, perhaps inadvertently, of a repressive attitude which drove Winston Churchill, a cadet of one noble house, to boisterous but illegal protest, and Lord Arthur Somerset, a cadet of another, into humiliating exile. The controversy surrounding the CD Acts raised important issues; the campaign against the Acts recruited supporters experienced in reform activity. By analysing the structure of the repeal movement during its 16-year progress to victory, this study will shed more light on the half-hidden army of Victorian reformers and their subculture of principled negative protest. It will have much to say about their conception of pressure-group strategy, their tactics and perception of the importance of good judgement and leadership, and of course the place of ideals and principles, for some an end in themselves, in the achievement of repeal.

Notes

1. See below, chapter 2, for further details of the provisions of each of the Acts. This is merely an introductory working definition of *aims* and *methods*. It ignores, for the moment, a whole range of ethical and practical considerations, and the embroidery of the argument by regulationists and repealers during the campaign. For regulation in Europe see Sheldon Amos, *Laws for the Regulation of Vice* (1877); Richard J. Evans, 'Prostitution, State and Society in Imperial Germany', *Past and Present* 70 (1976), pp. 106-29; Theodore Zeldin, *France 1848–1945*, 1 (Oxford 1973), pp. 303–10.

2. Edward J. Bristow, *Vice and Vigilance: Purity movements in Britain Since 1700* (Dublin, 1978), p. 5. Bristow's discussion of the campaign (pp. 75–85) relies too greatly on committed writers, and so tends to accept their view of the strength, success and wisdom of the campaign. Like most historians, he attributes to Josephine Butler the success of the campaign, at the cost of ignoring her less charismatic fellow-workers.

3. Feminist history has traditionally favoured the 'saints and martyrs' approach in which Josephine Butler is inevitably cast as heroine. See, for instance: Ray Strachey, *The Cause: A Short History of the Women's Movement in Great Britain* (1928); Millicent Garrett Fawcett, *What I Remember* (1924). The most recent semi-official history of the women's movement deals with the CD Acts campaign in a wholly biographical manner: Josephine Kamm, *Rapiers and Battleaxes: The Women's Movement and Its Aftermath* (1966), pp. 112–26. Marion Ramelson imposed a new interpretation on the standard material, which at least redressed the then usual middle-class bias of women's history, but did nothing to prove its point in 'The Fight Against the Contagious Diseases Acts', *Marxism Today* (June 1964); *The Petticoat Rebellion* (1967), chs. 10 and 11. Constance Rover, *Love, Morals and the Feminists* (1970), pp. 71–96, provides a brief sketch of a rather old-fashioned sort. There has been no rush of radical historians towards the repeal campaign in response to Sheila Rowbotham's call: 'an oppressed group . . . must project its own image onto history, In order to discover its own identity as distinct from the oppressor it has to become visible to itself.' (*Women's Consciousness, Man's World* (1973), p. 27). Nor does she herself manage to do more than raise the issue in her stimulating reinterpretation of women's history: *Hidden from History: 300 Years of Women's Oppression and the Fight Against It* (1973), pp. 52–3.

4. There are three illuminating recent approaches to the Acts: F.B. Smith, 'Ethics and Disease in the Later Nineteenth Century: The Contagious Diseases Acts', *Historical Studies* (University of Melbourne) 15 (1971), pp. 118–35; Jean L'Esperance, 'The Work of the Ladies' National Association for the Repeal of the Contagious Diseases Acts', *Bulletin of the Society for the Study of Labour History*, 26 (1973), pp. 13–16; J.R. Walkowitz, ' "We are not beasts of the field"; Prostitution and the Campaign Against the Contagious Diseases Acts, 1869–1886' (unpublished PhD thesis, Rochester University, 1974).

5. Keith Thomas, 'The Double Standard', *Journal of the History of Ideas*, 20 (1959), p. 199, an important contribution to discussion of the Acts.

6. See the *Shield* (the journal of the repeal movement) Mar. 1873, pp. 73–4, for a well reasoned leader on the assumptions underying the Acts. See also Alison Neilans, 'Changes in Sex Morality' in Ray Strachey (ed.), *Our Freedom and Its Results* (1936).

7. *Saturday Review*, 6 Oct. 1860, quoted in H.R.E. Ware, 'The Recruitment, Regulation and Role of Prostituion in Britain from the Middle of the Nineteenth Century to the Present Day' (unpblished PhD thesis, London University, 1969), p. 46. Dr Ware's comprehensive thesis is an essential starting point for anyone interested in nineteenth-century prostitution. See also J.R. Walkowitz, ' "We are not beasts of the field" ', chs. 1 and 2; E. Bristow, *Vice and Vigilance*, chs. 1–3 for more general background.

8. William Acton, *Prostitution, Considered in Its Moral, Social and Sanitary Aspects in London and Other Large Cities: With Proposals for the Mitigation and Prevention of Its Attendant Evils* (1st edn (1857). I have used the abridged Fitzroy edition (ed. Peter Fryer, 1968) of the second edition (1870). For Acton, see Fryer's introduction, and Steven Marcus, *The Other Victorians* (New York, 1966) ch. 1. Patricia Branca, *Women in Europe Since 1750* (1978), pp. 21–2 tends to disagree with Acton's view, and pictures prostitution as a desperate descent.

9. W.E.H. Lecky, *History of European Morals from Augustus to Charlemagne* (1869), 10th edn, 2 (1892), p. 283; for the debate in the 1850s and 1860s see E.M. Sigsworth and T.J. Wyke, 'A Study of Victorian Prostitution and Venereal Disease' in M. Vicinus (ed.), *Suffer and Be Still* (Bloomington, 1972), pp. 85–9.

10. If they were unfamiliar, Acton came to the rescue with an excellent

chapter on regulation abroad, which Fryer unfortunately abridges drastically.

11. For the navy in this period see Eugene L. Rasor, *Reform in the Royal Navy: A Social History of the Lower Deck, 1850–1880* (Hamden, 1976); for the army see, A. Ramsay Skelley, *The Victorian Army at Home: The Recruitment and Terms and Conditions of the British Regular, 1859–1899* (1977), pp. 21–84; and for its relationship to society see G. Harries-Jenkins, *The Army in Victorian Society* (1977), pp. 5–6.

12. Sigsworth and Wyke, ' A Study of Victorian Prostitution', is the best general survey of conditions in relation to VD. For conditions in two towns see J.R. and D.J. Walkowitz, ' "We are not beasts of the field": Prostitution and the poor in Plymouth and Southampton under the Contagious Diseases Acts', *Feminist Studies* (1974), pp. 73–106.

13. *Report of the Committee appointed to enquire into the pathology and treatment of Venereal Disease with the view to diminish its injurious effects on the men of the Army and Navy*, PP 1867–68 (4031), xxxvii, 425 Q6577; see also Q6749 (Supt. Guy).

14. For the changes within Liberalism see, John Vincent, *The Formation of the British Liberal Party 1857–1866* (1966, Penguin edn 1972), pp. 65–76; T.W. Heyck, 'British Radicals and Radicalism, 1874–1895: A Social Analysis' in R.J. Bezucha (ed.), *Modern European Social History* (1972), pp. 23–58; D.A. Hamer, *Liberal Politics in the Age of Gladstone and Rosebery* (Oxford 1972), chs. 1 and 2. For metropolitan radicalism see H.J. Hanham, *Elections and Party Management: Politics in the Time of Disraeli and Gladstone* (1959), pp. 138–40, 244–5; Brian Harrison, 'The Sunday Trading Riots of 1855', *Historical Journal*, 8 (1965), pp. 219–45; Gareth Stedman Jones, 'Working-class Culture and Working-class Politics in London, 1870–1900', *Journal of Social History*, 7 (1974), pp. 460–508, esp. pp. 464–6. The tension within reform movements is not difficult to uncover – even the Band of Hope was affected. See Lillian L. Shiman, 'The Band of Hope Movement: Respectable Recreation for Working-class Children', *Victorian Studies*, 17 (1973–4), pp. 49–74, esp. pp. 63–4.

15. Josephine Butler published two highly personal though not always accurate memoirs: *Recollections of George Butler* (Bristol *c.* 1893); *Personal Reminiscences of a Great Crusade* (1896). No recent biography is really satisfactory: A.S.G. Butler, *Portrait of Josephine Butler* (1954), is an attractive memoir by her grandson; E. Moberly Bell, *Josephine Butler, Flame of Fire* (1962), makes little effective use of her letters while rehashing her own works; Glen Petrie, *A Singular Iniquity: The Campaigns of Josephine Butler* (1971), adds nothing significant. Mrs. Butler tried to prevent biographies of herself: 'I hate the very appearance of egotism, I feel almost a *disgust* of speaking of myself.' Fortunately her pleas to correspondents to destroy her letters were often disobeyed, and a substantial archive remains. The largest collection is at the Fawcett Library, City of London Polytechnic (hereafter referred to as FLB) – it contains *inter alia* a letter refusing to write her autobiography for W.T. Stead, from which the above quotation is taken. An interesting collection of letters written to members of her family was deposited in Liverpool University Library by her grandson, A.S.G. Butler; and there are 24 letters from Mrs Butler in the Brotherton Library, Leeds (I have consulted photocopies of these at the Fawcett Library).

16. Liverpool University Library (Butler MSS) MS 8.4(3): Josephine Bulter to A.S. Butler, 12 Dec. 1896.

17. See Noel Annan, 'The Intellectual Aristocracy' in J.H. Plumb (ed.), *Studies in Social History* (1955) for the Butlers and their many connections.

18. Liverpool University Library (Butler MSS) MS 8.4(3): Josephine Butler to A.S. Butler, 3 June 1891.

19. See Butler, *Recollections*, pp. 182–3 for her own account of her espousal of voluntary work as therapy.

20. FLB 3010: a remarkable collection of copies of letters written by Josephine Butler in 1867; she describes her work in detail and reveals a deep concern for the fate of individual women, and a feeling of shared suffering.

21. FLB 3019: Josephine Butler to A. Rutson, 7 May 1868; 3020: Josephine Butler to F. Harrison, 9 May 1868; 3022: Josephine Butler to A. Rutson, 12 May 1868.

22. See also Margaret Simey, *Charitable Effort in Liverpool in the Nineteenth Century* (Liverpool, 1951), pp. 57–62, 74–80, for Mrs Butler's work in Liverpool, 1866–9.

23. See T.W. Bamford, *The Rise of the Public Schools* (1967), pp. 135, 248; D. Wainwright, *Liverpool Gentlemen* (1960), pp. 124–6.

24. Wainwright, *Liverpool Gentlemen*, pp. 146–54; H.J. Wilson Papers (at the Fawcett Library, City of London Polytechnic, hereafter FLW) Box 78 letter 620: J.E. Ellis to H.J. Wilson, 22 Feb. 1883, giving his (and James Stuart's) adverse opinion of George Butler at Liverpool College.

25. FLB 3884: Josephine Butler to Mrs Clark, 29 Apr. 1877; FLB 3909: Josephine Butler to Mrs Clark, 9 Oct. 1879; FLB: Josephine Butler to H.J. Wilson, 22 Apr. 1875; FLB 5108: Josephine Butler to Mrs Ford, 27 Dec. (1880?).

26. FLB 3922, 3923: correspondence relating to the 'Butler Fund', 1882. The operation was carried out very tactfully by two men of otherwise abrasive personality, R.F. Martineau of Birmingham and H.J. Wilson.

27. FLB 3707: Josephine Butler to H.J. Wilson, 25 July 1875.

28. FLB 3023: Josephine Butler to A. Rutson, 22 May 1868; 3858: Josephine Butler to Joseph Edmondson *c.* Feb. 1876.

29. FLB 3020: Josephine Butler to Frederic Harrison, 9 May 1868; see also her excellent *Paper on the Moral Reclaimability of Prostitutes* (1870).

30. FLW Box 82 letter 13: Josephine Butler to H.C.E. Childers, 12 Feb. 1873 (copy).

31. Josephine Butler, *Some Thoughts on the Present Aspect of the Crusade Against the State Regulation of Vice* (Liverpool, 1874).

32. FLB 3242: Josephine Butler to H.J. Wilson, 26 Feb. 1873.

33. Liverpool University Library (Butler MSS) MS 8.4(2): Josephine Butler to her grandchildren (n.d., probably 1890s).

34. See below chapter 6, for further comments on the LNA's activities; for other assessments of the significance of women's involvement see F.B. Smith, 'Sexuality in Britain, 1800–1900', *University of Newcastle (NSW) Historical Journal*, 2 (1974), pp. 30–1; Kathleen E. McCrone, 'The Assertion of Women's Rights in Mid-Victorian England', *Historical Papers (Canadian Historical Association)* (1972), p. 50; E. Bristow, *Vice and Vigilance*, p. 62.

35. FLB 3187: Josephine Butler to H.J. Wilson, *c.* Sept. 1872.

36. Bristow, *Vice and Vigilance*, p. 76, citing Henry Scott Holland.

37. H. Ausubel, *In Hard Times: Reformers Among the Late Victorians* (New York, 1960), p. 71.

38. The best modern evaluation of Mrs Butler is, Brian Harrison, 'Josephine Butler' in J.F.C. Harrison, B. Taylor and I. Armstrong (eds.), *Eminently Victorian* (1974).

39. There is a good biography of Stansfeld by J.L. and B. Hammond, *James Stansfeld: A Victorian Champion of Sex Equality* (1932). Stansfeld's contribution to the repeal movement is assessed below, chapter 4, p. 91; chapter 8, p. 206; see chapter 9, p. 248; for his position as a brewer.

40. *Review of Reviews*, 15 June 1895, pp. 504–21, published a character

sketch of Stansfeld, then on the point of retiring from parliament; it lays
particular emphasis on his advocacy of Mazzini. For the Italophile milieu of mid-
nineteenth-century London see, Derek Beales, *England and Italy, 1859–1860*
(1961).

41. Vincent, *Formation of the British Liberal Party*, p. 55; for Stansfeld's
important role as a mediator between labour and the Liberal party see, Royden
Harrison, *Before the Socialists: Studies in Labour and Politics, 1861–1881*
(1965), chapter 4.

42. Wilson's background and contribution to repeal is discussed below, chapter
4, p. 77.

43. T.W. Heyck, *The Dimensions of British Radicalism: The Case of Ireland,
1874–1895* (1974), pp. 9–10. Wilson's papers were divided into three parts
after his death and deposited separately. For the study of the repeal campaign, the
best collection is that preserved at the Fawcett Library. The other collections are
in the Sheffield Central Library and the Sheffield University Library. Wilson kept
everything, and despite the temptation to the historian of attaching undue
weight to those whose papers survive, Wilson's do show him to have been an
activist and organiser of the first order.

44. A point developed further in chapter 8, below.

45. D.A. Hamer, *The Politics of Electoral Pressure: A Study in the History
of Victorian Reform Agitations* (Hassocks 1977), provides this sort of approach
for one aspect (electoral) of pressure group activity, but unfortunately has little
to say about the Contagious Diseases Acts.

46. Historians not thus blinded include F.B. Smith, 'Ethics and Disease',
pp. 118–25, and W.L. Burn, *The Age of Equipoise, A Study of the Mid-Victorian
Generation* (1964), pp. 158–60. See below chapter 3, p. 59, for precisely this
argument being advanced by Lyon Playfair. The debate on the nature of intervention is usefully summarised by Valerie Cromwell, 'Interpretations of Nineteenth-
century Administration: An Analysis', *Victorian Studies*, 9 (1966), pp. 245–55.

47. Paul Smith, *Disraelian Conservatism and Social Reform* (1967), p. 20.

48. FLB 3136: Josephine Butler to Joseph Edmondson, 28 Mar. 1872.

49. Jean L'Esperance, 'Doctors and Women in Nineteenth-Century Society:
Sexuality and Role' in J. Woodward and D. Richards (eds.), *Health Care and
Popular Medicine in Nineteenth-Century England* (1977), pp. 105–27 is useful
on suspicion of doctors. W.L. Burn, *The Age of Equipoise*, pp. 202–11
discusses the medical struggle towards full respectability. For anti-vaccination see,
Roy M. MacLeod, 'Law, Medicine and Public Opinion: The Resistance to
Compulsory Health Legislation, 1870–1907', *Public Law* (Summer-Autumn 1967).
For anti-vivisection see, R.D. French, *Anti-Vivisection and Medical Science in
Victorian Society* (Princeton, 1975).

50. F.W. Newman, *The Coming Revolution* (1882) in which he blasts two of
his favourite targets, medical men and official centralisers.

51. *Shield*, 2 June 1883, pp. 168–72; see also FLB 3179: Josephine Butler
to H.J. Wilson, 23 Aug. 1872.

52. *Shield*, 27 May 1876, p. 175, reporting a speech by Sir Harcourt
Johnstone.

53. See Josephine Butler, *Address Delivered in Craigie Hall, Edinburgh, 24
February 1871* (Manchester 1871) a speech which presaged the foundation of
the ultra-individualist Viligance Association fo the Defence of Personal Rights.

54. *Shield*, 2 May 1885, p. 57, reporting a speech by Rev. C.S. Collingwood.

55. *Shield*, 1 Apr. 1875, p. 96.

56. I exempt Smith, 'Ethics and Disease', and Sigsworth and Wyke 'A Case
Study of Victorian Prostitution', from this criticism; but see R.L. Blanco,
'Attempted Control of Venereal Disease in the Army of Mid-Victorian England',
Journal of the Society for Army Historical Research, 45 (1967), pp. 234–41, for

an article which fails to consider the army's role in society.

57. Rasor, *Reform in the Royal Navy*, pp. 112–23; Skelley, *The Victorian Army at Home*, pp. 235–300; for the volunteers see, Hugh Cunningham, *The Volunteer Force* (1975).

58. This tentative suggestion owes much to H.J. Hanham, 'Religion and Nationality in the Mid-Victorian Army' in M.R.D. Foot (ed.), *War and Society* (1973).

59. For instance, *PP* 1867–68 (4031), xxxvii, 425 QQ1595/6, evidence of Dr W.H. Sloggett.

60. Josephine Butler, *Address Delivered at Croydon, 3 July 1871* (1871).

61. A point developed further in chapter 7 below.

62. FLB 3471: Josephine Butler to H.J. Wilson, 28 June 1875; 3130: Josephine Butler to Mrs H.J. Wilson, *c.* March 1872.

63. See Peter T. Cominos, 'Late Victorian Sexual Respectability and the Social System', *International Review of Social History*, 8 (1963), esp. p. 47 for changes in moral attitudes.

64. Bristow, *Vice and Vigilance*, chapter 5, pp. 94–121, is the best recent discussion of the NVA and the Social Purity 'wave' of the 1880s.

65. Respectively the Secretary of the NVA and the Empire Music Hall's fanatical enemy. Walkowitz, ' "We are not beasts of the field" ', pp. 23–4, 316–25, 369–75, discusses the tension between repeal and social purity attitudes.

2 REGULATING PROSTITUTION

In many respects the Crimean War began the steady march towards regulation. It prompted the reform of the Army Medical Department, brought British doctors directly into contact with their French colleagues experienced in the ways of the licensing system and at the war's end inflated the statistics for venereal disease as soldiers and sailors returned to the United Kingdom. Another post-Crimean reform — the annual reports of the Army and Navy Medical Departments made these statistics readily available, and the investigations of the Army Sanitary Commission spotlighted them while drawing attention to the primitive conditions endured by soldiers.[1]

The Sanitary Commission's improvements, although held by the official historian of the Contagious Diseases Acts campaign to have produced a fall of 40 per cent in the rate of venereal disease over six years,[2] failed to halt the regulationist zeal among the reformers of the Army Medical Department. In 1860 a pamphlet entitled *Soldiers and the Social Evil* by 'A Chaplain to the Forces' summarised the hygienic arguments for regulation,[3] and in 1861 Florence Nightingale despairingly noted:

> That the disease of vice is daily increasing in the Army — so that fully one half of all the sickness at home is owing to that . . . and it is to be feared that the present War Secretary who is totally ignorant of his business, considers that there is no remedy for this but the French plan . . . a plan invented expressly to degrade the national character.[4]

Her solution was to improve soldiers' conditions, for instance by providing day rooms, institutes, clubs — and thus to raise moral and physical standards simultaneously. The Sanitary Commission had, of course, proceeded on these lines and one of its measures to increase the soldiers' self esteem (and partly to accommodate the repugnance of medical officers) had been the abolition of periodical inspection throughout the army in 1859.[5] Regulationists could be pressed to admit that they would welcome its return, but did not force the issue, compared to their clamour for inspection of women. Florence Nightingale's protegé, Dr T. Graham Balfour, though converted to the Acts once they were in operation, remained resolutely opposed to periodical examination of soldiers; it was useless, ineffective, unpopular with officers and men and would reverse all efforts to improve morale by levelling up.[6] Reformers whose attention focused on the individual soldier rather than the 'state of the army' stressed the need for recreational alternatives to the pub/brothel, more 'leave to marry' and a humane attitude to the soldier as an individual: 'The great men in office', said Miss Nightingale, 'always look upon the soldier as an animal whom nothing can check — any more than i can check my cat from lapping milk — I don't.'[7] Whereas reformers more concerned with general conditions, with lines on graphs and with the sheer expense of a high level of venereal infection (often vividly expressed as so many battleships or regiments out of action) accepted the inevitability of prostitution around the camps and ports, and insisted on the importance of rendering identifiable prostitutes as healthy as possible.

In 1862 an Admiralty departmental committee under Samuel Whitbread considered the whole question but refused to recommend the stringent regulation which the doctors were arguing for. It found that regulation only really worked in Malta, a special case, and that the provision of hospitals and voluntary inspection would achieve all the benefits claimed for regulation without the need to employ a special police force or an elaborate system of examination.[8] Throughout the year, Florence Nightingale continued her vigilant oversight of the question, firing off letters to Gladstone drawing his attention to the 'strong influence' at work to introduce the 'French system', supplying evidence from India and from official statistics to prove the inefficacy of regulation and urging a moral approach for the sake of the soldier.[9] All she could ever draw from him was a wistful, self-deprecating 'I am in truth ignorant of military administration and my impressions are distant and vague.'[10]

But far from confounding the regulationists, Whitbread's report may have goaded them on. Certainly nothing was done to provide the recommended facilities, and the appointment of a new Secretary for War, Earl de Grey, in April 1863, meant that Florence Nightingale had to start the work of converting a sceptic all over again.[11] In August 1863 a campaign of letters and leaders began in *The Times*, carried on semi-officially by Higgins of the India Office using one of his pseudonyms, 'Jacob Omnium'.[12] It stressed the utility of regulation, the government's *duty* to act in the national (and the taxpayer's) interest: 'What may be the causes of danger to that health (of the forces) is an irrelevant question, whether they are or not connected with immorality; we must have our army, if we possibly can, healthy and not diseased.'[13] In reply to this campaign Miss Nightingale put up Miss Harriet Martineau, her regular and privileged mouthpiece, to counter-attack in the *Daily News*; again the memoranda and statistics were supplied, and the series of articles in September 1863 which resulted from this collaboration were predictably distinguished.[14]

But this skirmish simply aired the arguments (probably for the first time) without affecting policy. A committee of ministers and ex-ministers was now meeting to resolve the question, and Florence Nightingale though aware of the committee's existence found herself powerless to influence it. When she did receive a draft she was startled: 'I don't believe any Ho of C [sic] will pass this bill. Any honest girl might be locked up all night by mistake by it.'[15] But her detailed objections to the draft were brushed aside; she was told that the proposers had faith in the police — and the Bill was introduced by Lord Clarence Paget, Secretary to the Admiralty, on 20 June 1864.

The legislative progress of the Bill was to become a matter of notoriety amongst repealers during the next 20 years. Introduced in a thin house, late at night, a government measure with a title deceptively similar to an act dealing with veterinary rather than venereal disease,[16] the Bill passed silently through both houses, receiving the royal assent on 29 July without a word being said about it. How-ever the Bill was significantly amended in committee where Sir Harry Verney, Florence Nightingale's nephew, and the Radical, A.S. Ayrton, were the only non-regulationists in a committee of 19.[17] The peremptory powers of the police to take women suspected of prostitution and venereal infection before a JP were removed, a clause making the practice of prostitution while knowingly diseased an offence was dropped, and the numerous references to 'common prostitute' and 'prostitution' in the Bill were drastically reduced in the Act, the definition of prostitution disappearing in the process. A clause was added permitting a woman to avoid public appearance in court by voluntarily submitting to examination; this clause was to become the cornerstone of the system.

The Act as passed (27 and 28 Vict. cap. 85) provided for the certification of hospitals by an inspecting officer. Information that a woman was a prostitute with a venereal disease and had been soliciting in a public place could be laid before a JP by the police or certain doctors. The JP could then summon the woman before him and if satisfied that the information was correct, order her to be examined in a certified hospital. If she was found to be diseased, he could then order her detention for a maximum of three months (in the Bill the limit was 'until cured' which might have resulted in permanent incarceration for some). The woman might escape the interrogatory process by voluntarily submitting herself to examination. A controversial clause provided penalties for innkeepers, publicans, etc., who allowed their premises to be used by women, whom they knew to be diseased, for the purposes of prostitution. Thus the brothel keeper was enlisted as an informer, and in practice unofficially tolerated by the police, despite the Act's specific disavowal of this.[18] The Act was to apply to eleven garrison and dockyard towns but could not be brought into operation until a hospital within 50 miles had been certified.

The Act was limited to three years duration which led repealers to argue with some justice that it was designed simply to establish the principle, not to work.[19] Indeed even before it was first applied (at Portsmouth on 3 December 1864) the military departments had set up a committee of medical men under the chairmanship of a surgeon, F.C. Skey, FRS, 'to enquire into the pathology and treatment of venereal disease'. Florence Nightingale was asked to draw up its instructions and name the War Office member of the committee (she suggested T. Graham Balfour); she was also asked to name an army medical officer to work the Act but indignantly refused.[20] The instructions were limited in scope as might be expected with a medical committee; though this was surprising in view of Florence Nightingale's interest in the social causes of disease — perhaps she believed that the evidence would be sufficient to discredit regulation, and Balfour was her nominee. They were 'to discover a sound principle of treatment of the disease known under the name of syphilis'; special attention was to be given to the use of mercury. But in addition they were asked for 'Any practical rules which the Committee can suggest to the Naval and Military authorities to diminish the frequency of cases of contagion, and which are capable of adoption *in the daily life of the ship or barrack*.'[21] And it was on this inappropriate peg that the committee was to hang its recommendation for extending the 1864 Act.

The first phase of the regulationist campaign was over, and a great triumph had been achieved. The principle had been established and a prestigious committee of picked men had been primed to take it further.[22] Moreover this success had been achieved silently with only the 'inside' opposition of Florence Nightingale against it, parliament had not debated it, the public knew little of it. As a critic of parliament put it many years later, it was 'a law foisted in under a title calculated to blind, and virtually passed in secret, so far as the nation was concerned,

though passed by the representatives of that nation'.[23] But by airing
the subject in public and pressing the principle further, the committee
destroyed the monopoly of knowledge possessed by official men, by
doctors and by the military; the extensionist campaign would have to
'go public'.

Skey's committee began taking evidence on 6 December 1864 and
sat for just over a year, interrogating the last of its 63 witnesses on 11
December 1865. Since the discovery of principles for treating venereal
disease was one of its instructions, doctors were the largest occupational
group, but since many of them had been called as expert witnesses on
the question of treatment, a number of doctors had no firm views on
regulation and preferred to remain neutral, often in the face of quite
outrageous leading questions.[24]

Thirty-five witnesses were regulationist; military doctors and those
concerned with the operation of the Act were the most enthusiastic.
Thus Dr Peter Leonard, Inspector-General of Hospitals and Fleets
and Inspector under the Act, testified to the good being done under
the 1864 Act but noted the existence of loopholes and urged as the
real solution 'registration and regular inspection at stated periods'.
Dr W.H. Sloggett, his successor as Inspector of Hospitals but at that
time Ship's Surgeon of HMS *Edgar*, fiercely advocated registration
and inspection of prostitutes, comparing regulated Tahiti with un-
regulated Honolulu to illustrate the benefits conferred. He noted that
the better health of officers was due partly to better moral restraint
but partly also to their frequenting a different class of woman.
Among the regulationist witnesses opinions varied as to the
examination of men. Sloggett undertook it willingly, Surgeon Fraser
of the 10th Hussars only before and after furloughs, but Surgeon
Perry of the Royal Artillery felt degraded at having to examine
1,500 men: 'I thought that I was placed in an utterly false position
as a gentleman, and as a medical man.' Witnesses usually agreed on
the need to improve conditions as a way to improve morals, though
Peter Cowrie, Sloggett's assistant on the *Edgar*, was critical of the
moral, do-gooding tone of Sailors' Homes: 'the nature of the
publications that are provided by very well meaning people are not of
that light or amusing nature which the men generally like'. While Dr
Hardie of the 73rd Regiment was fatalistic about the good to be
expected from better means of recreation: 'I believe that it is a stronger
power that impels them [men] — stronger than any precautions of
that kind will repress.' Dr de Meric of the Royal Free Hospital must
have startled the committee when he announced that for the previous

four or five years he had been contracted by a London brothel keeper to examine her girls once a week. From this position of peculiar experience he observed that even more frequent examination was desriable and regular clients should be included in this — practical observations which the committee seems not to have taken up.

Twenty-five witnesses declined to commit themselves or were in-sufficiently knowledgeable about the Act to be counted as regulationists. Compared to the zeal of the latter group, their reservations and alter-native panaceas cannot have seemed impressive. Perhaps the most realistic of these dissenters was Admiral Grey who insisted, against a string of tough leading questions from the chairman, that sailors were wily enough to circumvent any prohibition of soliciting. Dr William Lawrence said point-blank that visual inspection of women could not be relied on; he had been unable to find evidence of disease in women he knew had infected men — the committee failed to press the point. This less well-informed group was typified by Dr Langston Parker who displayed astonishing faith in ablutions of a draconian nature as the best preventative.

Only three witnesses can be defined as anti-regulationist: two of them had no experience of it but were inclined to doubt its efficacy, but the third, Samuel Solly, FRS, Senior Surgeon of St Thomas's Hospital, offered a remarkable opinion (though one later to be found among the more fundamentalist repealers). He saw no reason to protect men from the consequences of vice:

> I think it is intended as a punishment for our sins, and that we should not interfere in the matter. I think that if every young man knew that he could have intercourse without the danger of syphilis there would be a great deal more fornication than there is. (Q3898)

He remained unmoved by the argument that the innocent suffered with the guilty, that was the way of the world. The most efficient means of protection and the right course was to influence others 'to avoid, as a sin, the act which produce the disease'.[25] Solly's moral stand was an isolated one as Table 2.1 shows.

A majority of the committee agreed with the official view and determined to recommend periodical inspection. Skey mentioned this to the penultimate witness, the Duke of Cambridge, who expressed approval though doubted whether the proposal was politically practicable;[26] as it turned out his doubts were premature. However

Table 2.1: Attitudes to Regulation of Witnesses before the Skey
Committee

	for	against	neutral
doctors (military)	16	–	3
doctors (official)	5	–	1
doctors (civilian)	8	3	19
policemen	2	–	–
military men	3	–	1
civil servants	1	–	–
miscellaneous	–	–	1
	35	3	25

an earlier witness had unconsciously pointed to a problem of execution
while arguing for regulation. Dr Walter Dickson, a naval officer, had
observed that regulation worked well on the island of Malta, but was
much more difficult to enforce in Hong Kong given ease of access to
the Chinese mainland. It was just this sort of detail that regulationists
were able to slide over, given the collusion of a partial committee and
the lack of aggressive opposition. Their good fortune was not to last
long.

In February 1866 the committee delivered an interim report
dealing solely with the fifth of its instructions — the prevention of
disease.[27] With T. Graham Balfour dissenting, they recommended that
'a periodical inspection or examination of all known prostitutes be
made compulsory, under a well-organised system of medical police'.
They urged extension to all naval and garrison towns and favoured
direct government control of both police and hospitals. They
correctly observed that these recommendations followed the evidence
of the majority of witnesses (they claimed 42), and they reflected the
division of opinion over inspection of males by failing to provide a clear
recommendation. Balfour's dissenting report argued that weekly
inspection did imply recognition of prostitution; he preferred a policy
of repression coupled with retaining hospital provision for diseased
women. He denied that reclamation of fallen women was necessarily
tied to inspection. He was wholly opposed to periodical inspection of
men, which went completely against all efforts to raise their moral
character. He was willing, however, to concede inspection of men
going on and returning from furlough (other than respectable sergeants
and married men) as a justifiable exception which would not degrade.

Balfour's dissent suggested a clearer grasp of what was practically possible than did the moralising report of the majority. Where they proposed a system of regular medical and police supervision (but not prosecution) of known prostitutes — and dressed the system up with references to the prevention of 'scandalous and barefaced immorality' and declarations that it in no way implied legalisation of vice — Balfour took the view that if the problem was really to do with the state of the forces (and not a generalised attack on venereal disease as was probably the real motive for many doctors) the answer was to raise their quality while simultaneously attacking prostitution, not just disease. Ironically Balfour's views (or were they Florence Nightingale's?) were ultimately proved correct, but their author changed his mind after seeing periodical inspection in action, and three years later was himself defending it before an investigating committee.

On 15 March 1866, only three days after Gladstone had introduced the Reform Bill which was to capture parliament's attention throughout the session (repealers suggested that this preoccupation explained the Contagious Diseases Bill's easy passage — as we have seen, the Duke of Cambridge expected quite another reception) Lord Clarence Paget introduced his second Contagious Diseases Bill. It came up for a second reading in the early hours of 22 March, when Paget introduced it as a renewal measure (which was true, though a year early) with 'additional powers recommended by a committee of medical men'. The veteran Tory, J.W. Henley, criticised such legislation as 'vicious' if unaccompanied by any effort at reclamation, and apparently a failure in operation; and A.S. Ayrton returned to the attack, stigmatising the measure as 'a Bill for the sustentation of vice'. This, the first parliamentary discussion of the subject, was wound up briefly and blandly by Gladstone who assured the House that the Bill simply proposed the continuation of a system which had already received parliament's sanction. By 1883 he had understandably forgotten this businesslike intervention when he said that although a member of the governments which had passed the Acts, he had no idea how or by whom they had been carried through the House of Commons — they had been passed 'almost without the knowledge of anyone'.[28]

The Bill was referred to a Select Committee of 17 members, 14 of whom had been on the 1864 committee.[29] Here Ayrton made attempts to reshape the Bill, and while he failed to have the wilful communication of a venereal disease to a woman made an offence,

he succeeded in adding a clause requiring hospitals to make provision
for moral and religious instruction of the women as a condition of
certification. It is noteworthy that this clause, which was later used as
a major defence argument, was actually carried by an opponent and
was not part of the original strategy. A number of minor amendments
were made and the Bill was sent back to the House where another short
debate took place during the committee stage on 26 April.[30] Ayrton
tried to restore the requirement that a police officer should proceed
against a prostitute only when he suspected that she was suffering
from a venereal disease. Ministers defended the Bill as a limited measure
to protect the forces, and insisted that no certification of vice was
intended; the amendment was soundly defeated by 76 votes to 5. This
was a respectable enough attendance for 2 a.m. to make one doubt
the repealers' claim that the Acts were smuggled through. It might be
better to say that although many may have known the terms of the
Act, few as yet had any knowledge of their administration or could
grasp the departure of principle involved. Later in the campaign,
parliament's dereliction had to be explained and the 'smuggling'
myth was evolved. Following this debate the Bill went through all
remaining stages without further discussion and received the royal
assent on 11 June 1866.

The 1866 Act (29 Vict. Cap. 35) replaced the temporary 1864 Act
but was itself of unlimited duration; it became the basis of the regulation
system in the United Kingdom. Its major departure was the power
given to JPs to order women to undergo periodical medical examinations for periods of up to one year. Together with clauses which
tightened up the legislation and closed loopholes, this enabled the
Skey Committee to pronounce the Act to be 'in entire accordance'
with its recommendations. The schedule of subjected districts was
increased to 12, by the addition of Windsor.

When the 1866 Act came into force in September, the earlier Act
had in fact been applied only to four districts (Plymouth/Devonport,
Portsmouth, Chatham and Sheerness — the latter two served by the
same hospital). The new measure could be speedily applied to them,
but the other stations had to wait until hospital accommodation
could be provided, and it was 1870 before the system was in full
operation. When the Act was applied to a district, a small force of
Metropolitan Police in plain clothes was provided for its enforcement.
In ports these were usually recruited from the dockyard or 'water'
police. Their direct relationship with the government, designed to
emancipate them from local influence and from too close a relationship

with brothel keepers, was to make them particularly odious to individualist opponents of the state in the repeal movement; the fact that they operated in plain clothes opened them to the slightly absurd charge of being a 'spy-police'. Although repealers monitored police behaviour closely, they were seldom able to prove allegations of mis-behaviour to the satisfaction of the courts.[31] This might, of course, indicate collusion between police and the bench, though the courts did discover, perhaps not surprisingly, that the police behaved towards the women in a brusque and authoritarian manner — far from the humanitarian attitude usually claimed for them. An Assistant Commissioner, Captain W.C. Harris, was given charge of the adminis-tration of police. His annual report of the results achieved under the Acts, though often highly tendentious, provided a mine of facts and figures from which both sides quarried eagerly; his own testimony in favour of the Acts was vigorous and effective. But the policeman to whom attention was most often called was the Inspector in charge at Devonport, S.R. Anniss, whose evidence to both the 1870—1 Royal Commission and the 1879—82 select committee was disowned by Devonport Borough Council and attacked by repealers, who tended to concentrate on Anniss and Devonport to the exclusion of other stations and officers.

The 1866 Act had scarcely been put into operation before fresh demands for its extension were made, and again medical men were to the fore. In 1867 the promoters of an international medical congress to be held at Paris proposed for consideration the question of measures which governments might adopt for the prevention of venereal disease. The Harveian Medical Society of London there-upon set up a committee to look into the question. This committee circularised the medical profession and discovered a serious shortage of Lock accommodation for VD cases; it also received the same sort of medical advice as that already submitted to Skey's committee (to which eight of its own members had testified). Its report, dis-cussed and adopted on 1 July 1867, called for extension of the 1866 Act to the civil population in London and other large towns.[32] It stressed that such a system would require the provision of more hospital beds at public expense, but that it implied no public recognition of prostitution. The Society resolved to form an 'Association for the prevention of contagious venereal diseases' and asked its VD Committee to act as a provisional committee for the purpose of organising this new association. The lack of opposition to regulation at this stage is reflected in the fact that Dr John Chapman and Dr C.R.

Drysdale, two later medical opponents of the Acts, were members of
the VD Committee. Indeed Dr Drysdale proposed both its formation
and the acceptance of its report.

The Extensionist Association (hereafter EA) got to work at once.
Two energetic doctors, Berkeley Hill, surgeon at the London Lock
Hospital, and J. Brendon Curgenven, secretary to the Harveian
Society, became its honorary secretaries and set about obtaining
support and collecting further information on the incidence of disease
among prostitutes. Within a year they had recruited about 400 members
including nearly all the prominent men in the medical profession, a few
peers, 30 MPs, a number of clergy including two bishops and many
officers. The Vice-Chancellors of Oxford and Cambridge were vice-
presidents. Dr Leighton of Oxford having consented to serve with the
express approval of the Council.[33] In 1868 the Association mounted
an effective campaign for extension. In May a memorial signed by a
distinguished collection of doctors (led by the Presidents of the Royal
Colleges of Physicians and Surgeons) and others (most notably the
Vice-Chancellors and the Dean of Westminster) was presented to the
Lord President, the Duke of Marlborough. This was followed by
letters in *The Times* and the *Daily Telegraph* and by a short debate in
the House of Lords on 15 May, brought on by Viscount Lifford, a
member of the EA Committee.[34] He asked about extension to London,
and Marlborough in reply, while doubting whether the expense (which
he estimated would be £25,000 per annum) could be justified, urged
Lifford to move for a select committee to consider the whole subject
of extending the Act. Given an official hint, Lifford moved quickly; the
committee was named on 19 May and at its first meeting on 22 May he
became chairman.

Of all the enquiries into regulation, the Lords Committee of 1868
was the most partial. It examined 18 witnesses, 17 of whom
pronounced definitely for extension; its questioning led witnesses
to the points the committee wished to hear; and its report conceded
no difficulties in the way of extension.[35] Lifford and his colleagues
had two aims. One was to demonstrate the good being done in the
subjected towns; they therefore summoned Thomas Woollcombe,
secretary to the Royal Albert Hospital Devonport, Dr Leonard the
Inspector-General of Hospitals, and two civil servants, Romaine of the
Admiralty and Veasey of the War Office. Veasey may have disappointed
the committee; he preferred to talk about administrative clashes
between Admiralty and War Office, and despite a barrage of leading
questions from Lifford, failed to show much enthusiasm for the Act.

He was soon dismissed, but the other witnesses did rather better.
Woollcombe in particular was a shrewd local worthy who produced
chapter and verse on the physical and moral benefits conferred on
Devonport by the Act, but could see problems about general extension,
especially the question of who would pay, which the committee
seemed inclined to brush over. Their other aim was to demonstrate
the practicability of and need for extension. Captain Harris obliged
with a paper on extension to London which provided for inspection
of brothels 'to enforce cleanliness and good order' and registration of
prostitutes who would have to carry cards. He insisted that this was
to be distinguished from a licensing system which he admitted would
be repugnant to the country. Hill and Curgenven were summoned
before this committee for whose existence they were largely responsible
and gave predictable evidence. Dr William Acton's expertise on
prostitution made him a less tractable witness. Nevertheless his
evidence, although complex, included a clear recommendation for
extension while avoiding the moral perils of a licensing system. (Q946)
An interesting feature of the evidence given by this *expert* was his
ignorance of the terms of the 1866 Act. He thought all submissions
were voluntary and when told about the powers of compulsion said:

> I have found it so difficult to get the public to give up the liberty
> of the subject, that I have been chary of recommending anything
> of that kind myself; but now that others have brought forward
> these measures, I shall be only too happy to carry them out; but
> hitherto we have not dared to interfere in that way. (Q1021)

That Acton should know nothing about compulsion helps to explain
the lack of public response to the Act; a response which he and other
witnesses obviously expected to be hostile given their repeated dis-
avowals of regulation as a system of licensing. The only witness to
stand out against leading questioning was none other than F.C. Skey.
Although a signatory to the memorial for extension, and a member
of the EA, he seems to have had a surprising change of heart; he
criticised the EA for exaggerating the horrors and extent of VD and
hesitated to recommend extension until the 1866 Act had been in
operation for at least two years. Although he was in favour of gradual
extension, he had been angered by the hard-selling approach of the
extensionists. The committee did not detain him for long.[36]
    The report was short and to the point: in so far as it could be tested
after a few year's operation, the Contagious Diseases Act was working

Table 2.2: Attitudes to Regulation of Witnesses before the 1868 Lords Select Committee

	(a) Before the 1868 Lords SC			(b) Before all Enquiries so far**		
	for	against	neutral	for	against	neutral
doctors (military)	1	—	—	17	—	3
doctors (official)	1	—	—	6	—	1
doctors (civilian)	8*	—	—	16	3	19
policemen	2	—	—	4	—	—
military men	1	—	—	4	—	1
civil servants	2	—	—	3	—	—
clergy	1	—	—	1	—	—
miscellaneous	2	—	—	2	—	1
	18	—	—	53	3	25

Notes: *Includes F.C. Skey who approved of the principle of regulation but disapproved of EA tactics.
**This cumulative total counts witnesses who testified to more than one enquiry separately each time.

well; extension would increase its efficiency by reducing the danger of importing disease, its initial expense might be heavy but this would diminish with success; no real problems would be encountered as long as the present tactful mode of operation continued. Those who drafted the report were aiming at the government and presenting a plausible, well-argued case for intervention, but the report had one serious defect — it required that its assumptions should continue to escape serious opposition. However this was no longer the position.

Opposition was first raised by the committee of the Rescue Society, an evangelical body engaged in the reclamation of 'fallen women'. In his report for 1868, its secretary, Daniel Cooper, denounced the 1866 Act under the heading 'A dear remedy.' Apparently this stimulated a sense of outrage amongst its readers, and the Society summoned a conference of similar bodies when the Lords Committee's report was published (2 July 1868) to protest against extension.[37] Following this conference a strongly worded protest was sent to all members of both Houses of Parliament; this was the warning shot of the campaign, for the moment a weak one, but nevertheless a signal to extensionists that the opposition they feared was materialising.

As opposition slowly built up, the last covert attempt to extend the system was essayed. In January 1869 the Admiralty put up a draft bill suggesting that the administration of the Act should be transferred to the Home Office and extension permitted to any towns willing to pay

the costs of the Act.[38] On 25 February Mitford and Lifford in their
respective Houses urged the government to action but were fobbed off
with promises. Two factors probably induced the government to resist
this pressure: opposition was now becoming significant; on 20 March a
deputation led by Cooper saw the Under-Secretary at the Home Office,
Knatchbull-Hugessen, who suggested that they prepare a memorandum
on the subject — this was submitted in April and, in effect, warned the
government of the trouble they could face if the Act was extended.[39]
Secondly, and possibly of more significance, the Home Office referred
the Admiralty Bill to Sir John Simon, Medical Officer to the Privy
Council, and in a memorandum of compelling force he dismissed
the arguments for extension. Simon, agreeing with Skey, believed that
the extensionists had exaggerated the extent of disease, but that if
their figures were correct, the expense would be enormous — £100,000
in London alone. He doubted whether venereal disease could claim
such a high priority in national health treatment; he could see that there
would be moral objections and considered the principle of *caveat
emptor* reasonable. Simon was willing to defend the system as it stood
because it was exceptional legislation designed to remedy a problem
related to the maintenance of the services; for this reason he opposed
transferring its administration to the Home Office as likely to be mis-
understood: 'infinite caution ought to be used against drifting into
positions which become pledges'.[40]

   This sort of argument had a telling effect on a Gladstone administration. On 16 April, Earl de Grey, the Lord President and an extensionist who had served on Lifford's committee, urged the Home
Secretary to bring in a Bill permitting local authorities who would
themselves bear the costs to have the CD Act. However even he
accepted the impossibility of government financing extension to the
civil population.[41] The Home Office returned a dusty reply to the
Admiralty's similar scheme, and on 13 May Bruce moved for a select
committee, this time of the Commons to consider the principles of
the Act before any extension could be contemplated.[42] The government had, in effect, torn up the Lords Committee's recommendations;
it was unwilling to face the appalling costs and fierce opposition
involved with only the one-sided 1868 report as its authority.[43] By
mid-1869 the smooth progress of extension had been halted; its
hitherto unresisted advance would now begin to encounter serious
opposition.

   The Commons Select Committee on the 1866 Act was appointed on
8 June 1869; it consisted of 21 members who sat for three weeks

interviewing 13 witnesses, all but one of whom had an official connection with the Act or with public health. The narrowness of this selection is perhaps explained by the way in which they disregarded their instructions — these were 'to consider whether, and how far, and under what conditions it may be expedient to extend its [the 1866 Act's] operation', but their report blandly announced that they had not discussed extension to the civil population as it was a question of too great a magnitude. Instead they had confined themselves to studying its operation in military towns and whether any further towns should be added. Their disinclination to consider one of the principal points at issue concerning the Acts looks even odder when one considers that two members, Sir John Simeon and W.T. Mitford, were on the EA Committee and all but one of them supported the Acts in divisions in the 1870s. Perhaps the sheer improbability of pressing general extension upon the government induced the committee to settle for an investigation which would cast a favourable light on the existing Act's operation in the hope that it might be gradually extended. This would explain their choice of witnesses — all men who had firm information to offer; it would also explain why, bias apart, they declined to call Dr Hooppell who offered to testify. Hooppell, the Principal of Winterbotham Nautical Training College, South Shields, was one of the earliest opponents of the Acts, and had protested against them as early as May 1868: experience of seamen he had, but experience of the Acts he had not.[44]

The minutes of evidence suggest that the atmosphere was intimate; the witnesses were, with the exception of Simon and Balfour, genuinely committed to the Act and were giving evidence to a committee which largely shared their views. Where the Lords committee had rather clumsily led its witnesses towards the objective, the Commons committee and its witnesses marched hand in hand towards their more limited goal. Thus Dr Sloggett, now visiting surgeon at Devonport, gave clear and practical evidence about the medical benefits of the Act without being too extravagant about moral improvements. He suggested examination of merchant seamen, an area within a 15 mile radius from Devonport to be included, and strongly opposed using borough police to enforce the Acts as local influences might work upon them. His attitude to the women involved was revealing. He wanted those who submitted voluntarily and were found to be healthy to be thereafter subject to the penal clause in the Act. The chairman correctly pointed out that this would deter women from voluntary submissions but Sloggett brushed aside this objection – the women were all prostitutes, why bother magistrates with applications for orders?[45]

His colleague at Aldershot, Dr J.C. Barr, was even more mechanistic in his approach to women. Where Sloggett boasted of a reduction in the number of prostitutes from 2,000 in 1864 to 770, Barr lamented their shortage in Aldershot where 320 served the needs of 13,000 troops. He too omitted to lay much emphasis on reclamation, his interest was with the health of women subjected to the Acts and he was confident that periodical inspection was improving it – as well as inducing the women to behave in a more decent manner. Barr's evidence suggests that he was unaware of the gathering opposition; he gladly handed out 'hostages' for the future – for instance, besides his concern for the 'market in vice' he described in some detail the co-operation between police and brothel keepers.[46]

Civil servants from the War Office and Admiralty argued for extension to further stations and proposed administrative improvements. Greene, the War Office representative, revealed that his department had already anticipated a favourable report by allocating finance for another eight stations, the principle of *virement* being thrown to the winds to achieve this.[47]

The two most distinguished witnesses, and also the two least connected with regulation, were Simon and Balfour. The latter spoke with some authority, both as Deputy Inspector-General of Military Hospitals and as a veteran of the Skey Committee; his evidence was able and exceptionally fair. He presented a long statistical survey of the results of the Act which, judging by the naive questions put to him, the committee digested with some difficulty. His general conclusion was that 'there has been a marked advantage but I do not think it has been so great as was anticipated', largely due to the inadequate duration of the experimental period and the fact that the whole population was not subjected to it. Balfour remained completely opposed to periodical inspection of men as ineffective, unpopular and likely to harm efforts to improve the morale of the army by 'levelling up', but he was now willing to tolerate inspection of women given that it was now the law and appeared to be having some effect – hardly an enthusiastic commendation but still a reversal of view by a disinterested witness. Yet Balfour could see that the moral objections still existed and admitted that prostitution was effectively legalised under the 1866 Act, precisely the objection soon to be levelled by repealers.[48] Simon's evidence was carefully given, presumably to avoid misunderstanding; he opposed extension to the civil population, but retained an open mind on the Act as applied to the military – it was simply too early to say, and indeed he would have approved an extension of the Act if its experimental basis could be thus improved. Like most perceptive witnesses, he argued that it was restriction of marriage in the forces which encouraged clandestine prostitution.

Simon's mild approval, Balfour's half conversion, and eleven committed supporters of regulation meant that this committee's evidence was as one-sided as that of its predecessors, though one or two reservations had begun to creep in. Yet the resulting report was more cautious; it rehearsed the benefits obtained, 'prostitution appears to have diminished, its worst features softened, and its physical evils abated', but where such results had in the previous year led the Lords committee to demand immediate extension, now they merely prompted the Commons committee to suggest a short list of additional stations which should be covered and to recommend a further select committee to consider extension.

Table 2.3: Attitudes to Regulation of Witnesses before the 1869 Commons Select Committee

	(a) Before the 1869 Commons SC			(b) Before all enquiries so far		
	for	against	neutral	for	against	neutral
doctors (military)	2	–	–	19	–	3
doctors (official)	6	–	–	12	–	1
doctors (civilian)	1	–	–	17	3	19
policemen	2	–	–	6	–	–
military men	–	–	–	4	–	1
civil servants	2	–	–	5	–	–
clergy	–	–	–	1	–	–
miscellaneous	–	–	–	2	–	1
	13	–	–	66	3	25

The report was clearly arguing for further though moderate legislation, if for no other reason, than to remedy operational defects in the 1866 Act; it was this cautious pragmatism which made the final exercise in extension politically and financially acceptable. On 23 July Lord Northbrook, Under-Secretary for War, introduced a bill which passed through all its stages in Lords and Commons without debate, receiving the royal assent as 32 and 33 Victoria Cap. 96 on 11 August. This

1869 Act amended that of 1866 by extending its provisions to six more stations, widening the areas affected at each station, lengthening the maximum period of detention to nine months and permitting the detention of women for five days if they were unfit for examination, i.e. menstruating. Visiting surgeons were given authority to relieve women from examination after consulting the police; finally, women were no longer handed their certificates of discharge from hospital, they were kept by the police to prevent misuse. The 1869 Act completed the system of military regulation of prostitution; no further amendments would be made during its 14 more years of life.[49]

Notes

1. M. Gregory, *A Short Summary of the Parliamentary History of State Regulated Vice in the United Kingdom* (1900); H.R.E. Ware, 'The Recruitment Regulation and Role of Prostitution in Britain from the Middle of the Nineteenth Century to the Present Day' (unpublished PhD thesis, London University, 1969), ch. 3; E.M. Sigsworth and T.J. Wyke, 'A Study of Victorian Prostitution and Venereal Disease' in M. Vicinus (ed.), *Suffer and Be Still* (Bloomington, 1972), pp. 89–94.

2. Benjamin Scott, *A State Iniquity; Its Rise, Extension and Overthrow* (1890).

3. Ware, 'The Recruitment, Regulation and Role of Prostitution', suggests that this was a kite flown by the army to test reactions.

4. BL Add. MSS 45788 (Nightingale Papers) f.127: Florence Nightingale to Harriet Martineau, 25 Sept. 1861.

5. *Report of the Committee appointed to enquire into the pathology and treatment of Venereal Disease with the view to diminish its injurious effects on the men of the Army and Navy*, PP 1867–68 (4031), xxxvii, 425 (hereafter *Skey Committee*). Opinions about the usefulness of inspections varied among MOs – they *were* enforced in some regiments, e.g. the Coldstreams where Asst.-Surgeon Trotter managed to examine 500–600 men in half an hour (QQ5658–9).

6. *Report from the Select Committee on the Contagious Diseases Act, PP* 1868–69 (306), vii, QQ1237–44, 1147 (hereafter Commons SC 1869). However soldiers were inspected when their regiments came into a camp and when returning from furlough.

7. BL Add. MSS 50134 (Balfour Papers), ff.90–3: Florence Nightingale to T. Graham Balfour, 10 Dec. 1860.

8. PRO War Office 1863 33/12, *Report of the Committee upon Venereal Disease in the Army and Navy*.

9. BL Add. MSS 44398 (Gladstone Papers), ff.213, 239.

10. Ibid., 44397 f.50.

11. BL Add. MSS 43546 (Ripon Papers), f.26: Florence Nightingale to de Grey, 2 June 1863; F.66: same, 13 July 1863.

12. Higgins was a compulsive pseudonymous correspondent; see Cyril Pearl, *The Girl with the Swansdown Seat* (1955), p. 102; William White, *The Inner Life of the House of Commons*, 1 (1897), p. 9.

13. *Times*, 25 Aug. 1863.

14. BL Add. MSS 45788 (Nightingale Papers), ff.208, 214, 218, 224: Florence Nightingale to Harriet Martineau, Aug. and Sept. 1863.

15. Ibid., f.267: Florence Nightingale to Harriet Martineau, 31 May 1864.

16. Scott, *A State Iniquity*, p. 14; Gregory, *A Short Summary*, p. 6 adds that the indexer to Hansard succumbed to the same confusion and put the two acts under the same heading in 1867/8.

17. Ayrton was in favour of efficient and economical armed forces, and he was also a firm opponent of centralisation, but his most obvious characteristic was an irascible temperament – the most thoroughly disliked member of the House of Commons until displaced by Lowe. See *Dod's Parliamentary Companion*, 1869; Henry W. Lucy, *Men and Manner in Parliament* (1919 edn), pp. 235–8.

18. PRO Home Office 45-9511/17273A-190 for Home Office asking Metropolitan Police why they are not prosecuting pubs they know to be brothels – the disingenuous reply is that it is the responsibility of the local police.

19. Gregory, *A Short Summary*, p. 6.

20. BL Add. MSS 45788 (Nightingale Papers), f.275: Florence Nightingale to Harriet Martineau, 31 Aug. 1864.

21. *Skey Committee*, i–ii (my emphasis).

22. Skey's later evidence to other enquiries showed him to be a regulationist, and four of the other members he selected were later to join the Extensionist Association; indeed Spencer Smith, the committee's secretary, became Treasurer of the Extensionist Association.

23. Dr William Arthur, *Hush or Speak Out* (1885).

24. E.g. QQ4800–2 where a Dr Watson firmly refused to agree to a number of regulationist statements put to him by Dr Donnet, the Navy Medical Board's representative on the committee. Equally, a few doctors were happy to offer opinions on regulation based on the flimsiest knowledge.

25. *Skey Committee*, Q562 (Dr Leonard), Q1513–4 (Dr Sloggett), Q479 (Surgeon Perry), Q1023 (Dr Cowrie), Q1912 (Dr Hardie), QQ4043–5 (Dr de Meric), Q5351 (Dr Lawrence), Q3374 (Dr Parker), QQ3898, 3914 (Dr Solly).

26. Ibid., Q7030.

27. The main part of the report which recommended mercury as the treatment for syphilis was delivered in May 1867, and the whole presented to parliament in 1868.

28. *Hansard*, 3rd series (7 May 1883) 279 Col.65.

29. *PP* 1866 (200), xi, 523.

30. *Hansard*, 3rd series (26 Apr. 1866) 182 Col.2176ff.

31. The only serious malpractice by a CD policeman was an embezzlement by Inspector E.P. Coffey, in charge at Dover. Although irrelevant to the operation of the Acts, it was nevertheless reported gleefully by the *Shield*, 13 July 1878, pp. 194–5.

32. Harveian Medical Society of London, *Report of the Committee for the Prevention of Venereal Diseases* (1867).

33. *Report from the Select Committee of the House of Lords on the Contagious Diseases Act, 1866*, Session 1867–68 (46) (hereafter *Lords SC 1868*), evidence of W.T. Mitford, MP, a member of the Extensionist Association's Committee.

34. *Hansard*, 3rd series (15 May 1868) 192 Cols.324–30.

35. See note 33 above.

36. *Lords SC 1868*, Q742 (Captain Harris), QQ946, 1021 (Dr Acton), Q617 (F.C. Skey).

37. Scott, *A State Iniquity*, pp. 84–5; *Licensing Prostitution* (reprinted from the 16th Annual Report of the Rescue Society for 1869, Nottingham, 1870), pp. 2–6.

38. PRO Home Office 45/9322/17273-5, 25 Jan. 1869; Romaine, Secretary to the Admiralty to Home Office.

39. Scott, *A State Iniquity*, pp. 85–6; J.L. and B. Hammond, *Sir James Stansfeld* (1932), p. 140.

40. PRO Home Office 45/9322/17273-236 Memorandum of 3 Apr. 1869; see also Royston Lambert, *Sir John Simon, 1816–1904, and English Social Administration* (1963), pp. 405-6.

41. BL Add MSS 43534 (Ripon Papers) ff.243–5: de Grey to Bruce, 16 Apr. 1869.

42. *Hansard* 3rd series (13 May 1869) 298 Col.808.

43. Gregory, *A Short Summary*, p. 14 argues that the government appointed the Commons SC to reverse the recommendation of the Lords SC.

44. Scott, *A State Iniquity*, p. 87.

45. *Commons SC 1869*, QQ60, 187-98, 215 (Dr Sloggett).

46. Ibid., Q104 (Dr Sloggett), QQ645-7, 584-5, 642 (Dr Barr).

47. *Commons SC 1869*, QQ787-90.

48. Ibid. QQ1123-4, 1127, 1137-44, 1147, 1162, 1247.

49. The Acts of 1866 and 1869, together with a minor revision of 1868, were usually cited as the 'Contagious Diseases Acts 1866–69'. See also, J.B. Post, 'A Foreign Office Survey of Venereal Disease and Prostitution Control, 1869–70', *Medical History*, 22 (1978), pp. 327–34, for further evidence on the changing climate of opinion.

3   THE ATTACK ON THE ACTS LAUNCHED

I

Until the autumn of 1869, opposition to the Acts had been confined to
Florence Nightingale and her associates, and, operating quite
separately, groups of philanthropists working for the reclamation of
prostitutes. Now, opposition began to assume permanent, institutional
form, and the pioneers gained reinforcements. Dr Hooppell of South
Shields, having successfully disputed the assertions of extensionists at
a meeting in Newcastle, managed to get his intervention into a newspaper where it was seen by a Nottingham doctor, Charles Bell Taylor.
The two men cooperated in organising a meeting in October at Bristol
during the period in which the Social Science Congress was convened.
The future secretary of the National Association for Repeal, F.C.
Banks, a Nottingham bookseller, handled the correspondence, and two
Bristol Quakers, Thomas Pease and Robert Charleton, paid the meeting's
expenses, the latter presiding. This initial meeting attracted a number of
future stalwarts including Professor F.W. Newman, then living at
Clifton, Miss E.C. Wolstenholme, an activist in the struggle for the
higher education of women and thus known to Josephine Butler, and
Dr Thomas Worth of Nottingham; it concluded with a motion
denouncing the Acts supported by all but six of the seventy present.[1]
After the meeting Miss Wolstenholme sent a telegram to Josephine
Butler which she received upon landing at Dover from her summer
vacation in Switzerland. It urged her to 'haste to the rescue', introduced her to the Acts and threw her into an agony of doubt as to the
correct course to take which lasted three months and was resolved by
an inner conviction that this was her divinely appointed task. With
her husband's consent, she had begun to take a leading role in the
agitation by the end of the year.[2]

Following the initial meeting, Bell Taylor found that he was down to
read a paper to the Congress, and at a session on 4 October with about
100 present, the Acts were debated and eventually condemned by a
2 to 1 majority. On the following day at a meeting in the Victoria
Hall it was decided to found a National Anti-Contagious Diseases Acts
Association (hereafter NA). Robert Charleton became Treasurer, Drs
Hooppell and Worth were the Hon. Secretaries, and F.C. Banks began
to set up an organisation, working initially from Nottingham. Due to a

misunderstanding there were no ladies present and although many later
joined the NA (which was in no sense a male organisation) this accident
seems to have helped to cause a separate Ladies' National Association
(hereafter LNA) to be founded.[3]

In the remaining months of 1869 the fledgeling movement did
what it could to arouse the public against the Acts: Banks began to
issue pamphlets and handbills from his Nottingham publishing office;
Dr John Chapman, the editor of the *Westminster Review*, published a
series of articles in late 1869 and early 1870 which reviewed the
evidence given to the three enquiries and thoroughly condemned
regulation.[4] Both he and Banks reprinted the section on treatment
of prostitutes in Simon's 11th Annual Report to the Privy Council
in which the government's chief adviser on health repeated his disapproval of the principle of extension; this constituted an enormously
important support in that it revealed a split within 'official' opinion.
The Rescue Society and Harriet Martineau returned to the fray, the
former with another denunciation in its 1869 report entitled 'licensing
prostitution', the latter with four letters in the *Daily News*, praised
by Josephine Butler in 1869 as the best yet written on 'our question'.[5]
Before the year's end 'the movement moved from its merely defensive
position and became aggressive in character'.[6] Mrs Butler had visited
the subjected districts with Cooper and R.B. Williams of the Rescue
Society and had made her first speeches on the subject, to audiences
of working men whom she found warmly sympathetic.[7]

On New Year's Day 1870 the *Daily News* published a Protest
against the Acts drawn up by Harriet Martineau and signed initially
by 124 women including Florence Nightingale, Josephine Butler, the
penal reformer Mary Carpenter and the suffragist Lydia Becker. It
attacked the Acts on eight counts; three illustrated a new feminist
concern with the position of fellow women, that the Acts put women
at the mercy of the police, that they unjustly punished the sex who
were the victims of vice and not the sex who were its main cause, and
that they cruelly degraded their female victims. Two stressed that the
state was easing the path of evil by withdrawing moral restraints
without trying to tackle the moral cause of disease. Two dealt with
the dangers to civil liberty posed by Acts passed by an ignorant
parliament punishing an ill-defined offence. Only one bothered to
attack the nub of the regulationist case by denying that the Acts
could diminish disease. This exclusively female manifesto caused a
storm. The press reprinted it and dealt with it at length, and its general
effect was to stimulate discussion while bringing blasts of obloquy

upon its signatories' heads.[8] It also aroused some consciences hitherto untroubled by the Acts. On 4 January, Gertrude Wilson of Leeds wrote to her brother Henry J. Wilson, 'I find there is a division among good philanthropic people on the subject and some say that any law is better than the present state of utter lawlessness and impunity.' She thought the police powers of the Acts were 'most fearfully un-English' and was inclined to join a branch of the LNA then being formed in Leeds. Her brother urged her to do so.[9]

Elsewhere the Ladies' Protest stimulated the formation of new committees: A London Ladies Committee in the first week of January, followed by ladies and working-class committees in Edinburgh and Glasgow, a Scottish Association for Repeal, and a Metropolitan Association. Within a few months all major provincial cities had repeal societies and many had ladies' committees as well.[10] On 7 March Dr Hooppell began publishing the *Shield* as a weekly repeal journal. The first 25 issues were published from South Shields but from 3 September publication moved to London and it became the official organ of the National Association. With little coverage from the London press (a change in editorship of the *Daily News* from 1870 meant that it could no longer be relied on) the *Shield*'s existence was vital if repeal was to project itself as a realistic national movement. Josephine Butler dashed about addressing public meetings and organising new committees — in her first year of campaigning she travelled 3,700 miles and addressed 99 meetings.[11]

The apparent strength of their young movement intoxicated repealers; their political inexperience encouraged them to believe that they could hope for a swift victory. When a repeal Bill was introduced in April 1870, the *Shield* declared itself confident of success if 'the champions of the cause are only faithful and firm'.[12] MPs were questioned by their constituents, memorials were sent to Gladstone, the support of foreign luminaries such as Victor Hugo and Mazzini was cited, and parliament was extensively petitioned — 600,000 signatures had been collected by the close of the 1870 session. Enthusiasm produced its successes: The government was eager to relieve the parliamentary pressure on Cardwell by adding a known military reformer to the ministry. The officer in question was Sir Henry Storks, a former High Commissioner of the Ionian Islands and commander at Malta, a man of real ability, once a collaborator of Florence Nightingale.[13] Storks had to be found a seat in parliament and here his troubles began. Few men had so emphatically declared their belief in regulation, indeed he had bluntly informed the Skey

Committee 'that very little benefit will result from the best devised means of prevention until prostitution is recognised as a necessity'.[14] Such a man invited attack when he appeared at the hustings. His first attempt was at Newark, conveniently close to Nottingham. Bell Taylor and Worth went over and campaigned against him, Banks placarded the town with posters replete with lurid quotations; Storks withdrew on nomination day and a candidate pledged to repeal was elected. The *Shield* exulted, 'It will go from end to end of the land that a great champion of this vile system has been rejected with scorn by a whole soulled English constituency, though small in numbers, and though the candidate was backed up by all the power and prestige of a popular government.'[15]

The campaign was now taken into parliament where a Quaker, William Fowler, MP for Cambridge City, had given notice of his intention to introduce a simple Bill for 'Total and Immediate Repeal', a formula which greatly attracted uncompromising repealers.[16] A conference of about 100 activists met in London on 5 and 6 May 1870 to bring pressure to bear. A deputation from it visited Bruce and presented him with a memorial to which he responded by admitting 'the necessity of a speedy, full, fair and searching enquiry into the operation of the Acts'. This was unwelcome news to the *Shield* which feared it as a disguised effort to favour the extensionists.[17] In fact their cause was withering, and it was recognised that they were pressed to hold their ground.[18]

On 24 May 1870, Fowler introduced his Bill, but the debate was a disappointment. Its publicity value was impaired when the member for Ayr, E.H.J. Craufurd, 'spied strangers', an archaic procedure which obliged reporters to withdraw. He later explained that this was his intention as 'he conceived it to be his duty to prevent the flooding of breakfast tables with an authoritative report of details utterly unfit for modest eyes'.[19] As a discussion of the issue the debate failed utterly. Fowler launched a three-pronged attack: the Acts were medically ineffective (yet he contrived to praise the notoriously unhealthy French army during this exposition), legally and constitutionally offensive given the enormous powers the CD Police had over frightened and ignorant girls, and morally vicious, based as they were on the necessity for prostitution.[20] Dr Lyon Playfair, 'the unofficial parliamentary spokesman of the medical profession', replied with a medical defence of the Acts which, coming from a sanitary reformer, was more convincing than Fowler's rambling attack.[21] He also rejected moral arguments against the Acts: since the policy of the state was to keep 90 per cent of the forces celibate, 'certain sanitary safeguards' were essential. But his most interesting contention (and one seldom repeated in later debates) was that the Acts reflected the spirit of improvement in public health legislation after the 'do-nothing policy of three and a half centuries.' Accepting this spirit meant that he was sceptical about libertarian attacks: every progressive measure infringed liberty to some extent.

Playfair's speech was one of the few attempts to defend the Acts in terms as comprehensive as those in which they were attacked. Unfortunately the debate got no further as the adjournment was moved, and to the evident surprise of many, Bruce got up to announce that the government was prepared to have a Royal Commission on the Acts. Sir John Pakington, a prominent defender, objected to such an offer as premature, and repealers like Duncan McLaren and Edward Baines were doubtful. However Gladstone made a conciliatory speech promising that the Commission should discuss the moral as well as the physical aspects of the Acts. The government then carried the vote on the adjournment by 229 votes to 88.[22]

For repealers the first full debate on the Acts had been a sad anti-climax; the Acts had hardly been challenged effectively and a potential delaying tactic had been thrown up. The *Shield* was quick to attack the offer of a Royal Commission as a delusion likely to blunt the attack — the Acts were to be repealed not debated.[23] However the failure of an attempt to challenge the payment of a sum for administering the Acts in the Army Estimates,[24] and of the resumed debate on the repeal Bill on 20 July,[25] meant that the campaign would have to be carried over into the next session and the Commission reckoned with. The movement therefore had to adjust itself to the needs of a longer struggle: the National and Metropolitan Associations amalgamated and the former moved its headquarters from Nottingham to London; local committees were advised to transform themselves into NA branches; offices were taken at 50 Great Marlborough Street, and a £20,000 Guarantee Fund was inaugurated.[26] It was now accepted that the Acts would not be repealed until the Commission had done its work, the *Shield* reminded its readers that the anti-slavery movement had not been ashamed to cooperate with Commons' committees and reassured them (and perhaps itself) that 'the appointment of the Commission was a practical confession that the legislation of previous sessions required revision'.[27]

The government's offer of a Royal Commission was probably genuine, despite some doubts among repealers. The terms of reference

were extremely wide (including extension, to the fury of some) and
Bruce took care to try to balance the membership, indeed he took so
long doing so that Gladstone had to urge him to move faster.[28] He tried
to recruit Rev. Thomas Binney, 'the bishop of the dissenters', without
success,[29] but obtained a number of members likely to appeal to nonconformists: Dr John Hannah, Vicar of Brighton, whose father had been
President of the Wesleyan Conference,[30] Charles Buxton, MP and F.D.
Maurice, both Vice-Presidents of the EA. The extensionist cause could
also boast Sir John Pakington, one of the authors of the system,
G.E. Paget, President of the General Medical Council, and G.W. Hastings,
Secretary of the Social Science Association. Two radical MPs, Peter
Rylands (welcomed by the *Shield* as 'heartily with us in the cause of
repeal') and A.J. Mundella, were known repealers, and as a significant
innovation, Robert Applegarth, Secretary of the Carpenters' Union
and the first working man to serve on a Royal Commission, was
appointed.[31] The chairman was W.N. Massey, lately finance member
of the Government of India. There were enough uncommitted members
to make a fair assessment of the Acts possible — a situation which had
not existed with the one-sided enquiries previously held.

Not all repealers recognised the achievement involved in obtaining
such an enquiry from a busy government preoccupied with larger matters.
The LNA held firmly to the view that the enemy could be overcome
only by frontal assault, and preached non-cooperation:

> The Commission will, we believe, be appointed in the interests of
> the upholders of the Acts, to support a foregone conclusion. To
> preserve a show of impartiality, one or two men known to be
> adverse to the Acts have been named upon it, but although this
> legislation is exclusively applied to women, no woman has been
> asked to take part in the "inquiry". It is hoped, indeed, that no
> woman would, by consenting to serve on such a commission, have
> admitted that the operation of Acts utterly corrupt and
> indefensible in principle could be a proper subject for enquiry.
> . . .
> We hold that the practical working of an Act, wicked in itself, is not
> a proper subject for inquiry.
> . . .
> Into this trap of a Royal Commission, so cunningly devised by the
> astute and unscrupulous clique who have succeeded in placing
> these laws on the statute book, the L.N.A. is resolved not to
> walk.'[32]

Even the *Shield* thought that regulationists were over represented when the names were announced in late November — the result was already a 'foregone conclusion' with army, navy, professional classes and the Church of England represented, but not nonconformity. It ignored Applegarth's appointment, strangely for a journal eager to denounce the Acts as class legislation.[33]

The Commission met on 14 January 1871 and held 45 sittings to take evidence from 83 witnesses (49 for the Acts, 32 for repeal, 2 neutral).[34] The NA employed a barrister, Douglas Kingsford, as its legal representative to watch the proceedings; he intervened at Easter when only 12 repeal witnesses had been examined compared to 48 witnesses in favour of the Acts and persuaded it to hear further repeal witnesses including John Stuart Mill.[35] Kingsford subsequently produced a widely circulated and tendentiously arranged 'Critical Summary' of the evidence. Thanks to his exertions and to the militant nature of the repeal movement by 1871, the Commission interviewed a more balanced selection of witnesses than had any of the earlier enquiries (see Table 3.1).

The number of witnesses, mostly clergy and civilians, called to testify about the moral and side effects of the Acts is particularly noticeable, and indicates repealers' success in shifting the argument to grounds of their own choosing. Although defenders of the Acts were still more numerous and remained more 'official', this was at least an approach to a balanced enquiry and if Mundella is to be believed,

Table 3.1: Attitudes to Regulation of Witnesses before the 1870–71 Royal Commission

	(a) Before the 1870–71 RC			(b) Before all enquiries so far		
	for	against	neutral	for	against	neutral
doctors (military)	4	1	—	23	1	3
doctors (official)	10	1	—	22	1	1
doctors (civilian)	2	6	1	19	9	20
policemen	7	1	1	13	1	1
military men	2	1	—	6	1	1
civil servants	1	—	—	6	—	—
clergy	8	6	—	9	6	—
matrons/nurses	4	2	—	4	2	—
miscellaneous	11	14	—	13	14	1
	49	32	2	115	35	27

the repeal witnesses carried the day, the most convincing evidence was
that against the Acts, and when it came to drafting the report, Buxton,
Maurice, W.F. Cowper-Temple, Sir Walter James and Dr J.H. Bridges
all abandoned regulation, the first two also resigning their Vice-
Presidencies of the Extensionist Association.[36]

Much of the evidence given to support the Acts covered ground
already well trodden. Dr W.H. Sloggett, by now in charge of the
hospitals used under the Acts, testified as to the splendid effects all
round, squashed attempts to suggest that innocent girls were being
examined, and repeated his desire to see the periodical inspection of
men.[37] Inspector Anniss, head of the CD Police at Devonport,
provided a detailed account of his method of operation and made
very broad claims as to the moral and physical good ascribed to
the Acts' beneficent operation — claims which attacks on his
evidence showed to be more enthusiastic than accurate.[38] The
visiting surgeon at Portsmouth, E.K. Parsons, announced that he
approved of the Acts even more than when he had testified before
the Commons' committee in 1869 — clandestine prostitution and
disease were diminishing and he could see no moral harm in the
Acts.[39] But since there plainly were moral objections, regulationists
were obliged to answer them. Here they made impressive use of
clergy: Anglicans from Plymouth, Devonport, Portsmouth and
Maidstone, a Catholic priest from Cork, a Wesleyan chaplain from
Aldershot and a Baptist minister from Portsmouth all testified
to the physical and moral benefits conferred by the Acts. The
evidence of Rev. J.G. Gregson, the Baptist minister, was to the point;
he preferred voluntarism, he said, but periodical inspection worked
better, and was generally accepted in the area as necessary for avoiding a greater evil. In his experience only the brothel keepers were
opposed to the Acts, and he suggested that ladies campaigning against
them had been duped.[40]

Few repeal witnesses dwelt on the physical effects of the Acts.
Eight of them were doctors and they did succeed in throwing some
doubt on claims for periodical examination and the extent and danger
of venereal disease; but even they preferred to stress the violation of
liberty and the moral degradation which inspection implied. Most
repealers stuck to this tack. Indeed some regarded the medical details
as irrelevant and disgusting. Josephine Butler spoke for them:

I know scarcely anything of the garrison towns . . . of the

operation of the Acts I neither can nor will speak, and I must
decline to do so because I have no interest in the operation of the
Acts. It is nothing to me whether they operate well or ill, but I
will tell you what you wish to know as to my view of the
principle of the Acts.[41]

This was an extreme statement. Many witnesses did know a great deal
about the working of the Acts and gave telling evidence against them.
The best of these was William Littleton, a naval clothier and registrar
of marriages at Devonport. He described a number of plausible cases
of abuse of the Acts, stressing that *he* did not always believe the
women but took pains to check their stories. Against the alleged
moral benefits he boasted that he reclaimed more prostitutes than
did the Royal Albert Hospital, and convincingly argued that
clandestine prostitution was increasing despite the alleged vigilance
of the Metropolitan Police.[42]

A second group of witnesses knew something of the Acts but were
more concerned with their adverse effect on the reclaiming of
prostitutes. Daniel Cooper of the Rescue Society referred to the
hardening effect of the Acts – creating a corps of 'government
women' and continually dragging 'partially chaste women' into
permanent prostitution.[43] He was supported by Thomas of the
Midnight Meeting Society, Krause of the London City Mission and
Miss Brown, the former Matron of the Colchester Lock Hospital. Her
faith in the voluntary principle was so strong that she had no interest
in the alleged reduction of disease which the Acts had procured at
Colchester during her period there. All she wanted to do was to
rescue fallen women and she resisted anything which obstructed this
work – the worst sort of repeal witness, ill-informed and dogmatic.[44]

The third group of witnesses opposed regulation because of its
faulty general principle. William Shaen, the chairman of the NA and
a solicitor, insisted that the Acts tidied up prostitution instead of
attacking the circumstances which encouraged it; he argued that the
Acts were flawed because of their surreptitious passage through
parliament and the excessive discretion they gave to the police.[45]
The most impressive witness of all was John Stuart Mill, whose
testimony was carefully constructed and authoritative.[46] He began
by admitting frankly that he had no practical knowledge of the Acts
but that since his arguments were of general principle this would
not matter. The basis of his case was the Acts' natural tendency to
do moral harm: the government was providing securities against the

consequences of immorality which further degraded the women involved (he defended their capacity to be outraged by examination against those who believed them incapable of sinking further) but absolved their male clients — who should be the objects of deterrence if anyone was to be. His other major objection was a powerfully argued attack on the Acts as infringements of personal liberty. Mill's moral and libertarian evidence undercut the medical claims of the other side, making them appear irrelevant compared to 'higher' objections of principle.

Mill appeared some days after Josephine Butler, and his sane, well-reasoned approach may have redeemed any damage done by her evidence, for however great her eventual contribution to the success of repeal, the overwrought, even hysterical evidence which she gave on 18 March 1871 can have done little good. Her appearance was in itself surprising. The LNA had set itself dead against the Commission and she agreed with this verdict — it was a scandal to find 'a number of men, with Bishops and clergy forsooth, in deliberation to consider whether it *answers* to violate women by hundreds!'[47] This attitude underpinned her evidence as she lectured the Commissioners about higher moral standards, insisting that not even a 90 per cent reclamation rate could justify the Acts: 'what is the use . . . to save women while you are stimulating the vices of men? For men will have their victims.'[48] She memorably dismissed the Acts as 'a regulating of vice for the facilitating of its practice. It is a lowering of the moral standard in they eyes of the people. When the moral standard is lowered the practice of vice will be increased.'[49] And as we have seen, she refused to discuss their application. She took the most extreme view of state inter-ference, arguing that the legislature should leave individuals to deter-mine their own fates — although she acquiesced in state suppression of outward forms of vice.[50] Not even perfect behaviour by the police would induce her to look more favourably on the Acts; it was the principle, not just the abuses (however dramatic) which she opposed.[51] Nervous and inexperienced, she allowed her bitterness towards parliament and the upper classes to determine the drift of her evidence: thus she insisted on conveying the views of respectable working men in the north of England and contrasted their simply honesty with the sophistry of university men.[52] Thus she launched into a fierce attack on the Commission itself; repealers would be 'wholly indifferent' to its decision. They

> consider it an absurdity, a mockery, that any tribunal of gentlemen, however wise and conscientious, should be set to inquire into a

moral question like this. We have the word of God in our hands — the law of God in our consciences.[53]

Mrs Butler was undeniably a poor witness. She harangued the Commission rather than attempt to reason with it, but she was under great strain; she found her appearance a severe ordeal and believed that she was in the presence of a hostile group — she noticed how the commissioners had all her writings before them with some pages marked and turned down as if they wished to trip her up in cross-examination.[54] She was harshly handled by some commissioners, especially G.W. Hastings, who cornered her into admitting that she had declined to correspond with Berkeley Hill about the Acts,[55] but the uncompromising nature of her evidence invited such an attack. It was fortunate for the repeal movement that most of its evidence was less erratic than that of its leading advocate.

The Commission's report (or rather, series of reports) testifies to the success of the repealers' moral counter-attack in disrupting the regulationist case. The commissioners found they could agree on very little. They therefore signed a report so anodyne that both sides could use it to support their contentions. In addition seven minority reports, dissents and provisos were appended to stake out positions for future argument.

Massey, the chairman, drafted a report which recommended that periodical examination be abandoned. In effect he conceded that the repealers had shown that the existing system was insupportable. But their concentration on moral criticisms had left the medical evidence in favour of the Acts looking strong enough to justify retaining as much of the system as was politically possible. So Massey advocated reverting to the 1864 Act, strengthening the powers of detention in hospitals, and giving the police additional powers to attack prostitution. The report was a judicious attempt to reach a consensus, but at the cost of sacrificing clarity and hedging its bets confusingly; for instance, its justification of the special provisions taken by the state in the case of the Acts was a masterpiece of evasive argument. After considerable discussion, all the commissioners signed this report. Mundella later claimed that he did so in the belief that the government would thus be forced to end periodical inspection, after which the whole system would collapse. When this failed to occur he saw his mistake in signing, for as he pointed out, almost any statement in the report could be paired with a contradictory one elsewhere in it.[56] The regulationist members of the Commission claimed that they signed the report because it agreed with their view of the need to make special provision for venereal disease.

Strung out after the chairman's report were the special pleadings. The regulationist hardcore led by Sir John Pakington produced a short report entirely in defence of periodical examination (which had just been abandoned by a report they had also signed). Six repealers signed a moderate dissent drafted by Cowper-Temple; it objected to compulsory surgical examination on the 1864 lines, especially as it would hinge on a policeman's acceptance of hearsay evidence. Four of them also signed a stronger dissent drafted by Mundella which challenged the statistical defence of the Acts and attacked the 1864 Act. In addition three short provisos showed that their authors (Sir Walter James, Charles Buxton and Dr J.H. Bridges) were effectively repealers, while a 'further dissent' revealed Timothy Holmes FRCS as an extreme regulationist.

Nobody could be satisfied with this indecision. The government had designed the Commission to discover in private a generally acceptable legislative solution and marshal the evidence to support it. Both sides of the argument had expected a report which would endorse their policies. Instead they had all been disappointed — a set of contradictory opinions and a mountain of evidence were the product of the Commission's labours. As Josephine Butler said, 'It is almost laughable, if it were not so terrible an exhibition of weakness — "a house divided against itself".' Mundella told her that when the commissioners had signed all their reports they 'looked at each other in a sort of astonishment'.[57]

Even before the Commission reported, repealers had some idea of its proposals and were preparing to reject those which they found unacceptable. Josephine Butler accurately predicted that it would favour reverting to the 1864 Act and urged an uncompromising hostility to 'any form of the obnoxious principle'.[58] The *Shield* feared the worst and resumed its hostile attitude:

> The Report, based upon the interested evidence of spies and paid officials will, we fully expect, be as thoroughly one-sided as it can be, and as partial as the Admiralty and War Office can make it.[59]

It believed the only advantage would be that all the extensionist arguments would be printed as evidence and would be thus exposed and rendered liable to attack. Throughout June it concentrated on the

1864 Act, taking up a leak published in the *Daily News* and devoting three successive leaders to violent denunciations. Publication in early July merely confirmed these forebodings. The LNA promptly issued a condemnation which declared that its earlier accusations of bias were fully justified by the Report — it ignored the moral objections and simply removed the grossest provisions of the system:

> In truth the subject is one which admits of no compromise. If it is right to inspect and cleanse women for base uses, it must be right to do so effectually. If it is wrong, it must not be attempted at all.[60]

The *Shield* was scarcely less critical, 'a more self-contradictory or illogical document was never submitted to the consideration of Parliament or the country'.[61] It printed the report in full so that repealers might the more easily dwell on its inadequacies. The culmination of this swift repudiation, by repealers assailed with feelings of guilt about their brief dalliance with moderation, was a conference on 19 July at which William Shaen criticised Mundella and his associates for signing the report, and the movement set itself against compromise.[62]

Supporters of the Acts were equally dissatisfied though less clear as to what to do. The *Times* practised editorial selection; it summarised the report unfairly, ignoring real dissents, and extolled everything which supported the Acts: fear of abuse had been disproved, sanitary benefits were attested.[63] The *Saturday Review* made fun of the morality arguments and of the inconsistency with which the report demonstrated the benefits of the Acts only to recommend their partial repeal.[64] The EA persuaded itself that the report was largely favourable to the Acts although it obviously regretted the attack on periodical examination.[65]

The government lacked clear guidance, so decided not to make its mind up in a hurry. As Bruce explained in the Commons on 17 July, no outrages had been discovered and as the report required much consideration, the government saw no need to push a Bill through. Josephine Butler had feared that the delays which had beset the Commission would result in this sort of maintenance of the *status quo*; the *Times* was delighted and welcomed Bruce's reluctance to propose legislation on the basis of a divided report.[66]

Thus the promise of the Royal Commission ended in muddle, and neither side emerged with much glory. The regulationists had suffered most. For years they had dominated, indeed monopolised the argument, and public enquiries had served only to lend official weight to their opinions. The creation of a militant opposition in 1869 and 1870 threw them off balance. Essentially a pressure group aiming at the decision-making elite (of which so many of them were members), they were ill suited to a popular campaign — driven to distraction by 'inflammatory harangues' and 'appeals to the passions' from the more spirited repeal camp, they withdrew from 'platform agitation' and gave up the struggle to capture public opinion.[67] Their failure to win over the Royal Commission — their sort of forum — must have been especially galling, but can again be ascribed to their incompetence in the face of new opposition. They were no longer united by a common purpose. Some argued the case for retaining the Acts in their existing form with little reference to wider claims for extension. Others continued to put the classic case for generalising the system. Many diverted their energies into making pathetic and inconsistent claims for the moral results of the Acts. Their impetus was fatally checked and they were driven onto the defensive.

The repealers hardly realised their success in this respect. So determined to overthrow the Acts immediately, they failed to see that obliging their opponents to meet them on their own ground was in itself a triumph which turned the whole debate in their favour. They had been able to demonstrate the force of their moral objections so clearly that the Commission had accepted them albeit with some regret. They had compelled a hearing from a busy and uninterested government which could not fail to be aware of their strength. And as Mundella emphasised when later he defended signing the report, they had succeeded in preventing any further extension and secured a condemnation which could become the deathblow of the system: 'don't assume that the Commissioners' report is *against* us. On the contrary it saps the foundations of the Acts, and judiciously handled will destroy them.'[68] By mid-1871 the arguments on both sides had been laid out as fully as they would ever be. The regulationists had stated their medical case, and would henceforth reiterate it with evident pain that so reasonable a position should be subject to fanatical attack.[69] Their 'secret weapon' was the annual publication of official statistics, drawn up, as repealers pointed out, in the most optimistic manner possible, and extensively quoted.[70] But they also responded to the moral pressures imposed upon them by their enemies; every improvement in the condition of the subjected districts was annexed and boasted of in the annual reports of the

Metropolitan Police. Mundella was outraged by such 'sophistry':

> Everything that is done, and very properly done to close public
> houses and save young girls from the streets is placed to the credit
> of the Acts, whereas they have no more to do with such useful
> services than the Licensing Bill or any other Police Act. They are
> . . . parading this partial work which might be done throughout
> the United Kingdom as the effect of the Acts in the subjected
> districts.[71]

Repealers based their claims above all on moral grounds. Mundella
urged Josephine Butler: 'For heaven's sake, let alone the statistics, and
leave off *diagnosing* the disease, and stick to the *principle*',[72] though
she hardly needed urging. True, it later became necessary to demonstrate the questionable statistical basis of claims made for the Acts, and
arguments based on their class bias and on the outrage done by them to
women were both effective and popular. But the superiority of
principle over expediency was common ground to all repealers. This is
the great difference between the Royal Commission and the earlier
enquiries. The impressive strengthening of the case for repeal had
come not from witnesses able to spar with official, expert testimony,
but from non-official, civliian witnesses simply opposed in principle
to the Acts.

But how to convey their sense of outraged principle to a wider
public? Repealers had no doubts about their opponents' access to
centres of influence. Josephine Butler was obsessed by the power of
the medical establishment; 'the doctors here are very powerful in
Parliament and are very determined for the "Acts" in some form
or other'.[73] Her anti-medical prejudices were shared by other
repealers, though they were usually less vehemently expressed:
Mundella suggested that doctors had an instinctive urge to cure
disease, which led them to 'entirely overlook the social and moral
consequences of such pernicious legislation',[74] and they provided
a connection with other movements opposed to medical pretensions:
F.W. Newman, an arch-libertarian with a predilection for opposition
to 'the medical clique' could denounce the manner in which
parliament surrendered to medical dictators over vaccination, using
arguments identical to those he used against the Contagious Diseases
Acts.[75]

When doctors were employed by the state, they compounded their
disgrace in Josephine Butler's eyes by demonstrating the rise of a

'salaried monster', a huge official machine dedicated to an ignoble end. She seized on the vested interest which all those employed under the Acts had in their survival: 'when a host of salaried, permanent officials is once established; the system to which they belong must be perpetuated for their sakes'.[76] Throughout her speeches and writings runs a deep suspicion of the growing power of the state — she was the first secretary of the individualist Vigilance Association for the Defence of Personal Rights — but other repealers were equally suspicious of those who had contrived the Acts and stood to lose by their repeal. Mundella spoke of 'a hard fight against military and naval officials' on the Royal Commission; and the *Shield* compared the pecuniary interest of official witnesses in maintaining the Acts with the reverse among repeal agents whose success would deprive themselves of a job.[77]

II

Against this constellation of vested interest, the repeal movement gradually developed a complicated organisational structure; but in the first three years this was still quite straightforward. The Ladies' National Association (to be discussed later) went its own way with Josephine Butler as its leader and mouthpiece, while all other local associations were treated and regarded themselves as branches of the National Association for Repeal (NA). This, as we have seen, was an amalgamated body formed in August 1870 to provide the resources for a longer struggle than had at first been envisaged.

From the first, the dominant influence in the NA was that of London and Londoners. The agitation was 'too important and too gigantic to be effectually worked in a provincial town', said the *Shield*, and so all activity was concentrated in the offices of the former Metropolitan Association,[78] to which came as secretary F.C. Banks, previously the organiser of the provincial association. In theory the NA was governed by a large General Committee which met monthly; the first Annual Report listed 128 members, but of these, 37 were nominated as members of the Executive Committee which met weekly, and all were Londoners. They were the real directors of NA policy. In 1872, a year of considerable activity, only 9 provincial repealers ever attended a committee meeting, and none attended more than one. In addition, four MP vice-presidents attended. This was quite exceptional and occasioned by crisis; in the main, a score or so of Londoners provided the NA leadership.

The chairman of the NA Committee throughout its existence was

William Shaen, a London solicitor. Assiduous in his duties — in 1872
he attended 42 out of 48 committee meetings and chaired all but one —
yet his biography offers no suggestion that repeal was in any way the
most significant of the many causes with which he was concerned.[79]
He was a Unitarian, educated at University College London (of which
he was later a Fellow), where he met James Stansfeld; articled to
William Ashurst, the radical solicitor (he was responsible for introducing
Stansfeld into the Ashurst household and thus to his future wife), and
like most London radicals a Mazzinian. He was also a university
reformer, active in women's education (chairman of the Council of
Bedford College; solicitor to the Girls' Public Day School Company),
a captain in the Middlesex Volunteers (Tom Hughes was his colonel),
believing this to be a step towards abandoning a regular army, a
temperance advocate, a friend of Garrison and the American anti-
slavery movement, on the committee of the Aborigines' Protection
Society, active on behalf of feminist causes, a champion of all social
purity and morality causes, a strong opponent of vivisection. The
list could go much further; what it shows is how active Shaen was in
every conceivable branch of reform activity, and thus how experienced and well connected he was. He was a friend of Stansfeld;
also of F.W. Newman, with whom he shared a catholicity of reform
tastes and a gradual loosening of his Unitarian ties. Shaen's strength as
a repealer, besides his diligence and ability as an administrator, lay
in his firmness of principle coupled with considerable legal ability —
he was thus one of the movement's principal apologists.[80]

When Shaen was absent the chair was taken, sometimes by Frederick
Pennington, the chairman of the Finance Committee, sometimes by
the barrister C.H. Hopwood; they became less active following their
election to parliament in 1874 — both for the borough of Stockport.
Another occasional chairman, W.T. Malleson, later became the NA's
vice-chairman; another was the academic lawyer Professor Sheldon
Amos who later wrote the standard and extremely useful legal history
of regulated prostitution, *Laws for the Regulation of Vice*. The
Rescue Society which had first opposed the Acts was diligently
represented on the Committee by its secretary, Daniel Cooper, and by
R.B. Williams. These men were all active in the NA's early years and
constituted a small collective leadership. But the NA was not a male-
oriented body: on the contrary, there existed for two years, until its
voluntary dissolution in November 1872, a London Ladies'
Committee which preferred to remain separate from the LNA and
whose members served automatically on the NA's Committee.

Mrs. F.R. Malleson was its secretary and Mrs W. Hargreaves its treasurer, both their husbands were on the NA Committee, Mrs Pennington and Mrs W.T. Malleson were members, so too was the editor of the *Shield*, Mme Emilie Venturi (née Ashurst), Stansfeld's sister-in-law. The impression one gets of the NA's Committee in the early 1870s is that it was effectively a small, tightly-knit body of men and women, connected by family ties, Unitarian background, education at University College, and devotion to humanitarian and moral reform movements — the Social Purity Alliance (formed by Mrs W.T. Malleson in 1873) and the Vigilance Association for the defence of Personal Rights (to which Shaen was legal adviser) claimed the allegiance of many.

Table 3.2: Most Active Members of the NA Executive Committee, 1872 (those who attended more than 20 meetings — maximum possible 48)

Mrs. F. Pennington	45	
Mrs. F. Malleson	44	Secretary of London Ladies' Committee
Mr W. Shaen	42	Chairman
Mr D. Cooper	42	Secretary of the Rescue Society
Mr R.B. Williams	42	Representative of the Rescue Society
Mrs Hampson	40	
Mr F. Malleson	31	Treasurer of the (defunct) Metropolitan Association
Mr W. Malleson	31	Later Vice-Chairman; also on Committee of Vigilance Association; a Mazzinian
Mr H.N. Mozley	29	also on Committee of Vigilance Association
Mr C.H. Hopwood	29	Penal, humanitarian and moral reformer
Prof. Sheldon Amos	29	Professor of Jurisprudence at University College London; also on Vigilance Association Committee
Mme E. Venturi	28	Editor of *Shield*; also on Vigilance Association and Ladies' National Association Committees
Mrs W.T. Malleson	27	founded Social Purity Alliance in 1873
Mrs King	25	also on Vigilance Association Committee
Mrs Sheldon Amos	22	sister of Percy Bunting, editor of *Contemporary Review*

The NA's increasingly elaborate administration was directed by its secretary, F.C. Banks, who adjusted with ease from bookselling and publishing in Nottingham to running a busy London office. He was a highly competent administrator, with a creative ability to seize the right moment for bringing his Committee to take action; in addition he was willing to take to the road himself and was a determined and successful orator. On occasions he seems to have overstepped the line which separated employee from independent member of the movement, and participated in decision-making. It is a measure of the esteem in which he was held, that such behaviour was usually tolerated.[81] He was not universally well regarded — Mrs Butler thought him pedantic and slow — but he was innocent of intrigue,[82] a sheet-anchor for the movement as a whole by virtue of his continuous tenure as secretary (even beyond the dissolution of the NA — he continued to be paid until Christmas 1886 while sorting out the records; he then transferred to the Vigilance Association) and a valuable, under-rated servant of his cause.

Banks was highly paid by the standards of the time: in November 1872 his salary was £250, by January 1874 it had been raised to £400.[83] By this stage there was an assistant secretary, Miss Emilie Harrison, who was paid £80 per annum and a male clerk who got between £1 1s 0d and £1 5s 0d a week; all these salaries were subject to reduction should income contract. Besides an office staff (which was augmented when necessary — usually at elections) the NA began to employ travelling agents from October 1872 and depending on experience, these men merited anything between £100 and £250. Finally, the NA maintained an office and refuge in Plymouth which required the services of a local agent. Thus its salary bill increased over the years: £242 in 1870; £957 in 1874—5; £1069 in 1884—5.

The NA's contribution to the movement was persistently undervalued by provincial repealers who grew angry at what they thought was the passivity or timidity of Londoners. They hardly ever considered that there had to be a London office of some sort and that a central headquarters was vital to a national movement. The NA provided an excellent office which handled an enormous correspondence, provided a venue for meetings, an assembly point for deputations, an administrative centre for the innumerable conferences and conversaziones with which repealers bolstered their morale. As Banks observed in a long moan about the perversity of provincial critics, the NA had given liberally to other societies, it acted as a stopgap in providing services no other body would undertake (indeed it often did work for other bodies), and it was responsible for work done in connection with parliament and enquiries such as the Royal Commission or the Select Committee.[84] In short the NA might justly complain that if its presence was not appreciated, its absence would be sorely felt. It was the movement's chief publisher, it sustained the loss-making *Shield* and in many ways it provided hidden subsidies to more dynamic rivals.

All this was possible because its income was relatively high and rich

contributors were not lacking. In the first two years of its existence
almost £5,000 was raised which the Committee considered excellent
given that other charities were experiencing difficulties and there
were the claims on charitable funds produced by the Franco—Prussian
war to be considered.[85] Three £20,000 Guarantee funds designed to
provide a regular income were collected during the NA's existence:
only the third, started in 1880, faltered and as the Annual Report
explained, income was by then badly harmed by the economic
depression, and by the transfer of subscriptions to associated bodies.[86]
In the years for which balance sheets are available, income only once
dipped below £2,000, and was usually nearer £3,000, making the NA
the richest of repeal bodies.[87] Why then, asked provincial repealers,
did it so often fail to give a vigorous lead? Some suspected that the
corrupting influence of parliament had seeped into the bones of
London repealers; a fear buttressed by the NA's attitude to the
question of parliamentary action as a means of following up the
Royal Commission.

The government's lack of urgency in the summer of 1871 infuriated
repealers but left them helpless. Mundella failed three times in attempts
to introduce a Repeal Bill, so the only occasion for a debate was an
attack on the Estimates. On 14 August 1871 Fowler moved to remove
the sum for the maintenance of the CD Police from the Army
Estimates, arguing that since 16 of the commissioners were opposed
to periodical examination there could be no grounds for continuing
to maintain the police. He was supported by Mundella and by two
Conservatives: Russell Gurney, the Recorder of London, denounced
periodical examination which he said was widely resented in
Southampton, his constituency; and J.W. Henley (who had opposed
the passage of the 1866 Act), who reiterated his moral objections to
the system: 'the tenor of their Report was how to make vice more
attractive and less dangerous'. The government's mind being unclear, it
relied on an official defence to get by. Cardwell asked the House not
to deprive it of the means of carrying out its obligations, and it
scraped through in a thin House with a majority of 12.[88] The *Shield*
was pleased with the debate: the government's majority depended on
22 Conservative votes and 22 of the Liberals voting were office-
holders; it had hard words for absentee repealers and considered that
the division could have been won if those who had made pledges had
kept to them. It noted but did not remark on the fact that the
Cabinet's two most radical members, W.E. Forster and James Stansfeld,
were present but did not vote.[89] A further analysis of the figures

revealed that the 58 MPs supporting the Acts represented only 287,000 electors as against the 677,000 for the 46 repealers — a common radical complaint, as Dilke argued:

> We are being destroyed on every question because of the falsity of representation. For instance the minority in Fowler's division on the contagious diseases acts; the minority on the Lords' amendments to the Trades Unions Bill, and the minority on the election expenses clause of the ballot bill represented as I am prepared to prove the *majority* of voters in each case.[90]

During the recess, a difference of opinion between MPs and extra-parliamentary repealers began to appear. The issue was what attitude to take to the government's proposals when they appeared. In November 1871 the NA Committee asked Fowler to introduce a Repeal Bill as soon as possible. He replied that he wanted to discover what the government intended before taking action, and to that end he consulted Bruce unofficially. But his soundings disappointed the Committee who insisted on a Repeal Bill, and when Fowler asked them what they would like in it, he was told sharply that the Bill should be 'nothing but a demand for repeal'.[91]

Relations between Fowler and his followers were strained. Although his parliamentary speeches were satisfactory, he lacked the zeal and drive for which some of them yearned. Josephine Butler told her followers, 'Mr. Fowler may be a little apathetic and he must be kept up to the mark.'[92] Another repealer was even more critical:

> it is sad to see a man in the position of a leader who, with all his sincerity and good intentions, thus requires the inspiration and encouragement of those who should be his followers in courage and steadfastness.[93]

Indeed in December 1871 the erratic and violent Dr Hooppell had written to the NA to urge the removal of Fowler as leader. But apathy cannot explain Fowler's conduct: more relevant was an MP's knowledge that the government could carry a Bill so much more easily than a private member, and his belief that it was worth waiting to see if they would produce an acceptable measure.

On 13 February 1872 Bruce introduced his Bill — the government's reaction to the Royal Commission report.[94] He made it clear that he personally favoured the Acts, but accepted that there was a difference of opinion about their moral effect and the Commission had decided that they could not be maintained. He therefore proposed to repeal them, thus satisfying public opinion, but to keep some measure of regulation by knitting together and strenuously applying Acts already on the Statute Book, the 1824 Vagrancy Act and the 1867 Poor Law Amendment Act (slightly extended). These Acts applied to the whole country, of course; as he put it, 'the mesh may be somewhat larger, but the net will have a far wider sweep'. His solution preserved some of the beneficial results alleged to come from regulation while abolishing all the CD Acts; furthermore it extended these results to the whole country by a slight amendment to an existing statute. From the government's point of view it was an ingenious solution which implemented as far as possible the confused wishes of the commissioners. Bruce hoped that it would enjoy the wide support which the CD Acts lacked; in his view their only failing.

Supporters of the Acts were appalled: W.T. Mitford, MP for Midhurst and member of the Extensionist Association Committee, 'looked with dread at the prospect of doing away with the wholesome legislation of recent years'; Sir John Pakington thought the Bill was the 'triumph of prejudice and clamour over reason and truth'. *The Times* hammered the government for giving way to a 'fanatical and unscrupulous agitation' and doubted whether public opinion really did oppose the Acts.[95]

Repeal MPs were pleased with the Bill: Rylands said so in the House, and on the following day, he Fowler, Jacob Bright and Duncan McLaren attended a special meeting of the NA Committee. It was quite exceptional for MPs to attend the Committee, so it is reasonable to suppose that four turned up to overawe the meeting and swing it towards the Bill. If so, they succeeded. The Committee decided to support its second reading 'with a view to amend its objectionable clauses in committee'. On 28 February the Committee approved five necessary amendments to the bill, and on the following day a conference of 250 repealers from all over the country agreed to support the new policy against the advice of Mrs Butler and Mme Venturi (who had already offered to resign her editorship of the *Shield*). All the MPs spoke enthusiastically for amending the Bill; indeed Cowper-Temple and McLaren went so far as to declare that the Bill itself was everything they could desire. A face-saving compromise resolution was proposed and when the vote was taken, only six voted against. On the face of it, Bruce's Bill suitably amended was now the policy of the repeal movement.[96]

Two factors overturned the new policy. The LNA refused to accept the decision and began to campaign against it with the greatest vigour, flooding the *Shield* with protests;[97] and Bruce having introduced his Bill showed no sign of proceeding to a second reading. The NA Committee quickly lost its nerve and began asking Fowler to bring on his own Bill to fill the gap. Throughout March and April its requests grew more insistent and Fowler's excuses more desperate as he struggled to avoid a rupture with the government.

Fowler's caution may have been unwise. Josephine Butler consulted MPs who thought he should go ahead since ministers were not keen on presenting their own Bill, 'in their present shaky condition', and Mundella came out against Bruce's Bill after being petitioned by his Sheffield constituents and pressured by H.J. Wilson.[98] On 8 April the NA Committee decided that Bruce's Bill should be for repeal only; the clauses for protection of women and young girls should go into the Bastardy Bill then being sponsored by W.T. Charley, MP for Salford, and the clauses for the suppression of brothels should be a separate measure. A deputation stiffened by Mrs Butler was sent to tell MPs about these wrecking amendments.

Still Fowler temporised. Josephine Butler urged an ultimatum to him as he was making no effort — did they need a better leader?[97] By 25 May the *Shield* (which had earlier only printed an LNA statement with an editorial disclaimer) was accusing the government (with one exception — Stansfeld?) of treachery and making strident, if rather guilty, calls to repealers to accept nothing but repeal. Eventually Fowler capitulated and gave notice of his Bill. Alas his wife died in early June (the *Shield* was so preoccupied with the 'crisis' that it spared him little sympathy) and seizing on this bereavement, he excused himself and removed to Italy. Bright and Mundella found reasons for not taking the Bill on. The NA Committee was reduced to sending a deputation down to the House of Commons to look for a willing MP.[100] They succeeded in persuading another Quaker, Charles Gilpin, member for Northampton, to undertake it. On 9 July, despite sending telegrams to all friendly MPs, a house of 34 was humiliatingly counted out when Gilpin tried to introduce the Bill; on 15 July Bruce withdrew his Bill, which never reached its second reading.[101]

And so nothing emerged from a year of the greatest hope. Bruce dropped his Bill because it lacked the broad-based support which was its sole *raison d'être*. The repealers had rejected it, against their MPs' advice, because it failed to measure up to the highest moral position, that of the LNA. But regulationists were also unhappy. The legislation which was to replace the Acts was optional — it had really been used only in Liverpool. It would be left to local authorities and their police to enforce the revised system, and they had not been making use of existing possibilities. Further, the agents of the government, the Metropolitan Police, were to be withdrawn, and entirely against the tendency of social legislation of the time, the government was to hand over to local bodies a public health responsibility it had always shouldered.[102] The military interest was simply not concerned with amending the Acts, which it found perfectly satisfactory in its own areas; it certainly did not wish to see them diluted for the sake of some sort of extension throughout the country.

The subject embarrassed the government, and the agitation was distasteful. First the government had shunted the problem off to a Royal Commission which had failed to produce a decisive report; next it had itself worked out a subtle proposal with attractive features for both sides; they had rejected it. Bruce had known the feeling before. Only the previous year he had been abandoned by the temperance reformers who had failed to support his Licensing Bill. The government had been firmly committed to legislate on drink, and when the temperance forces supported it in 1872, it went ahead again.[103] But it was in no way committed to doing anything on the CD Acts: rather it was responding to public opinion. So when that opinion seemed unclear, Bruce was perfectly happy to withdraw his proposals (which remained the government's policy) and permit the system, of which he approved, to continue — which it did for eleven more years.

The result for the repeal movement of this imbroglio was to sharpen the extra-parliamentary repealers' suspicion of the legislature. In a notably silly leader on Gilpin's motion, the *Shield* denounced the House of Commons as useless and MPs unreliable — 'our strength is in the people, not in them' it declared. Henceforth they would work solely for repeal.[104] Repeal MPs who were aware of the difficulty of interesting parliament in the issue were irritated by this ill-judged optimism. Mundella patiently explained to H.J. Wilson the problems of a private member competing for parliamentary time with the government; and excused himself from speaking in public against the Acts on the grounds that to do so would weaken his position in parliament and make his task there all the harder.[105] Rylands, another sorely-tried commissioner, entirely lost patience and abused those who so signally failed to understand parliamentary tactics. He refused to see Josephine Butler, disparaged her moral commitment and ceased to work for repeal.[106]

If MPs were angered by those who did not have to face a hostile House of Commons, repeal militants were confirmed in their suspicions of parliament; Josephine Butler was outspoken in her criticism, if perhaps exaggerating the disaster in the heat of the moment:

> What an *awful* thing tyranny is. A Bourbon or a Bonaparte are not the only tyrants. Burke's prophecy of the most awful of all tyrannies has come true — the tyranny of parliament. The upper classes in parliament desire and are resolved to obtain and keep a system of legal harlotry superintended by government and paid for out of the taxes paid by the people. The mass of the people rebel against it, have petitioned, have protested, even threatened. Their cry has been an exceeding bitter cry, but it is all unheeded. The people are treated with undisguised contempt, and 'on the side of the oppressors there is power'. For looking back to past history one sees that when things come to such a pass only one cure sufficed. *Revolution.* And every one of England's revolutions has been a *restoring reviving* crisis, not a destructive one.[107]

Henceforward it would be an article of faith among repealers outside parliament that the atmosphere at Westminster could only corrupt good men unless watched ceaselessly. MPs did not even do their jobs properly. The first issue of the *Shield* had set out the negligence argument: the Acts had been smuggled through parliament — 'every care has been taken to avoid arousing a slumbering nation' but that nation, now awake, will press its demands upon parliament.[108] When an MP claimed never to have considered the CD Acts, the *Shield* was outraged and pointed out the vast amounts of propaganda and the huge petitions with which parliament was deluged, 'it is too late for any member of the legislative body to plead ignorance on a subject of such vital importance to the moral and physical welfare of the nation, with any show of decorum'.[109] An attitude which ignored the lack of concern evinced by MPs for social issues in general and their distaste for this one in particular.

In the eyes of provincial repealers, the NA was almost as suspect of faint-heartedness. It had inclined to compromise and seemed to defer too much to parliamentary considerations. Josephine Butler spoke dismissively of the quiescent attitude of 'our central tyrants' while Mme Venturi, who had disagreed with her London colleagues over Bruce's

Bill, said of them:

> the majority of us are right in belief and intention, but silent and
> timid in the face of a tiny minority, which lives and moves and has
> its being only to obstruct anything like energetic action which
> might 'alienate our friends in parliament'.[110]

Certainly the NA's favoured tactics in the first three years of the
agitation were primarily designed to assist parliamentary action. Each
year Bruce was waiting upon by deputations of repealers who presented
memorials from large conferences and tried to reason with him. The
deputation which followed the publication of the Commission report
seems to have been carried away by its own enthusiasm. Over 200
repealers crowded into his office (causing Bruce to object that it was
not a public meeting) and proceeded to issue various threats to the
government and to Bruce's electoral position. His reply was tense and
hostile. *The Times* violently attacked the deputation and the presence
of women 'in these disorderly and indecent proceedings'. In contrast,
Mrs Butler thought the deputation courteous, well-prepared and well-
ordered, though Bruce was 'all flesh and blood and official haughtiness'
and tried to browbeat the deputation.[111] A year later, a smaller working
men's deputation was rebuffed and told that the majority of the
government approved of the Acts.[112] A great deal of effort went into
these deputations, but since they were poorly reported and Bruce was
unlikely to be moved by them, this was largely wasted. In any case,
this was the sort of tactic at which the opposition could better them:
in May 1872 150 MPs (87 Conservative, 63 Liberal — of which 77
were connected with the armed forces) saw Bruce in order to urge the
maintenance of the Acts — repealers could never muster that many
MPs.[113]

Sending petitions to parliament was something repealers could
manage better, and in the second year of the agitation, they improved
upon their total in the first. On 30 March 1871, Duncan McLaren
presented a petition from 250,000 women praying for repeal.
Josephine Butler described the surprise and interest which MPs showed
for such an impressive petition; she called it 'the dear fat baby' and
was amused to see that it bulked so large that the double doors into
the House had to be flung open to enable its sponsors to stagger
through with it. To Mrs Butler's indignation, press reports treated
the whole incident as a great joke.[114]

Again the problem was that petitioning, though important to morale in enabling repealers to register large numbers of supporters, and essential if repeal Bills were to appear credible, was still an activity oriented towards parliament. Petitions once presented were forgotten, and their impact rested on the interest of the press — at this stage not great. Three petitions from prostitutes for the maintenance of the Acts probably had as much news value, although the *Shield* was aghast and wondered if brothel keepers would be the next to be heard.[115]

III

By mid-1872, attempts to reach an accommodation with the government had ceased, and the movement began to practise a consistently militant strategy of confrontation and attack. There was nothing new in this; the *Shield* had been urging vigorous questioning of MPs and action at elections irrespective of party, and the extensionists had early felt pressure from their constituents as a result of outside agitation.[116] Hopes aroused by the Commission, and then by the parliamentary crisis early in 1872 had upstaged this strategy without completely replacing it. Indeed this was hardly possible, given the satisfaction to be obtained from putting pressure directly on MPs — something which simultaneously demonstrated the movement's virility and proved to the individual repealer his steadfastness and love of principle.

One of the most notable and successful examples of constituency pressure on an MP was curiously on James Stansfeld, in 1870 and 1871 still an undeclared member of the government. His Halifax constituents included a number of keen repealers, especially Joseph Edmondson and Edward Crossley, and at a meeting of between 6,000 and 7,000 on 19 January 1871 he was keenly questioned on his attitude to the Acts. He had already agreed to carry their repeal views to Gladstone. His determination to wait for the Commission's report disappointed his audience, although he pronounced firmly against extension. The *Shield* was delighted at the 'rebuke' he had received — significant because he was otherwise popular.[117] Gladstone's reply seemed to Stansfeld so satisfactory that he arranged for its publication — they both agreed that moral acceptability was the only real test of the Acts.[118] A year later, when Stansfeld was in the Cabinet, he was warned even more directly that his duty to his constituents (who were condemning Bruce's bill) was more important than his position.

If he could not lift up his voice against a bad measure because he

was a member of the Cabinet, his constituents ought to call upon
him to resign his place, in order that he might no longer be
tongue-tied when legislation required him to speak (loud cheers).[119]

Bruce was selected as a target for attack even before his measure was
announced. In September 1871 Scottish repealers sent agents into his
Renfrewshire constituency, and his autumn meetings were, as a
result, extremely unpleasant. The *Shield* attached great importance to
this lobbying and to the rough reception accorded to Bruce by his
constituents. Craufurd was given a vote of no confidence by his constituents because of his attitude to the Permissive Bill and the CD
Acts.[120]

In late 1872 and 1873 no MP was safe from the possibility of
interrogation by repealers: some refused to oblige their questioners
and were marked down as future targets, some gave uneasy pledges
of support, only to absent themselves when divisions were taken in
the House. There were of course those who needed no pressing:
thus a meeting of working men which filled the Glasgow City Hall
declared that they would oppose even School Board candidates who
supported the Acts ('they hold that a sound moral sense is essential
to fitness for any public office, and that the defenders of immoral
laws should be refused election to any office enabling the holder
to influence public morals') and then cheered their MPs, Graham
and Anderson, who readily declared their enthusiasm for repeal.[121]

The most obvious way to put pressure on a politician was to
threaten his electoral prospects. Two elections in the early years
became famous to repealers because of the violence used against
them. At Colchester in autumn 1870, the government tried for the
second time to get Sir Henry Storks into parliament, this time with
a greater chance of success as Colchester was a subjected district
where the Acts had allegedly brought about improvements. The
Shield denounced Storks — 'any borough that accepts Sir Henry as
a candidate accepts disgrace', and after cursory efforts to extract
assurances from him, announced that Dr J. Baxter Langley would
oppose him.[122]

Baxter Langley was a radical lawyer, also medically qualified, who
had some claims on the Liberal party's gratitude, having withdrawn
in Gladstone's favour at Greenwich in 1868. He was reluctant to
contest Colchester, but agreed when pressed, and on 22 October
issued his election address in the form of an enormous handbill
which was placarded throughout the town. In it, Langley made a bold

attempt to detach the 'advanced' vote from Storks. He pointed out Storks' more outrageous statements, then listed his own beliefs: he opposed the CD Acts, favoured religious freedom and equality and increased education, he was a vice-president of the Reform League and wanted further reform and the ballot, he looked forward to equality before the law for masters and men, direct representation of labour and reduction of hours, he wanted reduction of extravagance, a National Citizen Army as in Germany and arbitration for disputes.[123]

Armed with this manifesto, a small group of repealers led by Josephine Butler and James Stuart[124] descended on the town and conducted a short campaign, which thanks to their opponents was exceptionally violent. Meetings were disrupted and repealers threatened; Mrs Butler was driven from her hotel by threats and took refuge with a working-class family — the point much impressed her. Initially most Liberals were hostile to such wrecking tactics and only the Colchester Quakers helped. But the determination with which the repealers waged their brave campaign is said to have won many over; in particular Josephine Butler thought that many women obliged their husbands to vote against Storks because of his earlier attacks on military wives. Langley was under great pressure to withdraw — the government pressed him to do so. Storks wrote flatteringly and disavowed the roughs who had attacked repealers, and Langley, who was ill, had in fact intended only to harm Storks' chances, not seriously to seek election. He thus withdrew a few days before the poll having damaged Storks severely. Learmouth, the Tory, took the seat with a majority of 510.[125]

The election demonstrated the irreconcilable zeal which repealers brought to their cause, and the challenge which this might pose for the Liberals. Josephine Butler was sure she had won over the nonconformist vote by using moral argument and the effect would be to pressure the government into hurrying up the Royal Commission.[126] The press recognised that electoral work had made repeal a serious agitation, *The Times* listed it as the first of the reasons for Storks' defeat, the *Standard* attacked and mocked electioneering ladies and the *Saturday Review* tried to explain away the defeat by saying it had never 'doubted the value of the cry [repeal] for purposes of popular declamation'.[127]

In the following February Storks was at length found a seat; Earl de Grey slipped him in for his nomination borough of Ripon. The repealers found it difficult to do anything as the campaign was too short to put up a radical, and many while unwilling to support Storks would equally find it impossible to vote for a Tory; it hardly mattered, as the publicity had already been abundantly gained.[128]

At Pontefract in August 1872 an equally startling by-election campaign stimulated the growth of new election oriented repeal bodies. H.C.E. Childers, a former First Lord of the Admiralty, rejoined the ministry as Chancellor of the Duchy of Lancaster, and therefore had to seek re-election. A number of repealers decided to campaign against him. H.J. Wilson of Sheffield provided the money for Fothergill, the LNA's agent, to go there, and went himself.[129]

The object of this short campaign was not to defeat Childers — he was too popular in the constituency — but to embarrass him as a member of the government. Wilson issued a handbill to electors and non-electors suggesting questions about the Acts which they might ask Childers.[130] Mrs Butler and Stuart again campaigned, Wilson was joined by his wife and by Joseph Edmondson of Halifax. The campaign was short but violent, and in one notorious incident Josephine Butler and Mrs Wilson were trapped in a hay-loft by roughs who attempted to smoke them out. This attack coupled with the cheerful élan displayed by the repealers did much to swing opinion towards them. Childers was returned (against a very weak Conservative candidate) but with a majority reduced from 233 to 80. He was a relatively favourable Liberal (indeed he had tried to draw repeal fire off by asserting in a letter to *The Times* that he supported Bruce's Bill for its repeal clauses) who apologised for the unauthorised excesses of his supporters and offered to prosecute any who could be identified.[131]

The Pontefract election had a great effect on the course repeal would take in the next two years. The press was impressed by Childers' reduced majority. The hostile London press denounced repealers but gave them credit for it, whereas the *Manchester Examiner* preferred to denounce their assailants and the *Northern Echo*, then edited by W.T. Stead, treated the whole thing as a triumph for morality.[132]

But repealers were acutely aware that this success had been won by amateurs rushing into unprepared territory; there was only one professional among them, the LNA's recently appointed electoral agent, Samuel Fothergill. How much more effective they would be with a permanent organisation. As one put it:

The experience at Pontefract must stir us up in our efforts to establish machinery by which we shall be able to prepare *every* constituency *before* the occurrence of an election or re-election.

I know how extremely difficult it is to do it when the critical
period has actually arrived.[133]

Josephine Butler had in fact already suggested the formation of an
'electoral union' which could 'strike a heavy blow' at those MPs who
had urged Bruce to maintain the Acts. She told her followers that they
should now work towards the next general election; the list of MPs
on the regulationist deputation to Bruce could be used as a division
list, to identify enemies, the object being to 'make these fellows
afraid of us'.[134] The Pontefract result emphasised the need for better
organisation, which a group of northern radicals now set to work to
provide.

Notes

1. Benjamin Scott, *A State Iniquity; Its Rise, Extension and Overthrow*
(1890), pp. 87—90.

2. Ibid., p. 90; typescript *History of the English Repeal Movement* (1915)
in the Wilson Papers, Fawcett Library. These usually reliable sources indicate
that Miss Wolstenholme sent the telegram. Josephine Butler's recollections
varied. Towards the end of her life she attributed it to the Nottingham doctor,
Thomas Worth (Butler Papers, Fawcett Library, Josephine Butler to Charlotte
C. Wilson, Nov. 1905). Her confusion is explained in her *Personal Reminiscences
of a Great Crusade* (1896), p. 14, where she distinguishes between a telegram at
Dover and an appeal a few days later from Dr Bell Taylor and Dr Worth.

3. Scott, *A State Iniquity*, pp. 91—3; The precise date of the LNA's foundation
remains obscure, but it probably originated in Bristol.

4. Usefully reprinted in K. Nield (ed.), *Prostitution in the Victorian Age*
(1973).

5. FLB 3044: Josephine Butler to Mrs Ford, 31 Dec. 1869.

6. Scott, *A State Iniquity* , p. 100.

7. Josephine Butler, *Recollections of George Butler* (Bristol, *c.* 1893),
pp. 221—3; Scott, *A State Iniquity*, p. 109; FLB 3213: Josephine Butler to
H.J. Wilson, 27 Dec. 1872, 'the Leeds working men . . . were the first to take up
the cause and to answer my appeal in December 1869'.

8. *Shield*, 14 Mar. 1870, p. 12; 1 October 1870, pp. 235—8; Butler, *Personal
Reminiscences Of a Great Crusade* (1896), pp. 17—20; Scott, *A State Iniquity*,
pp. 101—4; *Pall Mall Gazette*, 25 Jan. 1870, for attack on repealers by Dr
Elizabeth Garrett, and reply by Justina (Florence Nightingale), 3 and 18 Mar.
1870.

9. Sheffield Central Library, (Wilson MSS) MD 2547, E. Gertrude Wilson to
H.J. and C.C. Wilson, 4 Jan. 1870, H.J. Wilson to E.G. Wilson, 5 Jan. 1870.

10. Scott, *A State Iniquity*, pp. 116—21.

11. M.G. Fawcett and E.M. Turner, *Josephine Butler: Her Work, Principles
and Their Meaning for the Twentieth Century* (1927), p. 59.

12. *Shield* , 18 Apr. 1870, p. 54.

13. J.L. and B. Hammond, *James Stansfeld, a Victorian Champion of Sex
Equality* (1932), p. 151; C. Woodham-Smith, *Florence Nightingale* (1950),

pp. 226–7.

14. *Skey Committee*, Appendix 2, Letter from Sir H. Storks to F.C. Skey,
22 Oct. 1865.

15. *Shield*, 4 Apr. 1870, pp. 38–9, 42.

16. *Shield*, 11 Apr. 1870, p. 46.

17. *Shield* , 9 May 1870.

18. *Saturday Review*, 21 May 1870, pp. 671–2; *Times*, 4 May 1870, p. 12,
reports a meeting of the EA which decided to concentrate on defending
existing Acts rather than to press for extension.

19. *Shield*, 11 Apr. 1870, p. 46; 18 Apr. 1870, p. 54.

20. *Hansard*, 3rd series (24 May 1870) 201 Col.1306. Fowler's speech, cols.
1309–24.

21. Jeanne L. Brand, *Doctors and the State: The British Medical Profession
and Government Action in Public Health, 1870–1912* (Baltimore, 1965), p. 14.

22. *Times*, 25 May 1870, pp. 7–9, broke its silence on the Acts but found
nothing to say in favour of Fowler; it defended 'a law which is successfully
battling against disease and depravity'.

23. *Shield*, 31 May 1870, p. 110; 6 June 1870, p. 118; 13 June 1870,
pp. 126–7. The *Saturday Review*, 28 May 1870, p. 701, welcomed the Royal
Commission which it expected would thoroughly vindicate the Acts.

24. *Hansard*, 3rd series (18 July 1870), 203 Col.431 – the first of many such
attacks.

25. *Hansard*, 3rd series (20 July 1870),203 Col.574; The *Shield*, 25 July
1870, p. 174, thought the debate was 'another very decided advance', a very
optimistic assessment since reporting was again stopped and three pro-Acts
speeches were reported to only one for repeal, that of Jacob Bright. The *Times*,
21 July 1870, p. 9, ranted against repealers in an extraordinary leader on this
debate.

26. *Shield*, 3 Sept. 1870, p. 206. The amalgamated body was slightly retitled to 'National Association for the repeal of the Contagious Diseases Acts'.

27. *Shield*, 17 Sept. 1870, pp. 223–4. It was defending itself against charges
by the LNA that it had indecently welcomed the Royal Commission.

28. Hammonds, *James Stansfeld*, p. 154.

29. H. Ausubel, *In Hard Times: Reformers among the Late Victorians* (New
York, 1960), p. 114.

30. I owe this reference to H.R.E. Ware, ch. 4, which contains an excellent
assessment of the Commission's significance.

31. A.W. Humphrey, *Robert Applegarth: Trade Unionist, Educationalist,
Reformer* (1913), pp. 248–57. Applegarth was forced to resign his Union
position as a result of his work on the Commission.

32. LNA, *Annual Report for 1870*, pp. 14–16.

33. *Shield*, 10 December 1870, pp. 322–3.

34. *Royal Commission upon the administration and operation of the
Contagious Diseases Acts, PP*, 1871, (408 and 408-1), xix.

35. NA, *Annual Report for 1871*, p. 8.

36. FLB 3200: Mundella to H.J. Wilson, 20 Nov. 1872; see also *Shield*, 25
Nov. 1874, pp. 249–53, a special report on a meeting at Bradford at which
Mundella broke his silence on the Commission and described the impact of
repeal evidence and the official pressure brought to bear on the Royal
Commission.

37. *PP*, 1871 (408), xix, QQ3991-4713.

38. Ibid., QQ433-1197 and 9107-420; for attacks see *Shield*, 14 Oct. 1871,
pp. 688–90, 4 Nov. 1871, pp. 717–18 in which statements made by Bruce as to
the condition of Devonport before and after the Acts were repudiated by the

bench and the town council and were stated to have been made on the authority of Inspector Anniss.

39. *PP*, 1871 (408), xix, QQ10511–959.

40. Ibid., QQ9586–817.

41. *PP*, 1871 (408), xix, Q12863.

42. Ibid., QQ8375–650.

43. Ibid., QQ17240–349.

44. Ibid., QQ17765–8036.

45. Ibid., QQ19526 – 699.

46. Ibid., QQ19920–20101.

47. FLB 3050: Josephine Butler to Miss Priestman, 12 Dec. 1870.

48. *PP*, 1871 (408), xix, Q12895.

49. Ibid., Q12871.

50. Ibid., Q12940 – 1.

51. Ibid., Q12962.

52. Ibid., QQ12921–30.

53. Ibid., Q12932.

54. Josephine Butler, *Recollections of George Butler* (Bristol, *c.* 1893), p. 234.

55. *PP*, 1871 (408), xix, Q13064; she also resented Applegarth's behaviour on the Royal Commission and thought he had 'some spite in him' (FLB 3250: Josephine Butler to H.J. Wilson, 1 Jan. 1873).

56. *Hansard*, 3rd series (14 Aug. 1871) 208 Cols.161–6, for a statement by Mundella describing clause by clause battles on the Commission; see also his revealing Bradford speech in Nov. 1874 reported in the *Shield*, 25 Nov. 1874, pp. 249–53.

57. FLB 5097: Josephine Butler to repealers, 8 July 1871.

58. FLB 3454: Josephine Butler to an unnamed South African correspondent, 9 June 1871.

59. *Shield*, 20 May 1871, p. 498.

60. LNA, *Annual Report for 1871*, p. 9.

61. *Shield*, 22 July 1871, p. 9.

62. *Shield*, 29 July 1871, pp. 383–90.

63. *Times*, 20 July 1871, p. 9 (leader); 25 July 1871, p. 4.

64. *Saturday Review*, 22 June 1871, p. 107.

65. Association for promoting the extension of the Contagious Diseases Acts (EA), *Fourth Report on the operation of the Contagious Diseases Acts* (1872), pp. 7–10; see also *Times*, 31 July 1871, p. 8.

66. FLB 3054: Josephine Butler to Bristol Ladies Committee, May 1871; *Times*, 20 July 1871, p. 9.

67. EA, *Fourth Report*, pp. 8–9.

68. FLB 3200: Mundella to H.J. Wilson, 20 Nov. 1872.

69. *Saturday Review*, 22 July 1871, p. 107; *Times*, 22 July 1871, p. 9.

70. *The Times* often printed extracts from Metropolitan Police reports with laudatory comments, e.g. 16 Apr. 1878, p. 8; 4 July 1879, p. 9; 23 July 1880, p. 5. An attempt to reply to one of these propaganda pieces was refused publication – see *National League Journal*, 1 May 1878.

71. Sheffield University Library (Mundella-Leader correspondence), Mundella to R. Leader, between 29 June and 2 July 1876.

72. FLB 3271: Josephine Butler to R.F. Martineau, 27 May 1873.

73. FLB 3454: Josephine Butler to a South African correspondent, 9 June 1871.

74. Sheffield University Library (Mundella-Leader correspondence), Mundella to R. Leader, 10 Feb. 1876.

75. F.W. Newman, *The Political Side of the Vaccination System* (1874), 16

page paper published by the National Anti-Compulsory Vaccination League.

76. FLB 3134: Josephine Butler to repealers, 12 Mar. 1872.

77. Sheffield University Library (Mundella-Leader correspondence), 18 June 1871; *Shield*, 26 Apr. 1873, pp. 129–30.

78. *Shield*, 8 Oct. 1870, p. 247.

78. M.J. Shaen, *William Shaen, A Brief Sketch Edited by his Daughter* (London, 1912).

80. Butler, *Personal Reminiscences of a Great Crusade* (1896), p. 195, for a tribute; Shaen's most widely circulated writings were papers delivered to repeal congresses and then reprinted as pamphlets: *Suggestions on the Limits of Legitimate Legislation on the Subject of Prostitution* (delivered at the Geneva Congress, 1877); *The Common Law in Its Relation to Personal Liberty and the State-Regulation of Vice* (delivered at the Genoa Congress, 1880).

81. NA EC Minutes, 17 May 1886; Shaen's warm testimonial to Banks emphasised that he had helped the EC 'with decided views on your own'.

82. Though in this respect greatly sinned against; provincial repealers came to suspect the NA of every possible perfidy, but Banks dealt with them civilly and honestly, e.g. his rather plaintive explanations of overwork when H.J. Wilson circulated criticisms of the *Shield*'s inadequacies without an initial approach to him – FLB 3268: Banks to H.J. Wilson, 28 May 1873.

83. To give some indication of the weight to be attached to these figures; Flora Thompson gives the salary of the Head Postmaster of Candleford in the 1880s as about £250 p.a. in *Lark Rise to Candleford* (World's Classics edn, 1954), p. 465.

84. *National Association Letter Book*, 1883–6; F.C. Banks to J. Stansfeld, 22 May 1884.

85. NA, *Annual Report for Years 1870 and 1871*, p. 12.

86. NA, *Annual Report for Years 1880 and 1881*, p. 19.

87. See Appendix B. To put the NA in the context of other pressure groups, in 1871–2 its income was £2,520 12s 2d that of the NEL £6,486 4s 8d. In 1881–2 the NA received £2,605 15s 9d, the Liberation Society £9,075 10s 11d, the UKA £17,332 6s 8d, but the NLF £1,944 6s 5d. The NA was small beer compared to the great nonconformist agitations (a point which will be taken further in chapter 9) but compares favourably with the NLF. Figures from NA Annual Reports and from H.J. Hanham, *Elections and Party Management* (1959), pp. 414–17.

88. *Hansard*, 3rd series (14 Aug. 1871) 208 Cols.1611–16.

89. *Shield*, 19 Aug. 1871, pp. 615–24.

90. Dilke to Mundella, Sept. 1871, quoted in D.A. Hamer, *Liberal Politics in the Age of Gladstone and Rosebery* (1972), p. 42.

91. NA EC Minutes: 27 Nov. 1871; 11 Dec. 1871; 18 Dec. 1871; 22 Jan. 1872.

92. FLB 3054: Josephine Butler to Bristol Ladies Committee, May 1871.

93. FLB 3228: Elizabeth Malleson to H.J. Wilson, 28 Feb. 1873.

94. *Hansard*, 3rd series (13 Feb. 1872), 209 Cols.330 ff.

95. *Times*, 15 Feb. 1872, p. 9.

96. Scott, *A State Iniquity*, pp. 151–3; Hammonds, *James Stansfeld*, pp. 167–77.

97. E.g. *Shield*, 23 Mar. 1872, contained a letter from a male repealer supporting the LNA, extracts from a long letter by Mrs Butler denouncing the bill, and a memorial to Gladstone from the Leeds LNA calling for repeal.

98. FLB 3138, Josephine Butler to H.J. Wilson, Apr. 1872.

99. Ibid. 3142: Josephine Butler to H.J. Wilson, 16 May 1872.

100. NA EC Minutes, 1 July 1872.

101. *Shield*, 20 July 1872, p. 1011.

102. See David Roberts, *Victorian Origins of the British Welfare State* (New Haven, 1960), p. 93. The Metropolitan Police also provided a division to administer the Common Lodging Houses Act, and in the previous year Bruce had himself proposed a special police in his Licensing Bill — criticised by Brewers in CD Acts' terms as a 'French Spy System'; see Brian Harrison, *Drink and the Victorians: The Temperance Question in England, 1815–1872* (1971), p. 266.

103. Harrison, *Drink and the Victorians*, pp. 269, 279.

104. *Shield*, 20 July 1872, p. 1011.

105. FLB 3151: Mundella to H.J. Wilson, 8 June 1872; 3200: Mundella to H.J. Wilson, 20 Nov. 1872.

106. Ibid., 3188: Josephine Butler to H.J. Wilson, Apr. 1872; Scott, *A State Iniquity*, p. 156.

107. FLB 3115: Josephine Butler to her sisters, summer 1872.

108. *Shield*, 7 Mar. 1870, p. 1.

109. *Shield*, 11 Jan. 1873, pp. 9, 10.

110. FLB 3205: Emilie A. Venturi to H.J. Wilson, 10 Dec. 1872.

111. *Times*, 21 July 1871, p. 12; 22 July 1871, p. 9. *Shield*, 29 July 1871, pp. 592–3. FLB 3060: Josephine Butler to George Butler, July 1871.

112. *Shield*, 3 Aug. 1872, p. 1034; 10 Aug. 1872, pp. 1036–39; Scott, *A State Iniquity*, p. 157.

113. *Shield*, 18 May 1872, pp. 939–43.

114. *Shield*, 8 Apr. 1871, pp. 450–3; FLB 3051: Josephine Butler to Mrs Tanner, 4 Apr. 1871.

115. *Shield*, 13 Apr. 1872, pp. 899–900.

116. *Shield*, 3 Sept. 1870, p. 207; *Times*, 4 May 1870, p. 12; *Saturday Review*, 28 Jan. 1871, p. 99.

117. *Times*, 21 Jan. 1871, p. 6; *Shield*, 28 Jan. 1871, pp. 367–8; *Halifax Courier*, 21 Jan. 1871.

118. *Times*, 9 Feb. 1871, p. 12; *Shield*, 18 Feb. 1871, p. 396. Stansfeld was subsequently accused of publishing the letter to influence the result of the Ripon by-election which he indignantly denied, *Daily News*, 13 Mar. 1871.

119. *Shield*, 6 Apr. 1872, p. 894: speech by Joseph Edmondson.

120. NA EC Minutes, 28 Sept. 1871; *Shield*, 7 Oct. 1871, pp. 676–81 (Bruce); *Shield*, 9 Dec. 1871, p. 757 (Craufurd).

121. *Shield*, 12 Apr. 1873, p. 114.

122. *Shield*, 22 Oct. 1870, pp. 266–7; *Shield*, 29 Oct. 1870, pp. 274–5.

123. FLW. Box 4: Address of J. Baxter Langley, 22 Oct. 1870.

124. Fellow Of Trinity College, Cambridge, and a pioneer of university extra-mural work, and of higher education for women (thus a pre-1870 connection with Mrs Butler). Later Professor of Applied Mathematics, later still a Gladstonian MP.

125. Butler, *Personal Reminiscences*, pp. 43–53; *Shield*, 5 Nov. 1870, pp. 254–6; *Shield*, 12 Nov. 1870, special issue on the election. See D.A. Hamer, *The Politics of Electoral Pressure* (1977), chs. 2 and 3, for a general discussion of the electoral policy of pressure groups.

126. FLB 8095: Josephine Butler to H.J. Wilson, 5 Nov. 1870.

127. *Times*, 4 Nov. 1870, p. 6; *Standard*, 4 Nov. 1870; *Saturday Review*, 12 Nov. 1870, p. 620.

128. Scott, *A State Iniquity*, pp. 139–40; *Shield*, 18 Feb. 1871, pp. 394–5, quoting *Daily News*, 'it is impossible to maintain them [the Acts] in the face of the strong popular feeling which has been voiced against them'. Hanham,

Elections and Party Management, pp. 218–20, discusses the Colchester election as the paradigm of those by-elections which wore down Gladstone's administration.

129. FLB 3105: Josephine Butler to·Mrs Tanner, 26 Aug. 1872.

130. Sheffield Central Library (Wilson MSS), MD 2540: H.J. Wilson to the electors and non-electors of Pontefract, 12 Aug. 1872.

131. FLW Box 82: Josephine Butler to H.C.E. Childers (copy), 12 Feb. 1873; *Times*, 13 Aug. 1872.

132. Scott, *A State Iniquity*, pp. 157–63; Butler, *Personal Reminiscences*. pp. 85–98 (the best account); *Shield*, 24 Aug. 1872.

133. FLB 3086: Dr Hooppell to Mrs H.J. Wilson, 12 Aug. 1872.

134. FLB 3139: Josephine Butler to LNA branches, May 1872; Ewing Whittle MD, Circular, 8 June 1872.

4 DEFEAT AND REGROUPING

The moving spirit of this group was Henry J. Wilson of Sheffield, who had been opposed to the Acts since 1870 and had organised the first Sheffield meetings against them in April 1871 — largely to avoid the shame of letting working-class activists take the lead. Wilson was always firm on the need for a middle-class leadership.[1] He was a tireless administrator and a born radical activist — although Mundella disliked him as an 'ultra-rabid Birmingham type' he had to admit that 'he is a capital fellow *in harness* and is only dangerous when he has nothing to do'.[2] Wilson was to be fully occupied for the next 14 years as a leading repealer, but like so many nonconformist radicals he spread his effort generously: in the early 1870s he was a pillar of the Sheffield Nonconformist Committee in opposition to the Education Act, he was a temperance advocate, a liberationist, active on the Eastern Question in 1876 and 1877, on moral questions in the 1880s (he was treasurer of the National Vigilance Association formed to enforce the 1885 Criminal Law Amendment Act), against the opium trade in the 1890s (the sole dissentient on the 1893 Royal Commission). His attitude to religion gloriously typifies his aggressive, independent cast of mind: brought up as a Congregationalist, he later took to attending Quaker meetings though without ever becoming a member; he explained that he did not care for chapel services because he so often wanted to move an amendment to the sermon.[3]

Wilson began to assemble experienced men for the new organisation, stressing the need to recruit those who had already been in 'some *national* political movement'. Dr Hooppell also played an important part in getting things going, offering sensible advice about securing the widest geographical spread at the inaugural meeting, while Mrs Butler laid down the law on how a firm chairman should be selected to ensure that the new body came down firmly against Bruce's Bill and the existing government.[4]

And so it did. The Northern Counties League for Repeal (NCL) was founded at a meeting in Sheffield on 29 August 1872 as a militant electoral body. Wilson became secretary in order to deny Hooppell the post; three days before the meeting, Josephine Butler warned Mrs Wilson off him quite emphatically — sound on Bruce's Bill, energetic and a good organiser, but fatally lacking in discretion — he had displayed the speculum at public meetings and minutely described its use to the disgust of many supporters.[5] Joseph Edmondson of Halifax bacame treasurer, and effectively Wilson's deputy. Edmondson's great strength was his talent for producing long and reasoned moral judgements whenever policy decisions had to be taken. He was one of the clearest thinkers in the movement, his opinions were authoritative. The chairman of the new League was a Quaker businessman, Edward Backhouse of Sunderland. Although sound on principle, he did not participate in the day to day running of the League; his great contribution was financial and until his death in 1879 he was the League's largest single contributor.[6]

Relations with London were difficult from the outset. Mrs Butler warned Wilson to brief Mme Venturi about the new League; she was friendly but needed to be properly handled lest she and the NA Committee took offence at its surreptitious foundation.[7] The *Shield* welcomed the NCL, and Mme Venturi — always one of the most militant Londoners — sent her personal good wishes, but the NA Committee seemed to have reservations and sent a rather frigid note asserting its supremacy:

> As the National Association was formed mainly for the purpose of combining the action of all the Associations of the country, in those things which can be efficiently dealt with by one Association, the Committee will be obliged by you informing them what part of the country the electoral league proposes to undertake.[8]

Though unenthusiastic, the desire to avoid collision was sensible, for the NA was itself about to appoint electoral agents. It had been asked to do so by those working men who had waited on Bruce on 1 August, and on 28 October its agents' subcommittee recommended the appointment of two men, Samuel MacDonald at £150 a year and William Charles at £100.[9] For the moment there was still only one agent at work, the LNA's Fothergill, who had been sent from Pontefract straight to Preston with instructions to harry the Liberal candidate.[10] By the end of the year, the NCL had two agents of its own in the field.

By then another electoral body had been founded. The Midlands had been an early centre of activity with two concentrations of repealers. In the East Midlands there were Charles Bell Taylor and Thomas Worth leading a flourishing local committee at Nottingham.

In the west midlands, the Birmingham Association for Repeal had been founded on 3rd March 1870 and had initially been vigorous and successful – in its first year it had collected 56,000 signatures to a petition, held numerous public meetings and sent two of its members, Arthur Albright, the Quaker industrialist, and William Morgan, a solicitor and a former anti-slavery activist, on a successful visit to Plymouth to investigate abuses of the Acts.[11]

By 1872 the Birmingham Association had subsided into mere subscription collecting. Josephine Butler told H.J. Wilson that Birmingham repealers were mostly Quakers, generous but timid, and suggested that the NCL might also run the midlands. The midlanders were rich enough for this not to be a financial burden, but it might be too much work for the NCL and it could anger the NA. Nottingham would be a better centre but the leaders were not religious and Bell Taylor repelled more serious people.[12] The most energetic of the Birmingham repealers, R.F. Martineau (Harriet's nephew), agreed with Mrs Butler and urged Wilson to take over the midlands, the financial saving compensating for the greater responsibility.[13] But Wilson prudently said no. A population of seven million in the six northern counties provided enough work and it would involve a collision with the NA which he wished to avoid. In any case, he did not want to get involved in local problems – the midlanders must be very dissatisfied with their present leaders to want to transfer themselves to a new and distant organisation.[14]

And so a marriage was somehow arranged between Birmingham and Nottingham, and the Midland Counties Electoral Union (MCEU) was founded on 11 December 1872. Josephine Butler thought the inaugural meeting a success and was especially pleased to see Anglican participation – the meeting was chaired by the Birmingham Broad Churchman, Archdeacon Sandford, who was the first president.[15] The new body worked better than was to be expected; Martineau became its leading figure, and while not as aggressive as Wilson or Edmondson, was yet a man of local political importance with useful experience and connections; while, unlike the NCL, the MCEU had paid officials capable of taking the initiative without direction – a useful facility if sometimes annoying to those who thought that men in receipt of salary should know their place.

The shift towards organised electoral pressure delighted Josephine Butler. She told Harriet Martineau that 'the quickened zeal of *men*, and the new electoral agencies have given us more hope than we ever had yet'.[16] This policy was aggressive and gave obvious proof of the movement's good health. In mid-1872 she had been depressed by the complete lack of progress after a three year struggle of an intensity unmatched since the anti-slavery campaign — even extension had seemed possible to her. But the electoral campaign uplifted her. When she was told that the Commons reporters' gallery thought that the repeal was making more rapid progress than any other in the House, she attributed this to the electoral work of the NCL and MCEU. [17]

The repeal movement was behaving in the same manner as the great nonconformist pressure groups — drink, disestablishment education — unable to persuade the government of the merits of their entire case (though as with repeal often successful at getting it to meet them halfway, which they then declared was not enough) and therefore seeking to intimidate it by demonstrating the strength of political nonconformity and its indispensable contribution to Liberalism's success. It was a risky policy — weakening one's friends to make them more constant — and at the time was disputed by a minority, e.g. Edward Baines or J.J. Colman. There is evidence that by April 1873 the Liberation Society, aware that this 'Nonconformist Revolt' simply demonstrated nonconformity's inability to maintain a separate political existence, was drawing back from the edge, but such moderation was unlikely to affect the more callow repeal movement. [18]

In fact repealers were proud of their improved organisation, and were convinced that their message must be getting across. They believed that if enough noise was made, if enough trouble was caused, then parliament must submit. The *Shield* reminded its readers that the great agitations — Anti-Slavery, Corn Laws, Suffrage, Ballot—had been advanced by tremendous petitioning effort; they should do the same — 'there must be a flood. Parliament is not likely to be moved by a feeble effort'. [19] Every opportunity was taken to question MPs, and by-elections were eagerly sought. The Butlers were quite shrewd about electoral tactics: Josephine discouraged her followers from spending time and effort on the big cities whose MPs were sound — better to work in small boroughs; George preferred contested elections to public meetings as the press could not avoid covering the former. [20] So agents were sent to Preston and Richmond in late 1872 — at the latter, Henry Wilson's wife made her first speech in public and met W.T. Stead working for repeal 'wearing a Scotch cap and giving useful information about the doings of the enemy' [21] — Liverpool, Dundee, Greenwich, Shaftesbury, Hull, Exeter and Bath (twice) in 1873.

The Bath election, of June 1873, illustrates the coooperation with other pressure groups which repealers thought natural. A radical candidate, J.C. Cox, was nominated to try to dislodge the official Liberal. He issued an address to the electors (from Belper!) which was a litany of nonconformist demands headed by National Education. Repeal was included and Coutts, an NA agent, was sent to Bath to help. However, Cox was displeased with Coutts' efforts and wired Wilson for help, hinting that Mrs Butler would be ideal. Wilson himself went down, and after checking on likely sources of support (temperance people, Republican clubs) concluded that Cox would have to withdraw or be badly beaten. He bullied Cox into withdrawing.[22] Cox was a professional 'forlorn hope' candidate, interested in demonstrations of principle rather than political reality; Wilson, while happy to support any candidate opposed to the Acts, was in another class — he argued that the Bath election showed it was preferable to threaten intervention rather than put up a candidate and reveal weakness.[23] But both men favoured joint pressure on government wherever possible, though Wilson disliked yielding first place to the National Education League and tried to wriggle out of paying the repeal share of the election costs when the bill came.[24]

Nonconformist radicals involved in different agitations were never closer than in 1873; they felt they were assaulting a hostile parliament — though in different branches of the same good cause. Repealers admired the superior organisation of the older bodies, while the clear moral position which the Acts required, appealed to other reformers: J.H. Raper of the UKA made a point of commending repeal to temperance office holders as a kindred movement.[25]

Whatever provincial repealers thought of parliament, they could not evade the awkward fact that parliamentary action was still central to their campaign. After the debacle over Bruce's Bill, the movement had shakily rallied round an attack on the Army Estimates on 22 June 1872.[26] The debate was a flop. The government refused to budge at all, and carried their vote by 140 to 74, a comfortable majority which, unlike 1871, owed nothing to Conservative support.

Repealers had to make use of such parliamentary strength as they had, now that they were left without official help. A threat to Fowler's leadership was dropped and he agreed to bring in a Bill in 1873 — though he warned the NA Committee that it was unlikely to succeed without government help.[27] Even the London Committee thought Fowler was weak; they organised a conference in February

1873 to stiffen his resolve, and in particular to bring him 'under the influence of the northern workers'.[28] Edmondson, shrewder and more honest than most, was not worried by Fowler's weakness as a leader; there was no chance of repeal this year, and anything less would be a disaster; better to spend the year strengthening one's forces.[29]

However a debate was an indispensable focus for activity, and Fowler was not allowed to avoid it — though he found his task disagreeable and was annoyed that extra-parliamentary repealers should determine parliamentary policy.[30] An impressive petition campaign was mounted, and a large conference was held on the eve of the debate (to bolster Fowler still further?).

The debate on 21 May 1873[31] was an improvement on the 1870 debate in two respects: the division was better, there were now 128 repealers (although regulationists slightly increased to 251), and secondly the government did not defend the Acts collectively. It failed to provide tellers, and of its 26 members with seats in the Commons only seven voted for the Acts; 14 abstained (including Gladstone and Childers) and five voted for repeal (Stansfeld, Forster, Shaw-Lefevre, the Secretary to the Admiralty and two others). John Bright also voted for repeal.[32] Edmondson was encouraged by the division — the government was now split and Bruce's Bill was thus no longer the policy of the ministry.[33]

The debate itself was a fair one lasting five hours.[34] Fowler opened in the usual manner by condemning the Acts as useless in practice (with a side-sweep at the accuracy of official statistics) and immoral in operation. He reminded the House that the much vaunted moral benefits of the Acts were either the result of an amendment not originally included by the Acts' sponsors, or were undertaken without any statutory authority. His speech neglected one of the major objections to the Acts — their affront to women — but J.W. Henley made much of this. In the course of a speech in which he said that no sanitary improvement could ever justify the Acts in his eyes, he stoutly defended the right of women to participate in the agitation — they alone suffered under the Acts, therefore they had to be free to tell men what this meant.

Bruce defended the Acts and left the House in no doubt that he preferred them to his own abortive Bill, but he spoke as an individual, and it was left to Sir John Pakington to move the rejection of the Bill. He criticised the government for not doing this, though as one of the sponsors of the original Act, he was as competent as any minister in

their defence. He discussed their history and gave his version of what
the Royal Commission had said. He was supported by J.D. Lewis, MP
for Devonport, whose fulsome praise of the Acts extended to the
rash declaration that it would be better that the borough be dis-
franchised than that it should lose the benefits of the Acts. Mundella
wound up for the repealers (he immodestly told Leader that he saved
the debate![35]) telling the House that from what Pakington had said,
he doubted whether they had been members of the same Commission;
he very much regretted signing 'the weak and contradictory report of
the Royal Commission'.

Josephine Butler was impressed by the vote; she told Martineau
that Stansfeld predicted the collapse of the government on the issue,
and gloated over the number of regulationists who had been
pressured into abstaining, though ominously the bulk of the Tory
leadership had opposed the Bill. Naturally she believed repealers
voted on grounds of conscience not pressure.[36] The *Shield* set the tone
of optimism:

We have baffled the 'conspiracy of silence', penetrated into the
very heart of the enemy's country; stormed, and for ever destroyed
their earthworks of false statistics, and laid bare the true centre
and key-stone of their evil position — THE NECESSITY OF VICE.[37]

It would be a mistake to take this sort of enthusiasm at its face
value. Ministers were undeniably being irritated by repeal action, but
apart from Stansfeld's emotional declaration (he spoke of a 'great
moral revival' with tears in his eyes) there is nothing to suggest that
they were shaken. Until the pressures were irresistible, Liberal
governments concerned themselves with sound administration, not
with reform agitations; if National Education could not impose itself
on the government, repeal was unlikely to do so. Indeed it was mentioned only three or four times in Cabinet during 1872, its most
eventful year. The Cabinet found the Alabama question far more
absorbing.[38] *The Times* treated the debate realistically — the Bill had
after all been defeated as had the rest of the year's 'sentimental
legislation', the Permissive Bill and disestablishment.[39]

In the summer of 1873 few repealers saw it that way. Prudent
advice from moderates about the necessity of working through the
Liberal party was brushed aside,[40] though with distinguished exceptions,
such as Henley or Gurney, the Tory voting record spoke for itself.
Still a violent policy was pushed to the embarrassment of repeal MPs

and with little hope of success in the weary 1868 parliament. At the conference on the eve of the 1873 debate, Fowler tried to explain the political background from the Commons' point of view: most repealers were Liberals (and of course he spoke as a loyal Liberal MP) — was it a sound plan to weaken Liberal strength and push them into the hands of a Tory government? He preferred to publicise an MP's vote in his constituency and let his electorate make the decision. ' "Members are beginning to see this", he said, "and I think some who have hitherto voted against me will walk out rather than say 'Aye' to that sentiment." (Cheers).' But most speakers wanted pressure to be put on MPs and candidates.[41] And the proof of this policy's success was said to be that of the 150 MPs who had urged Bruce to maintain the Acts in 1872; 45 failed to support them in the 1873 vote.[42]

Not all repealers were sure of the merits of aggression. Edmondson, though perfectly sound on principle, disliked the policy of forlorn hope candidates, arguing that it identified the movement too greatly with the NEL. He believed that the government was not definitely against repeal and so it was a risk to be seen as 'rank radicals'.[43] Fawcett warned Stuart about the danger of making a minority cause a test question — the opposition could do so much better. Stuart took the point but thought that particular men should be attacked.[44] Those who declined to accept an all or nothing position were bitterly criticised: thus when Applegarth commended W.N. Massey (who had chaired the Royal Commission) to the working-class electors of Tiverton, he was denounced as a traitor by the *Shield*, and was stung into a reply which observed that there were more things to campaign against than simply the CD Acts, and the Liberal party was a better instrument than the Tory party with which to fight them.[45] But for many repealers, the ideal position was that enunciated by R.F. Martineau — cooperation with the 'irreconcilables' of the NEL in a determined effort to force themselves upon the government: 'How different election matters look everywhere now! No candidate appears but has to mention the subject, and there is always respect for our views, and if not entire adhesion, always concession.'[46] At the end of 1873, Stansfeld told Josephine Butler that repeal was now seriously regarded in both cabinet and parliament.[47] But two questions remained unanswered: was it favourably regarded, and were the repealers correct in believing that the country had been aroused against the Acts?

The general election suddenly called in January 1874 gave the lie to all repeal hopes.[48] They had long believed that repeal 'involves issues so momentous that all considerations of party politics are as dust in the balance'. The *Shield* declared that 'at the next General Election, questions alike of party or place will be held subservient to the one great question of National Morality and National Justice'.[49] Indeed the situation did look promising, with prominent Liberals voting for repeal, greater activity than ever before, the forces of nonconformity flocking to the cause and repeal arguments 'treated with courtesy and respect'.[50] The Extensionist Association was lying low; its committee recommended it to 'confine its efforts towards maintaining the Acts . . . until a longer trial shall convince the public of the physical and moral benefits conferred by them'.[51]

The election came upon repealers too suddenly, yet they made vigorous efforts to put their case forward. The NA sent agents to the subjected districts and also to the constituencies of selected enemies: Sir John Pakington at Droitwich, J.D. Lewis at Devonport and W.T. Mitford at Midhurst (all of whom were defeated, though they refused to attribute this to repeal). It also advertised in all the leading dailies and some weeklies and printed 200,000 leaflets. A great deal of attention was paid to securing pledges from candidates, and Gladstone in particular was harried at Greenwich. The same sort of pressure which had been exerted throughout 1873 was intensively applied during late January and early February 1874; little more could have been done.[52]

The results cruelly disappointed heightened expectations. The *Shield* had compared repeal to Free Trade in being able to surmount party issues,[53] but repeal was not in the same league, it could not even compare with the fight for the Permissive Bill.[54] Political non-conformity was dragged down by the Liberal disaster to which it had so notably contributed.[55] Chamberlain's fear of too many sectional interests jostling to make theirs a test question had been justified and none could be satisfied by the Tory victory.[56]

At the most optimistic, the number of repeal MPs dropped to 144; an earlier, unofficial estimate had given the 1873 total as 173 repealers, but the *Shield* was quite prepared to admit that 60 repealers had lost their seats and about 100 known supporters had also gone.[57] Whatever the figures, the movement had suffered grievously. Conservative successes in the large boroughs, the most notable feature of their victory, struck at precisely those radicals who tended to support repeal.[58] Henry Lucy, who disliked radicals as parliamentary bores, was delighted to tell his readers that 'the ladies have lost a champion in Mr. Jacob Bright, miscellaneous causes an umpire in Mr. Fowler; and

the universe a guardian in Mr. Rylands'.[59] The debacle revealed a
gross misjudgement of repeal strategy — was it any consolation to
realise that older and more experienced agitations had suffered the
same fate?

II

The shock of failure after the general election produced a slump in
morale; Josephine Butler was in despair at the arrival of a hostile
Tory government and, seeking a new course, turned to prayer in the
belief that God must have intended the disaster.[60] Until the autumn,
the only significant incident was the final fling of the militant electoral
policy. J.D. Lewis, defeated at Devonport, tried to retain Oxford for
the Liberals; he impetuously declared that he would rather lose five
seats than vote for repeal, and was accordingly pursued and opposed
by repeal agents. Mrs Butler appealed to the women of Oxford, and
H.J. Wilson urged radicals to abstain (it was difficult to vote *for* the
Tory as he was a brewer). Lewis was defeated and the *Shield* rather
desperately welcomed this as the 'most signal triumph' since Colchester;
Lewis hastily denied that repeal had brough him down.[61]

This sort of campaign was on its last legs, resented by Liberals —
Mundella spoke of the 'infinite mischief' done by repealers at Oxford[62]
— and unlikely to be of any effect in a Conservative parliament. But
before the movement could find its way out of the doldrums it needed
a new parliamentary spokesman to replace the defeated Fowler.
Finding one proved exceptionally difficult.

On 16 February the NA Committee, reinforced by representatives
from the LNA, NCL, MCEU and Friend's Association for Repeal,
decided to ask a senior radical, P.A. Taylor, MP for Leicester, to take
on their bill. They prudently drew up a list of four alternatives should
he decline.[63] Not only did he do so (though he declared it an honour
to be asked) but so did the alternatives. Now began a search which
became increasingly desperate as MP after MP declined — perhaps mindful of the difficulties involved.[64] From established radicals, the field
was extended to include new members (S.D. Waddy), Conservative
(Russell Gurney, an early repealer, and Hugh Birley, who had never
voted for repeal and as a Manchester Tory was ironically one of Jacob
Bright's supplanters), and even a parliamentary candidate (H.R. Brand,
standing at Stroud). Mrs Butler made herself ill running round trying
to find someone; she thought a Tory would do well, but insisted on
firmness of principle — Mundella was rejected for lack of this, she
feared he would divide repealers.[65] The problem was eventually solved

in July: James Stansfeld, who had been helping in the search and had
himself declined the honour 'during the present session of parliament
at all events',[66] convened a meeting of MPs at the house of Sir
Harcourt Johnstone at which he proposed his host as leader. The
MPs present, some of whom had already declined, supported this
proposal and Johnstone 'readily consented to carry out the wishes of
those present'. The NA Committee met the following day, 23 July,
and ratified the proposal with a vote of thanks.[67]

The new leader was a Whig baronet, who represented the small
borough of Scarborough controlled by his family.[68] He had declared
for repeal in January 1872, had paired in favour of Bright's motion in
July 1872 and had presided at a public meeting in Scarborough in
April 1873. His first vote against the Acts was in 1873 (he had been in
parliament since 1869) and although his name had been mentioned in
the preliminary discussions about the leadership in February, it had
not been followed up. In short, he was a curious choice, but there was
not much of a field to choose from. He attended to his duties con-
scientiously, bringing in three repeal bills, speaking very occasionally
at public meetings (he used his position as leader as an excuse to
avoid engagements) and popularising the argument that the Acts
were examples of centralised despotism. His motive for accepting the
task was probably an altruistic sense of duty; he was uninterested in a
parliamentary career — he had unsuccessfully solicited a peerage
from Gladstone in 1873, and went readily to the Lords in 1880 to
make way for a defeated minister.[69]

Although Johnstone was the parliamentary leader, more important
in the public's eye was the movement's great new catch, James
Stansfeld, president of the Local Government Board in Gladstone's
Cabinet and one of the most prominent radicals. Since his introduction
to the Acts by his Halifax constituents in 1871, he had been the
Cabinet's unofficial repealer; the only vote he had ever given for the
Acts had been in support of the adjournment in 1870, a whipped vote.
Thereafter he had abstained until 1873 when he had voted for repeal.
Stansfeld's mind had been made up by the Royal Commission's
report; he became a private adviser to Josephine Butler, offering
tactical suggestions on how best to influence the government. She
responded warmly: 'Mr. Stansfeld has been like a kind, helpful
brother to me. His sympathy is *complete*. I am confident he cares little
for office in comparison with this question.'[70] In 1872 she was describing him as 'a truly Parliamentary friend to our cause' and he was
acting as intermediary between her and Gladstone.[71] In October 1873

he stayed with the Butlers who were impressed by his approach to
'the greatest of all subjects'.[72] His silence in public was attributed to
'official etiquette' and it was widely believed that he had stiffened the
repeal clauses in Bruce's Bill.[73] After the election, freed from the
responsibilities of office, he was able to take an open decision on his
position; he became an active repealer and in June 1874 accepted a
vice-presidency of the National Association. His refusal to become the
official leader was probably influenced by reluctance to sever himself
from the possibility of future office — he certainly realised the threat
to his career of too great an involvement in a disagreeable cause — but
decided to offer the languishing movement his undoubted experience
and ability.[74] Thereafter these very qualities propelled him to the
fore and pressed upon him the leading part he may not have desired.
He accepted this, and made a public declaration for repeal at the
beginning of October which cheered repealers. His first speech on the
subject was at the LNA Annual Meeting in the Colston Hall, Bristol,
on 15 October 1874; he declared:

> I have made my choice — I have cast in my lot with these men and
> women — for ever reverenced be their names — who hitherto have
> led a hope which too long has seemed forlorn, and never will I
> desist and never will they desist from this sacred agitation until
> these degrading laws are blotted out from the Statute Book for
> ever.[75]

Stansfeld and Johnstone were an enormous gain to the movement;
they provided determined leadership and a counterweight to provincial
extremism. After 1874, parliamentary considerations could no longer
be ignored as in the days of the indecisive Fowler's leadership. In short,
the initiative was now taken from the hands of those who had pressed
the unsuccessful militant policy. Instead, there began the process of
integrating the repeal cause into the general structure of Liberalism.
Mundella had foreseen that the Tory ministry would be 'a wholesome
discipline to the Liberal Party' and told Leader: 'A very distinguished
man of the moderates said to me today, "the next five years will be
spent in educating the Nonconformists." He meant in teaching them
to be tame and submissive. I don't believe this. I look forward to an
advanced and practical party with larger views and fewer crotchets.'[76]
The great nonconformist agitations: UKA, Liberation Society,
Education League, did indeed move closer towards the Liberal Party
in the aftermath of defeat, and under Stansfeld the repeal movement

followed suit, abandoning the non-partisan fanaticism of the early
years. Significantly, at the MCEU's Annual Meeting in December 1874
he warmly supported Fowler when the defeated leader inveighed
against 'endeavouring to split up parties into small sections by undue
pressure on candidates'.[77]

III

This more pedestrian policy necessitated changes in the movement's
structure and orientation. Quiet, behind the scenes pressure was not
the stuff of a great reforming agitation, nor was it likely to satisfy
Josephine Butler's crusading temperament. Fortunately she discovered
in foreign work an answer to both problems. On 25 June 1874, in the
middle of a period of depression and uncertainty, a conference was
held at York, at which the Rev. C.S. Collingwood, an Anglican repealer
of long standing and a former pupil of George Butler, referred to the
proceedings of a medical congress held at Vienna earlier in the year
which had proposed an international system of regulation. Mrs Butler
was inspired and outraged by this new challenge – the struggle would
be broadened and 'the unity of the moral law and the equality of all
human souls before God' preached throughout Europe. She flung
herself into organising foreign work, and spent the winter of 1874-5
on a famous European tour. Her day-to-day influence on the conduct
of the domestic struggle slackened, but her new contribution – to
turn repeal into an international movement, thus providing a
vicarious sense of cosmopolitan excitement for home workers, was
probably more important as a means of sustaining morale in the late
1870s.[78]

Unlike many of her insular repeal colleagues, Wilson especially, Mrs
Butler felt at ease working on the continent – her French was perfect,
her sister Hatty was married to an Italian merchant, the Butlers regularly
spent the summer in Switzerland,and, later in life, she was forced by ill
health to winter abroad. Her tour of Europe from December 1874 to
February 1875 convinced her that widening the battle against
regulation would revive the movement in Britain, and the challenge
posed by the continental system excited her. In France she visited the
St Lazare Hospital in Paris, and had a famous interview with Lecoeur,
the head of the *Police des Moeurs*, she enlisted the cooperation of
Edmond de Pressensé, a leading Protestant and a senator and of Yves
Guyot, the Radical journalist and politician; she even had
sympathetic interviews with Jules Favre and Jules Simon. In
Switzerland she recruited Aimé Humbert, a professor who had been
Chancellor of the Swiss Federation of ten years and who was

willing to work permanently for repeal if a salary could be found for him. She returned, determined to foster repeal activity on the continent.[79]

The first thing to do was to acquire support and money. To this end she enlisted H.J. Wilson's help in organising a small meeting to arouse interest. She had already received money from Quakers towards her tour, and she cannily impressed upon Wilson the need to invite 'those who are responsible for the money and who also have some faith in the necessity of not abandoning the work begun abroad'. They arranged a small meeting at the Euston Hotel on 3 March 1875 to consider privately her proposal to found a new organisation.[80] Evidently this meeting of financial supporters approved her proposals, as the inaugural meeting of what was to become the British, Continental and General Federation was held in Liverpool on 19 March; eight repeal bodies were represented and it was decided that the Federation's General Committee would consist of representatives of all societies subscribing at least £1 per annum, and it would elect an executive committee and officers. A subscription list was opened which, as Mrs Butler had predicted, was overwhelmingly filled up by internationalist-minded Quakers.[81] Josephine Butler handled the foreign work and Wilson temporarily acted as organising secretary. Although he helped to get the Federation started, and committed the NCL to supporting it, Wilson seems motivated more by concern for Mrs Butler's health (which did in fact break down by the summer) than by real interest in foreign work, and soon dropped out, to be replaced by James Stuart. The Cambridge don became the Federation's treasurer and, after Mrs Butler, its most committed adherent.

Stuart and Mrs Butler for a number of years *were* the Federation, indeed its international composition was suspect — initially the entire Executive Committee was British and foreigners seldom attended its first conferences held in Britain.[82] Despite generous references to continental workers, British finance was always crucial. The NA gave the Federation what Banks described as a 'generous start' which set back its own finances, and when the Federation opened an appeal fund for £1,500, it subscribed £250.[83] It also provided free administrative help; for instance, in 1877 it offered to undertake the Federation's fund-raising, so as to relieve Mrs Butler and Stuart, and in 1881 we find Banks doing all the administrative work for the Federation's London conference.[84] The two associations with which Mrs Butler was most closely associated, the LNA and the FA, subscribed generously. Despite all this, the Federation was a perennially poor body with few individual subscribers and high costs; Stuart regularly had to resort to begging funds from wealthier societies, and in 1876 naively proposed a central fund of repeal donations from which he presumed the Federation would be able to extract a larger share.[85] This suggestion prompted a violent reaction from the MCEU and NCL, who abandoned their earlier support and had to be chided by Stansfeld for thus taking too narrow an interpretation of their task — though the NCL's reaction is understandable as its president and largest subscriber, Edmund Backhouse, had just informed it that he would be reducing his subscription so as to give more to the Federation.[86] In its first three years the Federation raised £5,700. Only £400 came from the continent but £2,300 was spent there and another £1,850 went on the Geneva Congress.[87]

In its early years, the Federation was effectively run from Mrs Butler's Liverpool home; she drew £150 from its funds for the expenses of an office and one or two clerks. With these resources she conducted a massive correspondence coordinating the work of 24 affiliated organisations as well as isolated friends in Europe and America.[88] But at an early stage a continental office at Neuchatel was set up with Aimé Humbert in charge, and gradually this became an alternative headquarters, though never financially autonomous. Humbert was in a position to act against continental regulation — in Geneva, Paris, Brussels — and was supplied with the funds to do so. He also organised the first of the Federation's great Triennial Congresses at Geneva in 1877 — an enormous success which enhanced the standing of foreign work. The intermediate conferences and meetings of the Executive were still held in England and were British in composition, but the great events of the late 1870s and early 80s occurred abroad, and repealers implicitly acknowledged this by allowing their money to be spent there. From this handsome support for continental work the repeal movement derived three sorts of benefit.

Firstly, repealers were eager to demonstrate that they were part of a wider battle against immorality and that their movement was an international one — thus Mrs Butler's European tours, and that of the USA by Wilson and J.P. Gledstone in 1876. The support of foreign worthies — Mazzini, Garibaldi, Victor Hugo, Père Hyacinthe (a former priest and preacher of great power whose visit to London in 1876 was expertly handled by Mrs Butler to demonstrate to the English political establishment the international opposition to regulation,[89]) was received enthusiastically as evidence that correctness of principle knew no boundaries. Even Bebel was quoted, though with reservations about his views in general.[90] Secondly, foreign examples could be used to demonstrate the excesses to which the Acts might lead. In Hong Kong a similar system had led to great brutality and corruption, the details of which were eventually exposed by Sir John Pope-Hennessey when Governor.[91] Nearer home, the arrogant behaviour of the 'Morals Police' in France and Belgium, their disregard for morality in their haste to discipline prostitution, was a warning to English repealers, already mindful of centralised police despotism, of what the Metropolitans might lead to. Thirdly, the rise of foreign work came at precisely the time it was needed — it helped fill the gap caused by the collapse of the militant strategy in 1874. The attention to foreign news in the *Shield* reflects this: by 1878 it contained more foreign than domestic news (other than dreary court reports), and although the 1880 election redressed the balance, we find foreign reports are again staple fare in 1881, and its Annual Retrospect of notable events gave more space to foreign than to British news. And if reports from exotic parts were always welcome, they were yet more so when there was progress to be noted. The MCEU warmed to foreign work again when the Paris Municipal Council moved against the *Police des Moeurs* in December 1880, and the exposure of the traffic in young girls to Belgium was a thrilling story in any terms.[92] A special issue was devoted to the apparent demise of regulation in Paris, though this proved premature when the government overturned the municipality's decision.[93]

In the early 1880s the continental movement began to acquire some independence: the initial advantage enjoyed by the well-organised British movement began to wear off, and its remoteness became a disadvantage — all congresses and most conferences were held on the continent and repealers there profited from these meetings rather more than British delegates. Although there were almost as many British delegates (43) as the others combined (45) at the Hague Congress in 1883, there were signs that the easy predominance of the former group was coming to an end. The president of the Congress was the Belgian, Emile de Lavelaye, and the Dutch government lent an official building for the proceedings — progress not likely to be matched on the other side of the Channel.[94]

In the following year Mrs Butler relinquished day-to-day control to a new permanent *bureau* set up in Neuchatel and run by Humbert's former assistant, Henri Minod. This was empowered to act between meetings of the Executive Committee and thus Minod was able to exercise powers of initiative.[95] Real independence for the Federation came in 1886 with the triumph of the British campaign; the NA was dissolved and replaced by a mere branch of the international body.

IV

Foreign work was at best a palliative. Although the years of Conservative rule postponed any hope of success, the movement had to be kept alive for the day when the Liberals would return. Only hard work at home could ensure this. Therefore the movement's structure was diversified in the years after 1874 and an elaborate network of organisations was constructed so as to tap every possible source of support: denominations, doctors, the working class, the City and the subjected areas all came to have their own repeal bodies.

The central activity for these repealers, as for most reformers of the period, remained the annual attempt to persuade parliament to meet their demands. All other activities depended on it, and to a certain extent the result was less important than the effort: thus the Friends' Association for repeal complained in 1878 of the difficulty of conducting the agitation without a repeal bill, even if the 'mechanical majority' would automatically defeat it.[96] The importance of the annual motion was as a focus for the year's activity – petitions, meetings, conferences and the like would all be devoted to its support. This was especially so in the years after 1874 when, with the abandonment of an active electoral policy, the repeal bill was the one great piece of hard news in the year. The *Shield* was expanded to a treble number (price 6d – normal price 1d) to accommodate exhaustive analyses of the debate and division. Each year repealers had a great event to work towards, and if success eluded them, the debate at least produced an up-to-date register of friends and enemies in parliament.

This emphasis was highly gratifying to the parliamentary leadership. Stansfeld took great care to arrange supporting action for the debate, and used repeal conferences to orchestrate extra-parliamentary activity, organising speakers, meetings and so forth.[97] More than Johnstone, he appreciated the interdependence of parliamentary and extra-parliamentary activity, and regretted Johnstone's refusal to bring in a bill in 1877 – the official leader's parliamentary preoccupations blinded him to the bill's wider role – as a means of airing the arguments and showing that the agitation was alive. This was a common enough feature of reform activity: Lawson's Permissive Bill, Miall's disestablishment motion, Richards' efforts for international arbitration were features of the parliamentary scene. Associated with repeal were P.A. Taylor's annual efforts to amend the Mutiny Bill to give more protection to soldiers' and sailors' dependants — nothing came of them, but still he battled on for a good cause 'demanding justice for the oppressed, and . . . speaking for those who cannot speak for themselves.'[98]

Such activity was in itself worthwhile, simply to show that a cause was not lacking support; a decent showing was usually possible, and if not obtained, simply made reformers all the more anxious in the following year. Thus in 1881 J.W. Pease opened the debate on the opium trade by saying that as a rule he did not like annual motions, but was bringing this one on simply to remedy an unsatisfactory debate in 1880.[99]

Yet indispensable though it was, the annual motion could not succeed in the face of a permanently hostile Conservative majority; it wearied them and gave its proponents a reputation for crankiness. Henry Lucy defined an empty House as one in which 'Stansfeld was on his legs delivering his annual speech on the rights of his fellow-women'[100] and the knowledge that persistence in the Commons simply exposed one to ridicule, produced despair among repeal MPs who were pressed to go on with bills which they knew could not succeed in the doldrum years of Disraelian hegemony. In fact, despite clever juggling with figures, the repeal performance in parliament worsened between 1874 and 1880 as demoralisation set in. The 1875 repeal bill's second reading on 23 June was preceded by the usual wave of petitions and meetings and many repealers were swept away with confidence, having just been campaigning over a sordid example of the Act's effect — the suicide of Mrs Percy at Aldershot.[101] H.J. Wilson was more realistic, admitting privately that the bill would not be carried.[102]

The debate lasted six hours, the longest until then, which at least suggested acceptance of the subject as a serious one.[103] Johnstone made his first parliamentary speech on the Acts, criticising their centralising and immoral tendency, but making it clear that he was not a wages-of-sin man: 'I am not going to say that because the disease is caused by immorality, therefore it ought not to be cured.' Henley reminded the House of his early opposition to the Acts 'on the simple ground — which I stated at 3 in the morning — that it was no business of the state to provide clean sin for the people'. Colonel Alexander, Conservative member for South Ayrshire, moved the Bill's rejection in very moderate terms. He defended the Acts as effective public health measures, well liked in the areas to which they applied and no more a denial of liberty than other health acts. This worldly, rather superior tone was taken up by another Conservative, Stephen

Cave, who extolled supporters of the Acts as realistic yet benevolent men of principle, and patronised repealers who he suggested were deceived by their good hearts about the difficulties in the subjected towns. The middle ground was staked out by H.C.E. Childers, who suggested implementing the Royal Commission's report: abandon periodical inspection and fall back on the 1864 Act; predictably he was supported by W.N. Massey, who reiterated the Commission's conclusion of the medical efficacy but moral impossibility of periodical inspection. However, the hygienic arguments for the Acts, ignored contemptuously by most repealers, *were* taken up by Stansfeld in his parliamentary introduction to the Acts. (He had spoken briefly in defence of women repealers during the Women's suffrage debate on 7 April.) He treated the House to an involved criticism designed to weaken the departmental use of statistics; however he did not shake the government's confidence in them, as Gathorne Hardy, the able Secretary for War, made clear in his brief defence of the Acts when winding up.

It was not an entirely satisfactory debate for repealers. Johnstone and Alexander had gone on for hours with mediocre speeches, while Stansfeld had been obliged to abandon his for want of time. Childers had introduced a red herring, attractive to moderates as Mundella admitted.[104] Above all, the Cabinet had carried the division with a majority of 182, the largest ever; the Prime Minister cast his first and only vote on the subject. Wilson reassured the Northern Counties' League Committee that although the parliamentary performance was disappointing, they were at least getting stronger in the country.[105]

To cheer themselves up, repealers noted 'the improved tone and temper of the discussion'; at 126 the repeal vote was maintained surprisingly well. But the one really encouraging feature was the fact that the Liberal party was becoming identified with repeal. Gladstone, Bright, Childers, Forster and W.P. Adam had all voted for it, which suggested to the *Shield* 'a time, perhaps not far distant, when the Liberal leaders of the day will make the repeal of the Acts a part of their political programme?'[106] Although professionally optimistic, the *Shield* was looking in the right direction: 109 Liberals had supported the Acts in 1873, but in 1875 only 72 did so; whereas the number of Conservatives, increased by the election and whipped in by the government, had risen from 153 to 238. The moral was obvious: nothing at all could be expected from a Conservative majority, at least there was hope with a Liberal one.

The debate on the 1876 Bill was, if anything, even worse than

that of 1875.[107] It was dull, repetitive, overlong — and when it came
to the division, just as negative. Johnstone, Stansfeld, Mundella and
Henley repeated arguments made in previous years and were supported
by Samuel Whitbread, who had more experience of regulation than
most, since he had chaired the 1862 committee. Ward Hunt, the First
Lord of the Admiralty, defended the Acts in a brief, 'official' winding-
up, and the Bill was thrown out by the large majority of 122 (224
for the Acts, 102 against).

The *Shield* made what it could of the debate: only two speakers
had spoken in favour of the Acts, the absentees (100 members less
voted in 1876 than in 1875) had *all* been pressured by their constituents,
only the government's majority was maintaining the Acts 'in defence
of public feeling' — all this was designed to cheer the readership.[108]
But the futility of the debate could have kept away just as many MPs
as were subjected to pressure. However Colonel Alexander was a
notable victim of local agitation. After the 1875 debate repeal agents
had been sent to Ayrshire to organise petitioning, and as a result of
their efforts, the Colonel agreed to take no part in the debate, although
he voted for the Acts.[109] As in the previous year, the only hopeful sign
was the continued decline in the number of Liberals prepared to vote
for the Acts, now only 43 with only two ex-ministers, Hartington
and Lyon Playfair. While reassuring itself that its cause was one of
principle not party, the *Shield* pointed out 'that the feeling of the
country is better understood and more respected by Liberal than
Conservative members'.

In 1877 the repeal cause reached its nadir. The country was preoccupied with foreign affairs and many repealers were themselves
active supporters of the Eastern Question Conference. H.J. Wilson was
struck by the mighty Liberation Society's decision not to hold meetings
in so unfavourable a climate, while Stansfeld admitted that not much
could be done at home, so urged a concentration on foreign work, and
on reclaiming women in the subjected districts.[110] But alternatives
could not satisfy the repeal organisations. The NA summoned a
meeting of all repeal bodies on 5 February to discuss the form of action
for the session; it unanimously pressed for a repeal Bill.[111] But
Johnstone had no stomach for another heavy defeat and declined to
introduce a Bill. This rift between the two sides of the agitation was
based on their different preoccupations; MPs knew that the Bill would
be useless and would simply result in loss of face, but they failed to
appreciate its central importance to repealers outside the Palace of
Westminster. The *Shield* lamented the decision as a matter for

'universal regret', even if a Bill stood no chance it would have shown that the movement was still active. It suggested that there would be 'various attacks upon the system in its details' until 'the pitched battle in the next session'.[112] In fact the only signs of activity in the Commons were a tribute to women repealers by C.H. Hopwood (during a suffrage debate) and a question about the number of CD Police.

The absence of a Bill proved a disaster; activity slackened as repeal committees fumbled for substitutes. All this is evident if the *Shield* for 1877 is compared with volumes for other years; it discussed other Bills and reported almost any meeting at length but still had difficulty in filling its pages with interesting copy. At the beginning of 1878 in its annual 'retrospect of the year's activity', it could not select any notable happening or sign of progress in 1877, rather it concentrated on foreign news. The NA's subscriptions tailed off so that in November Banks was forced to send out an urgent begging letter as the NA was quite without funds.[113] In short, while parliamentary action had always been a focus for repealers, by 1877 it had become quite indispensable, and the parliamentary leadership had the initiative.

Towards the end of the session the NA convened a conference to discuss the promotion of 'a great revival of the movement'. Shaen urged a repeal Bill for 1878 on the MPs; the absence of one in 1877 had produced 'in appearance at least, a certain lull in our agitation', but a Bill next session would make repealers redouble their efforts. Stansfeld now thought it had been a mistake to have no Bill, and the conference warned that the movement would languish further without parliamentary action. Johnstone had to agree to introduce a Bill; he defended himself by listing the distinguished advisers he had consulted, including Gladstone, Bright, Childers and Forster, but he could only bow before the weight of demands.[114]

There was instant relief. The LNA Committee promptly and enthusiastically thanked him, and instructed its members to prepare their petition for the next session.[115] They produced a women's petition with over 100,000 signatures, and in general the movement made a special effort to support the Bill. A new, milder approach was evident — the *Shield* advised its readers that the best way to influence MPs was by constituents seeing them personally and laying out their arguments — a far cry from the days of barracking at meetings.[116] But no amount of judicious influence could alter the composition of the House or its procedures. On 22 May the Bill came second on the Orders of the Day, but the preceding measure took so long that there could be no time for a division; moreover an Irish member wasted time by attempting to have the galleries cleared (this had not happened during a repeal debate for eight years and the rules had been changed — the speaker reproved him for trifling with the House's dignity). The result was a crammed excuse for a debate: Johnstone made a long and boring speech, taking up so much time that Stansfeld could only formally support him. The government replied briefly and the debate ended.[117] Had it been divided upon, it would certainly have been defeated; as it was it did not even merit a special number of the *Shield*.

Tactically the movement was at a loss. The Bill had been a disappointment, as all MPs must have known it would be, but it would have to be mechanically repeated to avoid another slump in activity — the supporters of the Acts were ever watchful and eager to allege that the agitation had fallen off. Repeal had ceased to be an agitation capable of fixing its own course. It had come to be dependent on its parliamentary supporters, and they had no solution to offer as long as the Tories remained in office.

V

Working-class opposition to the Acts was to be expected — as obvious examples of 'class legislation', lack of it would have been a serious weakness. Josephine Butler's first appeals were to working-class audiences, and in early 1870 she circularised Trades Councils seeking their support. The Birmingham Trades Council held a special meeting to consider the matter and unanimously pledged its assistance. William Gilliver, its secretary, became a firm repealer. The TUC reply recognised that the Acts 'would affect the working classes more than any other class' and urged united action against them.[118] Rather obscurely the LNA claimed that until 1870 opposition to regulation had been confined to the working class and only now was the middle class taking up the struggle.[119]

In the early years, repeal speakers asserted without contradiction that the working class supported them; regulationists never dared to boast as did the *Shield* in 1873 that 'our strength is in the working classes of this country; when appealed to, they have never given an uncertain sound and many of their leaders, for instance Messrs Applegarth, Howell, Burt, Arch and Kane are among our most earnest supporters'. Particularly in the north, agents reported strong opposition to the Acts at well attended meetings.[120] Yet repealers were slow to arouse working-class feeling directly; that the potential was there is suggested by a Leeds workman, Algernon Challis, who acted as secretary to the Leeds Committee, despite having to work long hours, and walked to Pontefract and back in 1872 to help at the election.[121] However, when Bruce received a deputation of workers in 1872, it was led by a middle-class radical, a Brighton cab proprietor who 'exercised considerable influence amongst working men'.[122] Only Josephine Butler displayed any awareness of the need to enlist the distinctive support of workers; she selected agents for the LNA on ability to communi ate with working-class audiences, and claimed to find in one old artisan more consistency of principle than in many clergy.[123] But to reach large audiences of working men she believed it was necessary to recruit 'the upper class, trades union Leaders' and the breakthrough here came in January 1873 when she held two successful meetings when the TUC met at Leeds. George Howell presided at a public meeting of over 1,000; Arch and Broadhurst also spoke and a unanimous motion for repeal was carried. A 'tea-meeting' specifically for delegates was also held, and she made a point of trying to see Arch and other leaders privately. After this ardent wooing, the trade union leadership was reliably pro-repeal.[124] Even so not all repealers shared Mrs Butler's belief in the importance of recruiting leading trade unionists. The NA Committee declined to accept offers of paid work from both Broadhurst and Howell (though it gladly accepted both as members), exhibiting the same reluctance as the Liberation Society to entrust responsibility to (while welcoming the support of) men of independent standing.[125] Certainly there was room for disagreement; even Howell, with his predilection for working with the middle class, crossed swords with the *Shield* when he announced that one of his reasons for opposing the Acts was that they reversed the trend (instanced by the Factory Acts) of affording women greater protection. But middle-class reformers, beyond any need for industrial protection, failed to see his point. To the *Shield* there was a difference between real and ostensible protection. The Factory Acts offered the latter; by depriving women of 'honest industry' they caused prostitution — the only real protection was 'freedom and the right to responsible self-government'.[126]

When the question of founding a working-class auxiliary body arose, the impetus came not from London, but from Liverpool. A series of meetings organised by William Burgess, the LNA's agent, in the winter of 1874—5 resulted in the foundation of the Working Men's National League (WMNL) on 23 February 1875. Edmund Jones, a local basket weaver and old Chartist involved in various reform movements including temperance and peace for over 30 years, who had been speaking for two years for repeal, became its president, and, as he had to give up his shop, received a small salary from the League. Mrs Butler assured a sceptical H.J. Wilson that the new movement owed nothing to her (she had been abroad at the time) and insisted that it was genuinely spontaneous and thus far likelier to win working-class support than the efforts of middle-class organisations — including her own.[127] But despite her firm support, Wilson doubted the wisdom of having a separate organisation for workers; he particularly suspected anything to do with Burgess, and when Mrs Butler's health collapsed he began to work against the WMNL, initially by suggesting that Burgess was acting without authority. Burgess defended himself by getting Stansfeld to pronounce in favour of the new League — which he did most decidedly.[128] Wilson then turned on Jones and began investigating his abilities — the replies he received, though sometimes condescending in tone, were again satisfactory.[129] Finally Wilson issued a circular to the NCL Executive Committee questioning the whole idea of a separate workers' body; he urged the need for the classes to work together and said that in Sheffield this produced the best results. He also reverted to his theme that expanding a committee in Liverpool, 'of which a salaried President is the principal feature' would not win other working-class leaders.[130] This circular produced a mixed response: two members supported the WMNL, with George Butler pointing out the inconsistency of calling the Acts class legislation without enlisting the support of the class affected, and even more pertinently answering Wilson's standard complaint, 'It is the privilege of the wealthy to labour gratuitously for the public good. If we are to say that we cannot be served efficiently and faithfully by anyone who receives remuneration, we must close our ranks against all who are not in an independent position.'[131] But against this, two members replied in terms which showed that some middle-class reformers did not value the working-class contribution; as one put it, 'I do not think working men as a section, should be organised in any way, neither do I think they are likely to be got to support the cause in any special way. I have far more confidence in the middle class, who have hitherto been the *working* class in the cause.'[132] The issue was eventually decided at a conference in London called by Stansfeld; given his experience of working-class cooperation, and the support of the NA, LNA and MCEU, the foundation of the WMNL was greeted cordially — though unlike the generality of unanimous resolutions, three neutral votes were recorded. Wilson still felt unable to come to terms with independent working-class activity.[133]

The WMNL's aims were ambitious: it was intended as a large organisation, and hoped to recruit 50,000 members within a year. The sole condition of membership was acceptance of the principle of total repeal, so no particular demands were made — cards were available for the collection of small sums. Spreading the word amongst the working class was to be the chief activity — thus discussions would be promoted in clubs, trade unions and temperance societies, and all would be invited to affiliate to the League. A monthly paper, the *National League Journal*, was founded in August 1875 and freely distributed; it promised to keep the busy workers informed of the agitation's progress, to be decent in tone (so young and old of either sex could read it) and to print the names of all members — the National Roll.[134] Initially the *Journal* was a lively, distinctively militant paper, its content directly geared to its working-class readership; it continually stressed the force with which the Acts bore on working women, it linked them to the existence of a standing army, it liked to fill up space with little self-help aphorisms and paid particular attention to material conditions in the subjected towns. The Percy case provided a recent example of tyranny to point up, and Jones made the most of it; he addressed 70 meetings in the first year, 40,000 copies of his statement of principle were distributed, 5,000 in large poster form. Some successes were registered — Trades Councils at Glasgow, Bristol and Leeds condemned the Acts — but by July 1876 the National Roll contained only 10,000 names (and probably never reached 50,000, though this was claimed in 1884) and financial problems were beginning to delay progress.

It had always been clear that a generous recruitment policy would cause such problems and the League Committee had hoped to trust 'to the liberality of all classes to support their efforts'. A number of middle-class bodies did contribute to the first year, but individual subscriptions were said to be poor, and lack of money prevented the League from employing a full time agent to canvass support and get them to the promised 50,000.[135] At the first annual meeting, it was faced with the immediate question of how to pay off a debt of £100 and the longer term one of how to break out of the vicious circle of inadequate finance restricting membership. The solution reached was to compromise its independence and seek a permanent subsidy from the Friends Association, which had plenty of money (it doubled its subscribers in 1876) but little to spend it on since almost all Quakers were repealers.[136] The banker, George Gillett, advised the League on its future organisation, the *National League Journal*'s

publisher, Alfred S. Dyer, placed a London office at the League's disposal, and a Quaker flour-miller, William Catchpool, became the
Journal's editor. The debt was paid off by five wealthy repealers led
by P.A. Taylor, MP.[137] In January 1877 the League office was moved
to London to share the premises of the Friends Association. A new
constitution was adopted creating the post of chairman, filled by A.S.
Dyer, P.A. Taylor, (a Unitarian) became treasurer, and Edmund Jones
followed to London where he was occupied holding meetings on
behalf of the FA and the WMNL.[138]

Thus its financial weakness had driven the WMNL into the arms of
well-meaning middle-class Quakers; Banks described Dyer as the
League's 'chief' and told Stansfeld that the FA was its backer. A
Quaker writer described supporting the League as one of the FA's
main activities and henceforth grateful references to its generosity
were heard at all WMNL annual meetings.[139] With a largely middle-
class hierarchy, the League became exactly what Josephine Butler
had feared — a rather tame, careful auxiliary; in 1880 it was said of
the *Journal* that 'while ostensibly the monthly periodical of the
WMNL, [it] has really become a powerful and representative organ
of the movement'.[140]

Money still remained a problem; even Quaker pockets were not
bottomless, and the WMNL's history was one of appeals to the NA and
other bodies for small sums to tide it over crises, or pay exceptional
expenses. Once the Acts had been suspended, such assistance
diminished, and its usefulness at an end, the League virtually collapsed
in December 1884, The *Journal* merged with Dyer's social purity
periodical, *The Sentinel*, the secretary was dismissed and the League
moved into Dyer Bros.' offices, where it continued a moribund
existence until its final dissolution in 1886.[141]

After the 1877 changes, WMNL activity boiled down to keeping
the National Roll growing to its 50,000 target (and progress was slow
— 12,000 in 1877, 22,000 in 1879, 35,000 in 1881) and holding
meetings in London in conjunction with the NA and FA, rousing the
network of metropolitan clubs with speakers like Jones, the Hackney
radical F.A. Ford or A.S. Dyer's brother George, the author of many
penny biographies including one of Jones himself.[142] Any additional
activity could only be undertaken if a subsidy was forthcoming —
thus when Banks suggested to the WMNL council that they hold a
conference of London working men, they hung back, until he promised
that the NA would pay for it, whereupon their doubts disappeared
(in the event, the meeting was paid for and presided over by Samuel

Smith, MP).[143]

Yet, despite its decline into penny-pinching localism, the League could still attract impressive support. Among its officers, only the honorary secretaries were genuinely workers, but they were significant – Benjamin Lucraft, the first working-class member of the London School Board and a reformer of many years standing was one, the other was William Gilliver, the former secretary of the Birmingham Trades Council.[144] Arch, Broadhurst and Howell were members of the National Council, 1,600 office holders in unions, clubs and societies were members, and the aged William Lovett bestowed his blessing on Jones, 'a fellow labourer in the Chartist Movement', calling the Acts 'infamous and unjust', the product of 'Aristocratic power and influence'.[145]

The evidence that leaders of the labour aristocracy were repelled and insulted by the Acts is considerable – as the secretary of the Leeds Trades Council said:

Class legislation was un-English. He did not know how working men with daughters of their own could sit quiet under these Acts, knowing that they had the power to repeal them. But they did not understand them. Once let them understand them, and they would sweep them away.

The *National Reformer* condemned the Acts, the *Bee-Hive* came out against them in 1876, popular papers such as the *Echo* were equally 'sound', and when prominent labour leaders were approached, they were readily recruited into the League.[146] Had it received the finance to canvass really widely its impact would have been much greater and thus its value to the cause as a whole enhanced. In fact it was inadequately funded even to perform limited tasks; middle-class reluctance to give money to an organisation unable to raise it itself was probably responsible – a suspicion of those unable to prosper through 'self-help' exemplified by Wilson's contempt for a 'salaried President'.

Most distinctive ideas proffered by the WMNL were submerged in the broad attack led by middle-class repealers: nothing came of a proposal by a member of the National Council (and endorsed by the *Journal*) that the movement concentrate on one subjected district in order to bring home to the public the evil of the system – diffusion of effort continued as before; and a petition signed by the officers in 1882 was a very ordinary piece of repeal protestation with no emphasis on class solidarity.[147] Only two differences of opinion with the rest of the movement can be found: the WMNL supported a Habitual Drunkards Bill which the *Shield* condemned in terms of high principle, as an attack on personal rights; to the *Journal* the Bill appeared to be a humane attempt to deal with the practical evils of drunkenness familiar to its readers. While in 1880, when middle-class organisations decided not to make repeal a test question at the election, the WMNL Executive Committee took the view that the Acts were too offensive to the working class for them to forbear pressing their point home.[148] Otherwise there was little special about WMNL activity. Yet there was a clear difference in emphasis which it could have put forward; working-class speakers recognised that the Acts affected their class alone, but the WMNL never succeeded in stirring up the battle in those terms. Instead, its middle-class financiers steered it towards the sort of activity they knew well — petitions giving equal weight to constitutional objections to the Acts, 'tea meetings' of respectable working men patronisingly managed by wealthy repealers, collaboration with middle-class effort (as the junior partner) rather than exerting independent pressure. Edmund Jones did not even preside at his own annual meetings, the chair always being taken by a middle-class luminary. Leaders of the WMNL were aware of their failure to rouse their class and knew they were impotent where they should have been strong — Lucraft did not believe that working-class support had been tapped as it might have been, and another WMNL member believed that the Acts would not have lasted two months if applied to all classes.[149]

The WMNL was thus colonised by middle-class repealers as the price for its survival; they meant well and were clear on the need for working-class support, but were not quite sure of what to do with it. Like others schooled in the traditions of the Anti-Slavery and Anti-Corn Law campaigns, they viewed working-class support as a moral advantage rather than a practical need,[150] and failed to seize opportunities to bind recognised union leaders close to them — thus the NA was cautious about supporting Howell's parliamentary candidature for Norwich (they had to worry about the feelings of J.J. Colman, MP, a wealthy supporter) and declined to help Broadhurst at Stoke in 1880.[151] When Lucraft stood as a radical at Tower Hamlets in 1880 the WMNL naturally supported him, and the Quakers contributed handsomely to his expenses, but the NA later took the view that he had been 'forced upon' the constituency and did not exert itself to secure the election of the most important working-class activist.[152]

The attempt to secure working-class opposition to the Acts was not a failure: in the early 1880s the TUC regularly condemned the Acts — indeed in 1884 over a third of the delegates were connected with the League,[153] and on the eve of suspension the *Pall Mall Gazette* could say that

> in no constituency where the vote of the workman is decisive would any candidate stand a shadow of a chance if he were to defend the Acts. The working class, rightly or wrongly, are imbued with the idea that this law is unjust, because it affixes a stigma on the woman (who has most commonly come out of their class) and makes things easy for the man, who had done the original mischief, and who is — again, rightly, or wrongly — supposed to come in most instances from the classes above.[154]

Rather the WMNL is best seen as an opportunity missed; with so many leading working-class figures interested, only a pronouncedly middle-class value system can explain the attention paid to the adhesion of a wealthy MP such as P.A. Taylor — the *Shield* saluted this in a long article entitled 'Good news for working men' — compared to the relative lack of attention paid to Arch, Howell and Broadhurst.[155] When, towards the end of the campaign, a repealer paid tribute to the support of the working class, it was in the remote, missionary style which typifies the gulf between the two sides of the movement:

> we have . . . every reason to believe from past experience, that the great heart of the nation beats responsive to our principles, and we may fearlessly carry our argument once more to the masses of the people of England.[156]

Notes

1. Sheffield Central Library (Wilson MSS), MD 2479: Wilson's reminiscences, taken down 9 June 1912.

2. Sheffield University Library (Mundella-Leader correspondence): 25 May 1872, 2 Mar. 1876.

3. There are two hagiographies of Wilson, which make use of his papers deposited in Sheffield, but not those in London: Mosa Anderson, *H.J. Wilson, Fighter for Freedom* (1953) and W.S. Fowler, *H.J. Wilson. A Study in Radicalism and Dissent, The Life and Times of Henry Joseph Wilson, 1833–1914* (1961).

4. FLB 3152: H.J. Wilson to Ewing Whittle, 11 June 1872; 3171: Dr Hooppell to H.J. Wilson, 20 Aug. 1872; 3179: Josephine Butler to H.J. Wilson,

23 Aug. 1872.

5. FLB 3175: Josephine Butler to Mrs H.J. Wilson, 26 Aug. 1872.

6. E.g. FLB 3773: Backhouse to H.J. Wilson; gives £400 'by way of greasing the wheels'.

7. FLB 3172: Josephine Butler to H.J. Wilson, 25 Aug. 1872.

8. *Shield*, 7 Sept. 1872, p. 1074; NA EC Minutes, 2 Sept. 1872.

9. NA EC Minutes, 5 Aug. 1872, 28 Oct. 1872.

10. *Shield*, 14 Sept. 1872, pp. 1076–7. The Liberal declared for repeal.

11. Birmingham Reference Library 63018: *Report of the Birmingham Association for Repeal* (1870).

12. FLB 3187: Josephine Butler to H.J. Wilson, *c.* Sept. 1872; 3188: Josephine Butler to H.J. Wilson, 6 Oct. 1872.

13. FLB 3189: R.F. Martineau to H.J. Wilson, 10 Oct. 1872.

14. Ibid., 3307: H.J. Wilson to Josephine Butler and Joseph Edmondson, 4 Oct. 1872.

15. Ibid., 3207: Josephine Butler to Mrs Smyttan, *c.* Dec. 1872; *Shield*, 5 Apr. 1873, p. 111.

16. Birmingham University Library (Harriet Martineau MSS), HM 119: Josephine Butler to Harriet Martineau, 22 Dec. 1872.

17. FLB 3115: Josephine Butler to her sisters, summer 1872; 3249: Josephine Butler to H.J. Wilson, 1 Apr. 1873.

18. On the Liberation Society's move see S.M. Ingham, 'The Disestablishment Movement in England, 1868–1874', *Journal of Religious History*, 3 (1964), pp. pp. 38–58. On the revolt's failure see D.A. Hamer, *Liberal Politics in the Age of Gladstone and Rosebery* (Oxford 1972), ch. 1; D.A. Hamer, *The Politics of Electoral Pressure* (Hassocks 1977), ch. 7.

19. *Shield*, 11 Jan. 1873, p. 10.

20. FLB 3209: Josephine Butler to H.J. Wilson, 23 Dec. 1872; 3210: George Butler to H.J. Wilson, 24 Dec. 1872.

21. Sheffield Central Library (Wilson MSS), MD 2479: Wilson's reminiscences taken down 9 June 1912.

22. Sheffield University Library (Wilson MSS), Box 1, envelope 2, Box 4, envelope 1; Sheffield Central Library (Wilson MSS), MD 2479; Wilson's reminiscences.

23. Ibid., Box 4: H.J. Wilson to R.F. Martineau, 2 Aug. 1873.

24. FLW, Box 82: F. Adams (secretary of NEL) to H.J. Wilson, 26 Aug. 1873. See also Hamer, *Politics of Electoral Pressure*, pp. 132–3.

25. FLB 3292: Joseph Edmondson to H.J. Wilson, 16 July 1873.

26. *Hansard*, 3rd series (22 June 1872) 212 Col.1522 ff.; *Shield*, 3 Aug. 1872, pp. 1027–297.

27. NA EC Minutes: 28 Oct. 1872 (asking other repealers for their views on the leadership); 18 Nov. 1872 (reporting that no one wanted Fowler's dismissal); 25 Nov. 1872 (Fowler's views on his bill's chances – a circular designed to exert pressure on him to introduce a bill was withdrawn).

28. FLB 3228: Elizabeth Malleson to H.J. Wilson, 28 Jan. 1873.

29. Ibid., 3232: Joseph Edmondson to H.J. Wilson, 10 Feb. 1873.

30. Ibid., 3255: Josephine Butler to H.J. Wilson, early May 1873.

31. *Hansard*, 3rd series (21 May 1872) 216 Col.218 ff.; *Shield*, 24 May 1873, pp. 161–71.

32. *Shield*, 7 June 1873, p. 188.

33. FLB 3252: Joseph Edmondson to H.J. Wilson, 23 May 1873.

34. FLW Box 82: NCL handbill signed by H.J. Wilson, 26 May 1873.

35. Sheffield University Library (Mundella-Leader correspondence), 26 May 1873. Mundella was encouraged by the split in the government with under-secretaries voting against their chiefs.

36. FLB 3271: Josephine Butler to R.F. Martineau, 27 May 1873; 3275: Josephine Butler to H.J. Wilson, 1 June 1873.

37. *Shield*, 31 May 1873, p. 177.

38. BL Add. MSS 44640 (Gladstone Papers) cabinet minutes: ff.20, 148, 164 (subjects for 1873 − *not* including repeal) f.206. On cabinet business see J. Vincent, *The Formation of the Liberal Party* (Penguin edn, 1972) pp. 50−1.

39. *Times*, 22 May 1873, p. 9.

40. H.J. Wilson was regularly warned about this by Sheffield moderates, e.g. Alfred Allott in 1871: 'First get influence, then take up the questions you care about' − advice he was to take up in the 1880s (Sheffield Central Library, MD 2479: Wilson reminiscences); Mundella told him 'our only hope is on the Liberal benches' (FLB 3200, 20 Nov. 1872).

41. *Shield*, 24 May 1873, pp. 172−5.

42. LNA *Annual Report for 1873*, pp. 5−6.

43. FLB 3292: Joseph Edmondson to H.J. Wilson, 16 July 1873.

44. Ibid., 3312: James Stuart to Josephine Butler, *c.* 1873.

45. *Shield*, 16 Nov. 1872, pp. 1147−8; 30 Nov. 1872, p. 1166.

46. FLB 3293: R.F. Martineau to H.J. Wilson, 20 July 1873; 3298: R.F. Martineau to H.J. Wilson, 25 July 1873.

47. Birmingham University Library (Harriet Martineau MSS), Josephine Butler to Harriet Martineau, 21 Dec. 1873.

48. Benjamin Scott, *A State Iniquity: Its Rise, Extension and Overthrow* (1890), pp. 167−8 referred to the suddenness of the dissolution as 'one more grudge against Mr. Gladstone'.

49. *Shield*, 4 May 1872, p. 923.

50. *Shield*, 15 Nov. 1873, p. 370.

51. *Circular Letter from the joint secretaries of the Extensionist Association*, May 1873.

52. NA EC Minutes, 26, 29, 30 Jan., 2 and 9 Feb. 1874; *Shield*, 31 Jan., 7 and 14 Feb. 1874.

53. *Shield*, 31 Jan. 1874, p. 33.

54. The Permissive Bill had been widely discussed during the 1868 election, see Paul Smith, *Disraelian Conservatism and Social Reform* (1967), p. 120.

55. J.L. Hammond, *Gladstone and the Irish Nation* (1938), p. 133; but see Hamer, *Politics of Electoral Pressure*, pp. 137−8, for a milder estimate of non-conformity's influence.

56. Before the election he had tried to persuade repealers to support the NEL's prior claim so as to unite radicals (Sheffield University Library (Wilson MSS), Box 4: R.F. Martineau to H.J. Wilson, 3 Aug. 1873 − Wilson refused to give the NEL such support). After the election Chamberlain made the same point, though favouring Disestablishment as the unifying issue this time, in an important article in the *Fortnightly Review*, Oct. 1874, pp. 413ff.

57. *Shield*, 24 Oct. 1874, p. 194; 12 July 1873, p. 230; 14 Feb. 1874, pp. 49−50.

58. Smith, *Disraelian Conservatism*, p. 191; H.J. Hanham, *Elections and Party Management: Politics in the Time of Disraeli and Gladstone* (1959), pp. 119−22, show that other nonconformist groups who had been pursuing the same tactics, suffered the same fate.

59. Henry W. Lucy, *Men and Manner in Parliament* (1919 edn), p. 254.

60. FLB 3323: Josephine Butler to Miss Priestman, 28 Feb. 1874; 3334: Josephine Butler to friends, 15 Apr. 1874.

61. *Shield*, 21 Mar. 1874, 28 Feb. 1874, 14 Mar. 1874; *Manchester Examiner* 18 Mar. 1874, 21 Mar. 1874.

62. Sheffield University Library (Mundella-Leader correspondence), 18 Mar. 1874.

63. NA EC Minutes, 16 Feb. 1874.

64. Ibid., 27 Feb. 1874 – 23 July 1874. The Committee met almost every week to consider names during this period.

65. FLB 3323: Josephine Butler to Miss Priestman, 28 Feb. 1874; 3334: Josephine Butler to friends, 15 Apr. 1874.

66. NA EC Minutes, 20 Apr. 1874.

67. Ibid., 23 July 1874. Only 14 MPs were present although 64 had been invited. Stansfeld told the Committee that the suggestion for the meeting had come from Archbishop Manning!

68. Hanham, *Elections and Party Management*, pp. 80, 411.

69. BL Add. MSS 44439 (Gladstone Papers) f.290: Johnstone to Gladstone, 9 Aug. 1873; 44442 f.175: Johnstone to Gladstone, 7 Feb. 1874.

70. FLB 3058: Josephine Butler to friends (circular letter), 8 July 1871.

71. FLB 3130: Josephine Butler to Charlotte C. Wilson, *c.* Mar. 1872; J.L. and B. Hammond, *James Stansfeld, a Victorian Champion of Sex Equality* (1932), pp. 178–9.

72. FLB 3316: Josephine Butler to Joseph Edmondson, 1 Dec. 1873.

73. B. Scott, *A State Iniquity*, pp. 173, 176.

74. Hammonds, *James Stansfeld*, pp. 188–9; Josephine Butler, *Recollections of George Butler* (*c.* 1893), pp. 280–1.

75. *Shield*, 1 Nov. 1874, pp. 211–214.

76. Mundella to Leader, 7 Feb. 1874, cited in W.H.G. Armytage, *A.J. Mundella 1825–1897, the Liberal Background to the Labour Movement* (1951), pp. 140–1.

77. *Shield*, 1 Jan. 1875, pp. 2–6; see H.J. Hanham, *Elections and Party Management*, pp. 121–4 for the general movement.

78. *Shield*, 1 Aug. 1874, pp. 158–9; Scott, *A State Iniquity*, pp. 193–4; Josephine Butler, *Personal Reminiscences of a Great Crusade* (1896), pp. 108–14.

79. Butler, *Recollections*, pp. 281–94.

80. FLB 3119–3122: Josephine Butler to H.J. Wilson, 22 Feb.–28 Feb. 1875.

81. *Shield*, 15 Mar. 1875, p. 65; 1 Apr. 1875, pp. 102–3. M. Gregory, *The Crowning Crime of Christendom* (1896).

82. *Shield*, 1 Jan. 1876, p. 1; 4 Nov. 1876, pp. 341–2; 8 June 1878, pp. 154–6; 31 May 1879, pp. 91–3.

83. Fawcett Library, *Letter Book of N.A.*, F.C. Banks to James Stansfeld, 22 May 1884.

84. NA EC Minutes, 3 Dec. 1877; 9 and 16 May 1881.

85. FLW Box 2: Stuart to H.J. Wilson, 21 Nov. 1876.

86. Ibid., Box 2: H.J. Wilson to NCL, EC (circular letter), 29 Nov. 1876; *Shield*, 16 Dec. 1876, pp. 371–2.

87. FLW Box 5: Stuart and Josephine Butler to repealers (printed circular), 27 Apr. 1878.

88. FLB 3884: Josephine Butler to Mrs Clark, 29 Apr. 1877.

89. FLW Box 2: Josephine Butler to H.J. Wilson, 18 May 1876.

90. *Shield*, 16 May 1885, p. 66, citing Bebel's 'Woman in the Past, Present and Future'.

91. *Shield*, 24 May 1879, special issue on Hong Kong.

92. *Shield*, 5 Mar. 1881, pp. 36–9. Annual Report of MCEU arguing that foreign progress was one of the high spots of 1880.

93. *Shield*, 3 Feb. 1883, 6 Sept. 1884, pp. 146–9.

94. *Shield*, 6 Oct. 1883, pp. 244–51.

95. *Shield*, 4 Oct. 1884, p. 159.

96. *Shield*, 2 Mar. 1878, pp. 43–4.

97. *Shield*, 10 Nov. 1875, pp. 289–91 on two conferences in 1875 dominated by Stansfeld and devoted to very practical arrangements for supporting parliamentary debates.

98. *Shield*, 1 May 1875, pp. 127–8; the Vigilance Association emphasised Taylor's efforts in its reports from 1874 to 1877.

99. *Hansard*, 3rd series (29 Apr. 1881) 260 Col.1451.

100. H.W. Lucy, *A Diary of Two Parliaments. The Disraeli Parliament 1874–1880* (1885), p. 328 (for 23 Jan. 1878).

101. See below chapter 5.

102. FLB 3165: H.J. Wilson to Saul Solomon, 21 June 1875.

103. *Hansard*, 3rd series (23 June 1875) 225 Col. 351 ff.

104. Sheffield University Library (Mundella-Leader correspondence), 28 June 1875.

105. FLB 3468: H.J. Wilson to NCL EC (circular letter), 24 June 1875.

106. *Shield*, 17 July 1875, pp. 222–3; see also NA, *Annual Report for 1874–75*, pp. 18–19.

107. *Hansard*, 3rd series (19 July 1876), 230 Col.1556 ff.

108. *Shield*, 29 July 1876, special (treble) issue on the debate, p. 245.

109. LNA, *Annual Report for 1876*, pp. 13–14.

110. FLW, H.J. Wilson to NCL EC, 29 Nov. 1876 (circular letter); I. Whitwell Wilson to H.J. Wilson, 29 Nov. 1876.

111. *Shield*, 10 Feb. 1877, pp. 28–9.

112. Ibid., 24 Feb. 1877.

113. FLB 3888: F.C. Banks to repealers, Nov. 1877 (circular letter).

114. *Shield*, 7 July 1877, pp. 185–9.

115. LNA EC Minutes, 16 July 1877; LNA, *Annual Report for 1877*, p. 22.

116. *Shield*, 16 Mar. 1878, pp. 57–8.

117. *Hansard*, 3rd series (22 May 1878), 240 Col.474 ff.

118. Birmingham Reference Library, *Minutes of the Birmingham Trades Council*, vol. 1, p. 69 (12 May 1870); *Shield*, 27 June 1870, p. 142.

119. INA, *Annual Report for 1870*, p. 19.

120. *Shield*, 15 Nov. 1873, p. 370; 15 Mar. 1873, p. 84 (W.T. Swan speaking at Bolton, 3 Mar.).

121. FLB 3213: Josephine Butler to H.J. Wilson, 27 Dec. 1872.

122. *Shield*, 16 Nov. 1874, p. 233.

123. FLB 3238: Josephine Butler to Miss Priestman, 15 Feb. 1873.

124. Butler, *Personal Reminiscences*, p. 98; *Shield*, 25 Jan. 1873; p. 25; FLB 3220: Josephine Butler to H.J. Wilson, 1 Jan. 1873.

125. NA EC Minutes, 5 Oct. 1872, 8 Nov. 1875; S.M. Ingham, 'The Disestablishment Movement in England 1868–1874', *Journal of Religious History*, 3 (1964), pp. 47–50.

126. *Shield*, 1 Nov. 1874, p. 215, reporting a speech made by Howell, 15 Oct. 1874, welcoming Stansfeld's public adhesion. For Howell's earlier collaboration with Stansfeld and middle-class politicians, see Royden Harrison, *Before the Socialists, Studies in Labour and Politics 1861–1881* (1965), ch. 4.

127. FLB Josephine Butler to H.J. Wilson, 22 Apr. 1875; 3378: letter of recommendation for Jones from Josephine Butler, 20 Apr. 1875.

128. FLB 3435: Burgess to H.J. Wilson, 20 May 1875; 3441: Burgess to H.J. Wilson, 31 May 1875.

129. Ibid., 3701: Fielden Thorp to H.J. Wilson, 22 July 1875. He thought Jones was an adequate speaker, but as a working man 'might perhaps in consequence

carry more weight with men of the same station in life'.

130. Ibid., 3711: H.J. Wilson to NCL, EC, 26 July 1875.

131. Ibid., 3718: George Butler to H.J. Wilson, 27 July 1875.

132. Ibid., 3708: Hudson Scott (Carlisle) to H.J. Wilson, 28 July 1875.

133. NA EC Minutes, 9 Aug. 1875; FLB 3723: H.J. Wilson to NCL EC, 3 Aug. 1875..

134. *National League Journal*, 1 Aug. 1875, pp. 1–2.

135. Ibid., 1 July 1876, report of first year's work.

136. LNA EC Minutes, 11 Nov. 1876. Stansfeld was also consulted about the reorganisation, and Bligh, an LNA agent, was to be released by the LNA to be the League's Secretary. See below, pp. 131, 133-4.

137. *National League Journal*, 1 Aug. 1876, 2 Oct. 1876; *Shield*, 20 Jan. 1877, p. 13.

138. *National League Journal*, 1 Feb. 1877.

139. *Letter Book of N.A., 1883–86*: F.C. Banks to J. Stansfeld, 22 May 1884; Gregory, *The Crowning Crime*; *National League Journal*, 1 Dec. 1877.

140. Friends Association, *Annual Report for 1880*.

141. NA EC Minutes, 3 Nov. 1884, 17 Nov. 1884; *National League Journal*, 1 July 1884, 1 Nov. 1884.

142. Reports of these meetings (all similar) helped to fill the pages of the *Shield* and *National League Journal* in the early 1880s. F.A. Ford seems to have been a particularly energetic speaker.

143. NA EC Minutes, 8 Jan. 1883, 28 May 1883; *National League Journal*, 1 June 1883, pp. 4–8.

144. Lucraft was another subject of a Dyer penny biography, published in 1879, probably to assist him as radical candidate for Tower Hamlets. He succeeded Jones as president of the WMNL when the latter died in 1882.

145. *National League Journal*, 1 Sept. 1877, p. 6.

146. *Shield*, 5 Feb. 1881, p. 24; *Bee-Hive*, 11 and 18 Mar. 1876. The articles were probably written by George Howell, and 1,000 copies of each issue were bought by the NA.

147. *National League Journal*, 1 Jan. 1879; 1 Aug. 1882.

148. *National League Journal*, 1 Aug. 1878; 2 Feb. 1880 (their decision produced no noticeable effect).

149. Ibid., 1 June 1883; *Shield*, 2 June 1883 (speeches at Samuel Smith's tea-meeting).

150. Thus the Liberation Society — S.M. Ingham, 'The Disestablishment Movement'; or the Lord's Day Observance Society — Brian Harrison, 'Religion and Recreation in Nineteenth-century England', *Past and Present*, 38 (1967), p. 107.

151. NA EC Minutes, 24 May 1875.

152. *National League Journal*, 1 Apr. 1880, 1 May 1880; NA EC Minutes, 20 Oct. 1884.

153. Ibid., 1 Oct. 1884, p. 3. The TUC also condemned the Acts in 1881 and 1883.

154. *Pall Mall Gazette*, 13 Apr. 1883.

155. *Shield*, 29 June 1872, pp. 987–8.

156. *Shield*, 2 May 1885, p. 57, speech by Rev. C.S. Collingwood at Manchester, 9 Apr. 1885.

5 THE REPEAL CAMPAIGN IN ACTION — ORGANISATION AND METHODS

Repealers recognised the impossibility of making any progress during the Disraelian years, and the elaboration of their organisation reflects their efforts to remain battleworthy under adverse conditions. This is, therefore, an appropriate point at which to pause and consider the methods employed, and the nature of their appeal as the movement diversified for survival.

I

Public meetings were the usual means of demonstrating support. A standard agitational method, they provided their audience with enlightenment and possibly entertainment, and usually rewarded their organisers with a vote of support, which the local press would naturally print in its report of the meeting.

The most common form of meeting was a single evening meeting in a town, held by a professional travelling agent. Here was the staple repeal activity, showing the flag, cheering local supporters and filling the columns of the *Shield* with identical reports. A typical one of the early 1880s read:

> Mrs. Olive Scatcherd gave an eloquent address on 'The Contagious Diseases Acts: what they mean and why we desire their repeal' to the lady members and friends of the Hunslet Unitarian Chapel. The address was listened to with marked attention, the indignant comments of the hearers showed how thoroughly they grasped the dangerous character and immoral tendencies of these laws. A petition in favour of total repeal was heartily carried.[1]

The tone of moral earnestness typifies such reports, and is perhaps attributable to the audience being a 'safe' one — of chapel-goers, again a common enough feature. However the speak was a lady volunteer rather than an agent, and meetings were increasingly held by amateurs in the 1880s — but seldom where opposition might be found.

Then there were more elaborate meetings with guest speakers — perhaps F.C. Banks, Baxter Langley (good with radical audiences) or

125

Dr Birkbeck Nevins. These could sometimes be spectacular if, for instance, held during an election campaign or in a subjected district where local support for the Acts could be found. Thus in 1873, at Gravesend, supporters of the Acts gained control of the chair, let off fireworks and passed a pro-Acts motion; at Weston-Super-Mare they were beaten off in 'a disgraceful scene of disorder and confusion' thanks to the determined and partial chairmanship of F.W. Newman; at Croydon a meeting to be addressed by Baxter Langley was disrupted by a mob.[2] Violence was a danger in the early 1870s when the agitation was novel, thought to be salacious, and definitely challenged the Liberal Party; later it receded, although meetings at Devonport in the 1880s were still being challenged. Experienced agents and well respected local worthies in the chair were the best defence against disorder.

The safest meetings, and the most impressive were the annual gatherings of repeal bodies; the NA, LNA, NCL and MCEU all held day long or sometimes two-day meetings to which came large numbers of the faithful. Naturally such meetings were enthusiastic and well attended; agents usually canvassed the town in which they were held for weeks before, the mayor would usually be asked to attend and in the midlands and north, often did,[3] and the platform was packed with repeal dignitaries. All friendly MPs would be asked to such meetings, and if unable to attend (as was usually the case) they at least sent telegrams of support. A great deal of business was crammed into the day. At the NCL Annual Meetings on 16 November 1875 the timetable was: 10.00 a.m. Executive Committee, 10.30 a.m. General Committee, 12.30 p.m. Annual Meeting, 3.00 p.m. Conference, 5.30 p.m. Tea, 7.30 p.m. Public Meeting. The Conference and Public Meeting were packed out and successful with speakers like Josephine Butler, Joseph Edmondson, A.J. Mundella and James Stansfeld.[4] Meetings such as these always concluded by petitioning parliament for repeal.

Petitioning complemented the holding of public meetings, and was just as traditional a means of conducting an agitation. Petitions were relatively easy to get up as long as correctly printed forms were supplied (nonconformist chapels were ready petitioners), they were newsworthy, and they attested to extensive public support. Certainly the opposition could not match them. Between 1870 and 1886, 18,068 petitions containing 2,657,348 signatures were presented to parliament against the Acts; only 83 petitions with 3,883 signatures were in their defence.[5] Petitioning was so normal a part of pressure group activity that the absence of petitions would be thought a weakness. Josephine Butler preferred to memorialise MPs, i.e. to talk directly to them, but she accepted that it would be difficult to switch to memorials as it was expected that a repeal Bill would be supported by petitions — MPs took note of them and *The Times* printed lists.[6]

But most provincial repealers preferred the direct approach and thought mass petitioning a waste of effort — in the early 1870s this was a corollary of their preference for militant pressure. In April 1873 the provincial societies told the NA they were memorialising MPs and urged it to do likewise, and in October the Northern Counties League bluntly warned the NA that it intended to stop petitioning.[7] However the NA clung to peitions even though the MCEU also abandoned them in 1874, obliging the NA to work the midlands as well as the south. It refused to allow memorials to replace petitions as the standard means of publicising strength of feeling, and begged those who persisted in memorials to collect petitions as well. It would be a blow for repealers if their petition totals fell too greatly.[8]

This disagreement over tactics raises a broader question: how did different repealers think their aim was likely to be achieved? Broadly speaking, the London based NA believed in the power of public opinion; demonstrate that it opposed the Acts and parliament must surely repeal them. Thus the petition was a means of convincing parliament that repeal was a serious issue; it followed that petitioning *had* to be sustained at a regularly high level — and when F.C. Banks told Wilson that he favoured dropping petitions for a year, it was on the understanding that this was because it was becoming a stale tactic and that a year's break would enable petitioning to be resumed all the more vigorously thereafter. He also stipulated that petitioning should entirely cease, so as to avoid any suspicion of weakness.[9]

Provincial repealers believed in constant and diligent pressure on MPs; the Acts had been carried by parliament, so it must be *made* to repeal them. Of course they agreed with the Londoners on the need to mobilise public opinion, but having less contact with parliament (until the 1880s) they underestimated that institution's resistance to their social and moral attitudes. Thus a member of the NCL Executive Committee preferred memorials to petitions precisely because MPs disliked them; it was better to be 'a thorn in the side of obstinate and indifferent men'.[10] For similar reasons they had launched their electoral onslaught before 1874 (and traces of it continued in the later 70s; repeal agents were at by-elections at south Shropshire in

1876 and Oldham in 1877). After then they modified their tactics, but still preferred to pursue the individual MP who would have to cast a vote rather than make generalised appeals. It was a difficult and time consuming policy — it had to be dropped in favour of petitioning when H.J. Wilson visited the United States in 1876 because each memorial demanded individual attention.[11] But ultimately it strengthened the repeal position far more than impetuous assaults on the Liberal Party ever had. The argument about petitions was never resolved: a conference in 1875 fudged the issue, Johnstone and the NA clung to petitions, Stansfeld and the northerners preferred memorials but to avoid a split Stansfeld stopped the matter coming to a head.[12] In 1877 the NCL and MCEU tried to stop petitioning since there was no bill to support; the NA did nothing to encourage it, yet over 100 petitions were presented by those who simply found it a convenient way of bringing their view before the public.[13]

In the end, both sides got their way. Petitions were automatically collected each session to show the continuing strength of repeal. To Wilson's great annoyance the NCL became the backbone of petitioning whereas those Associations which had forced 'a comparatively useless expenditure of energy and money' on it did little to support their own views.[14] But all organisations contributed to the elaborate lobbying of MPs which characterised activity in the 80s and which ultimately helped to make parliament amenable to repeal.

II

Routine work was carried out by a small corps of salaried workers. Each association employed such servants as its purse could manage and level of activity required; there was no formal coordination of effort though if an agent was urgently required by one association, another might loan an employee of theirs provided that his salary and expenses were met.[15] At the height of the 1870s agitation, there were 13 to 14 secretaries, agents and clerks employed by the various bodies,[16] and even in the later 1870s there were at least eight paid workers not purely engaged in clerical work. Roughly speaking, the NA usually employed a secretary (F.C. Banks), an assistant secretary to run the London office (in the 1880s it was his wife), at least one travelling agent and an agent permanently resident at Plymouth (until 1880). The LNA employed at least one agent, sometimes more; the MCEU had a secretary and an agent, the NCL at least one agent, sometimes more; the Scottish National, Working Men's National and National Medical Associations each had paid secretaries by no means confined to office work. In addition the bigger associations had copying clerks and took on extra clerks at busy times; the NA in particular had to maintain a large establishment to be able to organise repeal conferences, distribute literature and publish the *Shield*.[17]

Apart from the obvious clerical work, paid staff did much of the campaigning which middle-class subscribers preferred not to do themselves. Although the paid agent was relegated to a supporting role at the great annual meetings, for much of the year it was he who tramped the country whipping up support and holding meetings. Agents were particularly important in the early years in making the agitation known; later on their number shrank as repealers began to undertake tasks previously left to their employees. Indeed, amongst some there was a suspicion of those who took money to labour in a good cause; H.J. Wilson was notorious for his peremptory treatment of those who received salaries.[18] From this point of view, the more work done by amateurs, the purer the movement seemed — it was, after all, a common argument against official doctors and CD Police that they were defending their salaries.[19] The comparison was made explicit by a wealthy Quaker repealer who objected to paid officials meddling in policy matters: 'Those secretaries play much the same part on the side of Repeal as Sloggett, Anniss &c. do on the other and it is about time they were set to healthier employment.'[20] In 1882 the new Parliamentary Committee explicitly forbade associations to nominate salaried officers as their representatives, a decision which at least one agent took badly.[21]

The secretaries (as opposed to honorary secretaries) of the bigger associations were the elite of the staff. In daily contact with their employers, well paid and respectable, they were able to contribute to decision-making, even if resented for so doing. The MCEU's secretary in the 1880s, of whom Ellis complained, was the Rev. William Wastell, an indefatigable organiser, keen on uniting the more vigorous provincial repealers and ignoring the NA. He wrote to H.J. Wilson on terms of equality, and Wilson accepted this; indeed he thought highly of Wastell and at one time hoped that he would go to London to breathe life into the NA.[22] The Working Men's National League (WMNL) employed a Quaker carpenter, Joseph Joyce, as its secretary. F.C. Banks's influence on the NA has already been noted. All these men hovered above the line separating employer from employee, for instance, representing their associations at delegate conferences. Significantly, H.J. Wilson, the honorary secretary of the NCL never shared his authority with an employee. The NCL office was built onto his home in Sheffield (beyond the billiard room) and from there a succession of clerks did the routine work under his supervision. That the title of secretary was coveted is shown by a petty intrigue in 1874 by which William Burgess, the NA's agent succeeded in persuading his employers to give him the title 'organising secretary' — he took advantage of Mrs Butler's absence abroad to wheedle it from her less experienced deputy, then had his name and title printed on LNA stationery and began corresponding with an outraged Wilson on an equal basis. Wilson would not tolerate this, especially as he had once employed the slightly sinister Burgess, and thundered against 'the assumptions of our "permanent officials" '.[23]

Burgess was in fact one of the more experienced agents; he had previously worked for the United Kingdom Alliance in Liverpool and had impressed Josephine Butler by building it up from nothing.[24] Used to working independently, he soon fell foul of Wilson who suspected him (justifiably as later events proved) of laziness and dishonesty. The NCL also hired a former Alliance man, W.T. Swan, who proved entirely satisfactory and worked for the repeal movement for nine years.

The apparently large pool of nonconformist ministers without chapels was another useful source of agents — and reliable, conscientious ones such as Wastell himself, Rev. J.H. Lynn (a Baptist minister) who worked for the NA as agent from 1874 to final repeal, or perhaps the best of them, the Congregational minister, J.P. Gledstone who worked for the NCL for two years (1875–77) between pastorates.

By far the largest group of agents was made up of respectable workingmen. Opposed to the Acts and attracted by the promised 'liberal salary' (usually £100–£250) they learnt their trade and usually worked diligently, some moving on after a while to other agitations, e.g. the Band of Hope (an NCL agent), the Anti-Vaccination Association (an LNA agent). For some, acting as an agent was a means of social promotion. Thus the permanent agent at Plymouth, the Wesleyan lay preacher, John Marshall, exchanged a job as a dock labourer for one in which he was the colleague of ministers and the confidant of middle-class repealers (Marshall was particularly esteemed because he suffered a month's imprisonment in 1870 for helping prostitutes to evade the police — after that his repeal reputation was made).[25]

Two agents merit special attention as their experience made them particularly valuable to repealers. A former constable in the CD Police was recruited in 1874, the NA promising to ensure that his pension would not be jeopardised. But although he had expressed abhorrence for his duties, ex-PC Phillips's performance as an agent did not live up to expectations.[26] The other 'catch' was a better one. Henry Bligh was an artilleryman of 20 years' service who was bought out of the army in 1873 by Mrs Butler. A man of intense, moral character, his ability to condemn the Acts from experience was a godsend to the LNA. Furthermore he was an excellent worker, thought by both Wilson and Mrs Butler to be the most valuable agent.[27] He was used as a 'spy' in subjected districts, making sensible use of his military background, and it had been decided to put him in charge of the WMNL, another appropriate job, in 1876, a short time before his death.

A travelling agent's primary responsibility was simply to visit as many places as possible, spreading the word and attracting support. H.J. Wilson's instructions to the NCL's first agent stressed speed of coverage: sow the seed before cultivating. He wanted the agent to work three or four boroughs a week, visiting ministers, temperance men, etc., posting up bills, distributing literature and generally arousing interest. This process would be repeated for a month, after which the agent would return and start reworking the original boroughs. The NCL office would help by writing to local nonconformists, and by means of this dual approach, successful meetings could probably then be arranged.[28] The NA's agents were equally fast. A meeting each evening in a different town was the rule: during the 1885 general election campaign, John Marshall addressed 41 meetings in the north-east in a little over a month, while Rev. J.H. Lynn visited 55 places in the south.[29]

Before 1874, electoral work was hectically carried on, agents being diverted from ordinary work to by-elections. The first agent to be appointed, the LNA's Samuel Fothergill, worked at eight elections in his first year besides the usual meetings, and when Bligh and Burgess were sent into Wales in the winter of 1873–4, they were told to concentrate on hostile MPs in anticipation of an election.[30] After 1874 agents were again concerned with building up local committees and rousing repealers by holding meetings. The NCL was particularly well organised for this, issuing agents with registers of residents marked up as to denomination, attitude to the CD Acts, politics, etc. Towns were frequently revisited giving a thorough coverage of the north which had a telling effect at the 1880 election in terms of candidates pledged to repeal.

It is clear from agents' reports to both the National Association and the Northern Counties' League that cultivating local clergy was an important part of their duties. The support of the minister of a chapel could bring with it weighty petitions, deputations to MPs, the formation of local committees and the enlistment of 'respectable working-men'; the minister could be the key to an extremely large door. Thus an agent defending himself against charges of slackness reeled off a three-page list of clergymen visited, and Josephine Butler checked on another agent's religious beliefs before sending him to Scotland: 'For Scotland one must have a religious man of Bible views — Evangelical.'[31] A Wesleyan local preacher applying to the NCL for part-time work stressed his acceptability to the religious community by providing numerous references from clergy and ministers; furthermore as an itinerant preacher he was used to reaching a large population in County Durham.[32]

A further duty required of agents was in effect to collect their own salaries by soliciting subscriptions and donations as they travelled. Josephine Butler was convinced that a good agent could attract more money than his salary, and was driven to distraction by Fothergill, her first agent, who felt that agents should not be fund-raisers:

> He never gets us a penny of money, and he solemnly declares that one person cannot combine in himself the vocation of a lecturer and a collector of money. He has driven me almost mad about this! He won't even *ask* for money; he says it would 'do harm'. So I have to do *every bit* of that myself.[33]

The NA bluntly instructed its staff 'that if they wish to keep their appointments, they must endeavour to increase the income of the Society'.[34]

The ideal agent seemed to elude repealers though the nonconformist ministers, if they stayed long enough, usually gave satisfaction: J.H. Lynn was often commended for initiative during his long service, while J.P. Gledstone was more a repealer who happened to be filling in time by working for the cause — H.J. Wilson regarded him as a friend (they went on a mission to the USA together in 1876) and after 1877 he became once more an 'amateur'. But many of the agents were poorly educated and could not be trusted to address middle-class audiences with any chance of success.[35] Indeed most agents were treated patronisingly by their employers, praised when they held an effective meeting, sternly taken to task and obliged to account for their actions if meetings failed; a definite gulf existed between the two sides, the one struggling to earn a living, the other intent on achieving its aim —

which would of course render its employees redundant.

Agents were not trusted to be industrious: the NA received weekly reports from its men; Wilson, the harshest taskmaster, required daily reports and prepared printed forms for his agents, while Josephine Butler in a less systematic manner supervised her employees effectively (at any rate, things slipped when she was away). Nor were they allowed much latitude — those who were slipshod or insufficiently diligent were promptly dismissed; Wilson warned one agent on his appointment that he would have to defer to his (Wilson's) views, and when the agent proved independent in spirit and unwilling to supply daily reports of his activities, he was warned and then sacked — this despite generally favourable reports on his work. He left, saying that it was impossible to satisfy Wilson who wanted the agitation run to a 'commercial standard'.[36] Wilson's action was thoroughly approved by Mrs Butler who urged him to exercise even stricter control, and herself dismissed an agent for smoking and drinking, 'habits which naturally do not commend him to people'.[37]

A number of incidents suggest that this wariness about agents was justified. In 1874, for instance, two societies had cause to investigate the conduct of an agent: the NA finding the reports of one of its agents, Johnson, to be too vague, sent a member of its Executive Committee to observe one of his meetings. He discovered the audience to be about 40 whereas Johnson reported to the Committee an audience of 400 — he was immediately dismissed. It turned out that his oratorical triumphs were products of his own imagination; he supplied local newspapers with optimistic accounts of his meetings before they occurred, then spoke wildly to whoever turned up to the meeting itself, relying on the falsified press report to reassure his employers.[38] Later in the year the NCL had to hold an enquiry into an alleged mismanagement of funds at the Oxford election by their agent Swan. They found him guilty of slackness but had to clear him of the more serious charge since Johnson, already dismissed for untruthfulness, was the only available witness.[39]

An altogether more serious scandal which led to the suicide of one agent and the disgrace of another occurred in 1876 but was handled so discreetly as not to cause any embarrassment to the movement. It concerned the two Liverpool-based agents of the LNA, Henry Bligh and William Burgess. The latter as we have seen was an ambitious, less than scrupulous character whom Bligh came to suspect of financial malpractice. Other agents agreed that Burgess's style of life seemed to exceed his income, and one alleged that Mrs Burgess boasted that her husband's income was £500 when officially it was £250.

However, when these allegations came to light, Burgess counter-attacked distastefully but with great effect. He had discovered that Bligh had contracted syphilis while serving in the East Indies in 1863—4, and asserted that the ex-soldier had infected his wife and newly-born child. Bligh denied the accusation, insisted that he had been examined before marriage, and that his wife and child were healthy. Stansfeld investigated and found this to be true. Burgess apologised yet Bligh's mind was not at rest; he felt cheated of justice, and in what the coroner found was a fit of temporary insanity, cut his throat with a penknife on 1 December 1876.

Henry Wilson investigated this unsavoury incident and was unable to reach a firm conclusion; he found that Bligh's mind had been slipping for some time and that he felt himself to be persecuted by Burgess; in this context, Burgess's outrageous accusation may well have unhinged him. One wonders though whether this evidence of progressive mental deterioration does not tend to support Burgess. Yet the latter's conduct had been disgraceful, and the suspicion about his accounts remained. He was retired from the LNA and the WMNL and left to serve the National Medical Association where Dr Nevins would keep a close watch on him. Plainly the 'clean bill of health' which he had been given was of limited value.[40]

Nothing of this came to light; the local press put it down to the effects of sunstroke in India, though the *Liverpool Daily Courier* waspishly suggested that 'circumstances in connection with his vocation had troubled him a good deal, and probably led to the commission of the fatal act'.[41] The *Shield* and repeal organisations contented themselves with expressions of condolence. That two well respected agents had thus pursued each other was hardly to be made public knowledge.

Yet on the whole the movement received good value for money from its bureaucracy. Its servants were usually hard workers, zealous for the cause, and the more experienced ones were capable of acting independently, even though this may have sometimes irritated their employers. Given that most repealers had no inclination to take to the streets, and those who had, lacked the time to do so, a corps of paid agents was inevitable if the movement was to spread. In the event it did rather well in securing workers who believed that their task was morally justifiable and who could satisfy some very demanding taskmasters.

III

All the activities discussed so far, meetings, elections, lobbying, parliamentary debates, obviously depended on the printed word for their widest impact; thus the attitude of the press was a crucial one as nobody doubted. The NA urged its supporters to keep it informed of the attitudes of local papers and maintained a record of friendly ones; in 1874–5 it sent 13 different mailings to the entire UK press and paid particular attention to the metropolitan and leading provincial papers.[42] Repealers could always bear in mind the fate of one of their largest early meetings – one held in the Free Trade Hall, Manchester, on 16 November 1870 which attracted an audience of 5,000–6,000, mostly women, yet received little publicity because the London press failed to report it. The enormous progress made by the LNA in only one year was thereby kept from the public. As George Butler grumbled, 'if a conspiracy of silence exists among the chief organs of the Press, the practical advantage of a large public meeting is nullified'.[43]

It was an article of faith amongst repealers that the press was conspiring to ignore their efforts; the very first number of the *Shield* contained a letter from Josephine Butler and Harriet Martineau protesting against the suppression of letters by the *Pall Mall Gazette* and the *Daily News*, and repeal meetings often referred to the disadvantages under which they laboured. There were indeed papers firmly committed to the Acts that declined to give repealers the right to reply – the *Times* was an offender while the *Saturday Review* would no more have given space to the repealers than would the *Shield* have permitted Berkeley Hill free rein in its columns.[44] But not many journals fell into this category. Others such as the *Daily News* (after its change of editor weakened Harriet Martineau's influence) or the *Daily Telegraph* avoided the subject whenever possible, but when they referred to it, they satisfied repealers as often as they disappointed them.[45]

Yet the impression which most repealers formed, and which their histories reflect is that silence was an alternative to misrepresentation. Enemy journals such as the *Saturday Review* and the *Pall Mall Gazette* practised the latter, while the rest of the press tacitly supported them with the former.[46] Thus Scott implied that the daily press suppressed repeal views, Mrs Butler insisted that the conspiracy of silence lasted from 1870 to 1874 and obliged repealers to concentrate on public meetings (would they not have done so otherwise?) and the Hammonds followed this lead.[47]

One might imagine that the campaign was systematically blacked out, that favourable references were entirely absent. This is not so. There were metropolitan papers sceptical about the Acts and uncertain as to whom to believe; and there were a few, such as the radical evening paper the *Echo* and the weekly *Examiner* (from 1874) which were positively favourable.[48] In the 1880s, the *Pall Mall Gazette* first under John Morley, then W.T. Stead, reversed its attitude and became sympathetic to repeal.[49]

It is not suggested that such papers were typical; rather most were embarrassed by the agitation and uneasy about its effect on their readership. As with the Bradlaugh–Besant trial, they were faced with a subject they did not like and which might harm them. In 1877 such was the interest that they could not avoid covering that trial, but the long and sometimes dull campaign against the Acts often failed to provide newsworthy material.[50] Most papers simply exercised journalistic selection and chose not to report that which they found lacking in news interest and likely to offend their delicate readerships. Naturally this was not good enough for crusading repealers with an exaggerated sense of their cause's importance.

Thus instead of constant and favourable coverage, repeal tended to attract reporting in newsworthy fits and starts, much of it hostile – a defeat for repealers at a public meeting, complained the NA, would be made much of, but victories were ignored.[51] Every favourable notice was monotonously hailed as a breakthrough in the fight against 'conspiracy of silence'; the deputation to Bruce in 1871, the Colchester and Pontefract elections were reported (the latter with some anger by the very Liberal press which the *Shield* had praised in the previous year as 'on the whole, true to the people's cause and to the cause of morality and justice')[52] but the promised breakthrough never came. The national press was simply not as enthralled by conference reports and the latest pamphlets of William Shaen and F.W. Newman as were most repealers.

However, the press never neglected a real news story: Stansfeld's first public declaration for repeal on 15 October 1874 was fully reported by *The Times* and other metropolitan papers on the following day and subjected to ferocious criticism by some. Naturally the *Shield* jumped to the conclusion that what was simply a good story heralded the conversion of the press, and Josephine Butler told her husband (with her usual inability to understand that her priorities were not general):

Is it not a good thing that the conspiracy of silence in the London

Press has at last suddenly broken down? We have been labouring
now for over five years and have not got a paragraph into the
London papers; but when an ex-cabinet minister speaks it is
thought worthwhile to notice the fact.[53]

Similarly the shocking suicide of Mrs Percy at Aldershot in 1875
produced press criticisms of the Acts, especially from the *Telegraph*,
which Josephine Butler yet again seized on as proof of a general advance
when really they amounted to no more than an intelligent press
response to a scandal.[54]

The provincial press, though variable, seems to have been on the
whole less hostile. The Butlers suffered at the hands of an unsympathetic
Liverpool press, but against this a number of powerful provincial
papers, usually Liberal in politics, supported repeal.[55] Thus the
Northern Echo condemned Cardwell's new military depots because
of the immorality associated with the army; at Oxford the new depot
was equally feared, and the Liberal *Oxford Times* displayed a firm
opposition to the Acts.[56] While the *Manchester Examiner* denounced
regulation saying that 'the sympathies of the working class are entirely
with those who seek the Repeal of this obnoxious measure'.[57]

The *Shield* made much of the adhesion of any provincial paper,
regarding this as an extension of repeal's influence which would
produce favourable reports of meetings. Certainly local papers, eager
for events to report, treated repeal meetings very fairly; the *Shield*
regularly reprinted extensive accounts from all sorts of papers, which
became fuller as the subject was increasingly accepted as suitable for
discussion.

By the late 1870s repealers believed that the press was coming to
treat them more fairly: Josephine Butler told Henry Richard that the
London press was at last reporting repeal, and another lady wrote to
the *Shield* urging a rain of letters to editors to destroy the crumbling
'conspiracy'.[58] Again, one can only perceive this improvement if one
accepts the existence of previous injustice; little change in the consistency of coverage can be seen — it all depended on how newsworthy repeal activity was.

The sort of enthusiastic commitment repealers craved was found
only if a particular editor was won to the cause. Under John Chapman,
the *Westminster Review* supported repeal, as did the *Medical Mirror*,
which Josephine Butler commended as a response to the other (hostile)
medical papers.[59] Bradlaugh's *National Reformer*, valued for its wide
circulation among the working class was a loyal supporter, while W.T.

Stead (*Northern Echo* then *Pall Mall Gazette*) and Percy Bunting (*Contemporary Review*) provided sympathetic coverage.[60]

Most editors preferred to go along with the trend, which by the 1880s was towards straight, unworried coverage given the movement's growing respectability. There was some mellowing in tone (not found in *The Times*) and a reciprocal lack of their earlier hysteria among repealers. Some enjoyed good contacts and could themselves put pressure on the press; J.E. Ellis suggested using Newcastle influence on John Morley to get a good article into the *Pall Mall Gazette* on the eve of the 1883 repeal debate, and when the *Daily News* failed to report a repeal success, he went straight to the proprietor, Samuel Morley, to complain.[61] Once men of political ability and influence were prominent the press *did* take repeal more seriously, and rightly so, but this is not to say that earlier assumptions of persecution were justified.

Even had the press been favourable, this would still have been insufficient to maintain enthusiasm and keep repealers informed about activities. A separate repeal journal was clearly indispensable. Thus the *Shield* was founded in March 1870; in September 1870 it became the official mouthpiece of the NA. From 1871 until its closure in 1886 it was edited by Stansfeld's sister-in-law, Mme. Emilie A. Venturi, a difficult woman, often at odds with her committee and, surprisingly, given that she was more militant than most Londoners, not much liked by Mrs Butler and provincial repealers. Initially it was a penny weekly of about 16 pages, devoting itself to reports of meetings, surveys of press attitudes, long lists of repeal petitions, a correspondence column and interminable serialisations of evidence from Blue Books, of papers written by Shaen, Mrs Butler, etc., indeed of anything relevant — the impression one gets is of difficulty in finding enough repeal material to fill an issue.

Up to 1874, elections and political information kept it fairly lively, but thereafter it became much more turgid. From April 1874 it was transformed into a monthly, allegedly to give fuller reports, but the start of foreign work began to produce significant amounts of interesting news, and in 1875 no fewer than 21 special issues were produced to accommodate this. Thereafter from February 1876 it became a fortnightly during the parliamentary session (February–July) and remained monthly for the rest of the year. In the 1870s its domestic coverage was appallingly dull for the very good reason that there was little to write about; however foreign news rescued it from the doldrums, and indeed in 1877 and 1879 constituted the largest and most interesting part of its coverage. From 1879 it picked up, with evidence from the select committee to serialise, and genuinely interesting developments in the 1880s to cover.

The *Shield* was the backbone of the movement and its journal of record, but it was, perhaps inevitably, a rather flat one. Both Josephine Butler and Henry Wilson found it unsatisfactory, and jibbed at the subsidies which it required (it lost £470 in 1875 which the repeal societies had to make up, though it is fair to say that it was distributed *gratis* on quite a lavish scale, all MPs receiving it fortnightly) — indeed Mrs Butler candidly said in 1886 that she was glad to see it cease as it would save expense![62] From the mid-70s the *Shield*'s deficiencies were mitigated by the provision of more specialised journals. The Wesleyan Society for Repeal published the *Methodist Protest* from January 1876 to October 1883 (retitled *The Protest* in January 1878 when the City of London Committee began to share the costs); Josephine Butler preferred it to the *Shield*. The Working Men's National League had a monthly *National League Journal* from August 1875 to December 1884. The National Medical Association published the *Medical Enquirer* from 1875 to 1880, but it appeared erratically because of financial problems. Finally the MCEU published a monthly *Occasional Paper* from January 1877 to 1886. These papers along with the *Vigilance Journal*, the organ of the like-minded but more broadly aimed VA, extended the *Shield*'s coverage slightly and in the obvious directions indicated by their sponsors, but mostly they duplicated it; this was recognised by repealers such as J.P. Gledstone who wanted to supersede the *Shield* and merge the others into the reformed paper, but nothing was ever done.[63]

Periodical publications were crucial for maintaining morale and orchestrating protest, but their nature prevented them reaching much beyond the ranks of the faithful. To supplement them, there existed a mighty publishing effort, which, taking advantage of the relative cheapness of printing, poured out tracts and pamphlets: in its first year the NCL distributed 70,000 leaflets and pamphlets and 7,000 large posters, in the early 1870s the NA put up placards during municipal elections with apparent success, and even in the agitation's final stages it was still prepared to issue 250,000–300,000 tracts (translating the best into Welsh) for the 1885 general election.[64] All the significant speeches of repeal leaders were printed up as pamphlets and in the 1880s critical statistical appreciations seem to have been particularly popular.

Thus the movement hoped to reach the masses. But reaching

leaders of opinion was also thought vital, though the appeal to 'the people' always took official pride of place in their efforts.[65] Florence Nightingale and Harriet Martineau had shown the way in attempting to influence men in authority and other repealers were not loath to press their views home.

The best example of this is Mrs Butler's pursuit of her political hero, W.E. Gladstone, for whom, before the agitation began, her admiration was boundless. This caused her to read into his opaque statements about the Acts, intentions and views which were not really his. Thus in July 1871 she assured her followers that she had heard from a friend that Gladstone abhorred the Acts and thought that the country's future turned on this question. He was quick to deny this, and declined to answer correspondence on the matter, turning it over to the Home Secretary.[66] Nothing daunted, she tackled him again in 1872 when he visited Liverpool College as the Butlers' guest. Again he avoided a direct answer to her pleas and retreated into theological abstractions; she was unable to press home her points because of her duties as hostess, and reported miserably that though Gladstone was with them at heart, in practical terms they could hope for little. She excused this lapse as being due to harmful influences around him.[67] Despite his reiterated commitment to the principle of Bruce's bill, repealers never stopped trying with Gladstone. Thus in January 1874 F.C. Banks and others harried him at Woolwich but could only extract from him a disavowal of Bruce's violent language, but not of the bill.[68] Mrs Butler tried again in 1877, and this time her appeal for support made explicit the similarities between the horrors of the Eastern Question (so recently Gladstone's primary concern) and the 'abominations' of State Regulation of Vice:

> We, like you, have been driven from any dependence upon Parliament, at least as it is at present constituted, to base our hopes upon the awakened conscience of the people at large; we have alike made our appeal to the people, and their response has been true and persistent.[69]

No reply is to be found, though Gladstone did not allow his name to be used. The explanation for his behaviour is surely that although he may well have found the Acts distasteful, they were of relatively little importance to him as a practical politician, and did not excite his moral indignation (as Mrs Butler hoped they might) to the extent necessary for him to join a difficult agitation. He therefore stuck to the government's agreed solution while avoiding giving offence to repealers. James Stuart read far too much into this attitude; a kind word from Gladstone about Mrs Butler's *The Constitution Violated* had him drawing up reading lists for the GOM whose commitment he, as an ultra-loyal Gladstonian, was always prone to exaggerate.[70] However, persistence probably inclined Gladstone to repeal if only for the sake of Liberal unity; he knew that the Acts did not work and his family influenced him towards repeal.[71] By 1884 the tactful Herbert Gladstone was offering repealers useful tactical advice and assuring them of his father's support.[72] One can only surmise about Gladstone's motive for coming round, but it would be consistent with his concern for practical politics to suppose that the evidence of increasing Liberal support for repeal had something to do with it — Edward Hamilton recorded Gladstone's surprise at Stansfeld's majority for repeal in 1883 and his regard for the tone of the debate, and in 1886 his intervention secured time for the final passage of repeal at a particularly difficult time; yet there was no enthusiasm for the subject, rather as Kimberley noted, a businesslike determination to treat the question as a minor problem of government, not really worth taking a stand on.[73]

John Bright was another obvious target, both as the most prominent nonconformist in politics and because of his supposed influence with Gladstone. Yet although he voted for repeal, the style of the agitation appalled him and led to an outburst at the Friends' Yearly Meeting in 1875 in which he protested against his wife and daughters receiving offensive (repeal) literature through the post.[74] Thereafter he was lost to the cause though most of his family and coreligionists were active in it. In 1883, J.E. Ellis described him as 'a solitary old lion in his rooms' and no help to repeal.[75] Chamberlain was similarly a disappointment. When active in Sheffield politics as radical candidate in 1873 and 1874 he had opposed the Acts quite strongly, probably in deference to the strong feelings of H.J. Wilson. By 1876 he was telling Wilson that there were other issues of greater importance to which he was more committed and stipulating that his donation should be anonymous.[76] Thereafter apart from some advice on tactics in 1883 he drops from sight.

No other leading politicians were prominent — certainly no Conservatives after the demise of J.W. Henley and Russell Gurney. Liberal Home Secretaries, Bruce then Harcourt, were sorely pressed by repealers and both reacted adversely, the latter very intemperately, to constituency pressure exerted upon him. The front benches were so seldom involved that one can well understand the thrill with which Stansfeld's adhesion was greeted; of his fellow Liberals, only Childers ever seems to have been pressed into taking much interest.

This lack of success in arousing the world of 'high politics' might be a partial confirmation of repeal complaints about prejudice in high places. A new body, the City of London Committee for Repeal, was founded in February 1877 as a means of overcoming this. It differed from other bodies in that it never tried to expand membership beyond a relatively small group of friendly city magnates. The chairman was the millionaire Congregationalist MP, Samuel Morley, who had hither-to remained aloof; Benjamin Scott, Chamberlain of the City of London, was its honorary secretary and the 50 or so members included pillars of the dissenting establishment such as Alderman Sir Andrew Lusk, MP and Alderman Sir William McArthur, MP. The Committee had an uneventful life, directing itself towards the churches and sub-sidising the *Methodist Protest*; it does not seem to have succeeded in breaking through into the inner world of decision making.[77]

IV

Since their case rested on the evils of the Acts, repealers should have been strong in the subjected towns — subjected, in their eyes, to moral degradation and the outrageous official support of vice. The *Shield* strove to depict those affected by the Acts as united against them. Even more plausibly, those likely to be newly subjected were supposed to recoil from the horrors they were presently spared: when the workers at a government clothing factory in Pimlico petitioned against its removal to Woolwich, one of the reasons cited was their fear of the effect of the Acts on women; when members of the University of Oxford opposed the siting of a barracks there, fear that the Acts might thereby be introduced was reported as one of their motives.[78]

Alas, however hard the *Shield* might try to obscure the case, it has to be said that these military towns were, at the very least, indifferent to the Acts; but were more often decidedly in favour of them. Stansfeld recognised the occupational and social reasons for this:

The populations of those districts were largely either naval or military, or dependent upon those professions, and they were too much interested in the maintenance of the Acts. Their prejudices were too strong to make it an easy matter to hold meetings, or obtain a fair hearing in those districts.[79]

For those above such considerations, town councils, the bench, local clergy and the like, part of the attractions of the Acts lay in the provision of government money for keeping their streets respectable. Repealers did not deny this; indeed for Josephine Butler the 'cosmetic' approach was the really degrading thing:

> Everything is more like Paris — pretty, proper vice, all under Police control . . . the really Christian people there are silenced and discouraged, and have had to fall back on the narrow aims, common to good people in profligate foreign cities, of trying to shelter their own children.[80]

Despite the difficulties of rousing opinion in the towns, it was vital to try since weakness would give regulationists a powerful weapon, as is seen by the reaction in the subjected districts to suspension of the Acts. Chamberlain told H.J. Wilson:

> The universal opinion in favour of the Acts wherever they are now at work is the real difficulty which you have to face . . . The evidence of this local feeling has been so remarkable that I observe it has rather shaken some of those who voted with Stansfeld the other day.[81]

How best to set about opposing the Acts where they operated? Two strategies presented themselves. On the one hand the repeal movement could support and attempt to direct the opposition to the Acts among the women themselves. To some extent this was done at both Plymouth and Southampton in the early 1870s though activity soon slackened. By 1874 Stansfeld was criticising repeal associations as 'craven and spiritless' for their passivity. While agreeing with his approach, Josephine Butler realistically pointed out the difficulties which the activitist encountered in taking up individual cases:

> our lawyers and friends will be satisfied with *none*, except one which will embrace all the points, and the woman must be *sober*, truthful, brave, upright — an angel in fact, and the angel under the Acts is not to be found.[82]

She would gladly have instigated a campaign of resistance and non-submission herself given time and money, but the NA whose province it was, remained prudently on the sidelines — when a riot occurred in the Portsea Hospital in 1877 it did nothing despite Mrs Butler's plea for action.[83] Its problem was that to oppose and disrupt the law, however wicked, would conflict with the alternative strategy — to appeal to the philanthropic spirit, to the moralist ethic of like-minded middle-class inhabitants of the towns. This more congenial strategy could succeed only if carried out on a plane of irreproachable respectability; no hint of condoning sin or sympathising with the women could be allowed — the point was to blacken the police and cast doubt on the principle of the Acts. The first strategy supposed that the Acts would be insupportable if dogged by disturbances; the second supposed that they would be weakened if the forces of respectability could be made aware of their real nature.

Inevitably a compromise emerged: the National Association set up a Rescue and Defence Fund which aided women who wanted to leave the towns or to obtain relief from the Acts. They thereby attempted to diminish the pool of women under police surveillance; but they went further than this, and also kept watch on the conduct of the police themselves, eager to check abuses of power. In addition they solicited the help of local councils, churches, even borough police forces. Thus repealers found themselves in competition with other philanthropists and with the Metropolitan Police in rescue work, and mixing attacks on one form of authority and respectability with appeals to other forms for help.

Repeal strength in any district depended not so much on the way the Acts were administered as on the presence of a dedicated activist. Some places were never aroused: Aldershot was embarrassingly unworked except by visiting agents. Nothing happened at Windsor, while Colchester's reputation for rowdiness persisted over the years — as late as 1880 a meeting was broken up and the repeal agent flung off the platform.[84] In Cork there were committees for ladies and gentlemen yet both were inactive — this was the town where women referred to themselves as 'in the employment of Her Majesty' or as 'Queen's women'.[85] Southampton was initially very active, thanks to the efforts of a Unitarian minister, Rev. E. Kell and his wife, but in 1872 the repeal agent there was dismissed and the office closed — the local committee having failed to provide financial support.[86] Similarly in Portsmouth an office was maintained until 1877 and then closed because of lack of activity on the part of the moribund local committee; indeed J.P. Gledstone reported to the National Association that Winchester was apathetic and public meetings would be useless in Southampton, Portsmouth and especially in Aldershot.[87]

In only three districts was there consistent opposition to the Acts.
In Dover a prominent Wesleyan, Alderman Rowland Rees, resisted
them from the first — he helped Mrs Butler during her first tour of Kent
in 1870 — and was particularly effective on the bench in probing
police behaviour. In Rochester and Chatham the Quaker, Frederic
Wheeler, kept repeal work going — he had retired from business to
devote himself to philanthropic work, and besides repeal, was much
involved in the arbitration movement as one of the editors of the
Peace Advocate.[88] In Devonport, opposition to the Acts was led by
W.S. Littleton until his death in 1877; he was a naval clothier
(whose business suffered as a result of his activities) and also
Devonport's Registrar of Marriages. He promoted meetings in the
three towns, testified before the Royal Commission and supervised
the work of John Marshall, the paid agent from 1870 to 1880.
Littleton was highly regarded by all sections of the repeal movement
— his expertise matched that of the police, and although not
prosperous (on occasions his expenses for attending conferences were
paid by the NA) he worked voluntarily, animated only by distaste for
the Acts, invulnerable to the charge of being a salaried worker.[89]

The NA assumed the responsibility for working the subjected
districts, it paid all the salaries and expenses of agents and offices,
and members of its committee from time to time visited these areas
to urge the locals to greater efforts. Despite all this, the NA failed
to generate enthusiasm, so that when Stansfeld came to the fore in
1874, he insisted that work in the subjected towns should take the
highest priority, criticised the NA's record and asked the NCL to send
voluntary workers to help.[90] As a result of this appeal, Wilson himself
visited the towns, and later the League's agent Gledstone was sent to
work there. A more impressive indication of the shift of direction
induced by Stansfeld was the creation on paper of a Subjected
Districts' League (SDL) and a burst of activity by the NA in the
winter of 1874—5. Money was spent freely and agents concentrated in
the towns, holding meetings and setting up committees — 13 were
founded and Southampton revived.[91] These were all nominally
regarded as branches of the SDL, although they were run by NA
agents and no committee for the SDL as a whole was ever formed —
indeed the NA seemed reluctant to set one up, and objected when
the Plymouth branch of the SDL took it upon itself to issue an
independent statement of policy.[92] The SDL was no more than a
convenient front for NA activity; it never functioned autonomously
and its constituent branches were all too dependent on paid agents

who did the work; nor were these necessarily competent — a Mrs Ford engaged to work Portsmouth gave up after a month 'depressed by her duties'.[93]

Results achieved in the first few months of the SDL campaign did not last. Thus the Portsmouth Working Men's Committee founded in January 1875 as a result of a 'tea meeting' held by H.J. Wilson and F.C. Banks, lapsed once agents were withdrawn, while the similar Greenwich Committee, one of the NA's showcases, lasted from 1875 until 1882 only because its secretary, J.H. Killick, received a modest payment from the NA. When it was discovered that the committee had not met for over two years, the subsidy was withdrawn and the committee promptly dissolved.[94] Although the Greenwich Committee was always asking for money, Killick's observation that it was difficult for working men to spare the time unless paid to do so, rings true. For a number of years it gave value for money, several members were also members of the Liberal 500, and it had continued to meet fortnightly after the Gentlemen's Committee had collapsed.[95]

Satisfactory results continued to be obtained in Devonport, where a paid agent and office enabled a combination of rescue and legal work to be carried on. But Littleton's death in 1877 was a serious blow, leaving Marshall, a limited man, without effective supervision. He was quite unable to appeal effectively to middle-class supporters. Thus, while he was away from Devonport in 1879, a 'coup' took place which compromised repeal work there. Miss Ellice Hopkins (of the White Cross League), a rescue worker unconvinced of the paramount need to repeal the Acts, persuaded the Ladies' Rescue Committee, hitherto associated with the NA, to merge itself into her committee which enjoyed police cooperation. The ladies, who seemed lost without Marshall, and ignorant of the NA's various efforts, were swept away before W.T. Swan could get there and attempt to win them back. The NA Committee saw this as a 'coup' for Anniss and his ally, Mr Grocer of the *Western Morning News*; they decided to stop rescue work and, despite Marshall's genuine pleas to be allowed to continue, the agency was closed in December 1880 and he was transferred to other duties.[96]

The abruptness with which this happened is remarkable. Rescue work as part of repeal activity was almost entirely concentrated on Plymouth and Devonport. Marshall's home had functioned as both office and reception centre; women were given advice about their rights under the Acts, and if they wished to leave the area, were helped to do so. Marshall enjoyed their confidence (especially since he too had been imprisoned) and the office was well used — in 1873 there were 126 applications for assistance by 62 women and girls, in 1876 222 applications by 80, in 1877 193 by 88, 29 of whom had been 'rescued'.[97] Here was successful philanthropic effort, yet it was suddenly stopped once semi-official agencies seemed to have the advantage. Perhaps there was little point in persisting in rescue work with repeal overtones when Ellice Hopkins had captured those to whom such efforts might appeal.[98]

Legal defence work was another activity pursued. In 1870 George Butler had suggested that solicitors should be retained in all subjected districts; this far-sighted aim was never achieved, but the 'three towns', Southampton, Rochester and Chatham, and the Kent coast towns eventually had solicitors experienced in handling CD cases. For important test cases, the chairman's firm, Shaen and Roscoe, were sometimes used. In part, solicitors checked on police interpretations of the Acts, and often found that they altered the provisions to suit their convenience, for instance putting up notices warning women of the penal consequences of non-submission, when none existed; or even extracting submissions from illiterates without explaining what they were. When it was discovered that the women were using examination tickets as certificates of cleanliness, the police, quite without legal sanction stopped issuing them.[99] The *Shield* pertinently wanted to know why, if the police could thus suspend part of the Acts, periodical inspection could not be as easily suspended.[100]

The main thrust of legal work lay in defending those women who were prepared to bring their cases into the open by refusing to submit, or who wished to apply for relief from examination. Most women went quietly, but when the police were challenged their evidence was often found to be carelessly prepared despite Captain Harris's assurance that:

No girl is considered a Prostitute unless there are several concurrent proofs. Solicitation in the Streets, residence in a Brothel, association with Prostitutes, frequenting places where Prostitutes resort, and lastly the Woman's own personal admission. The Police cannot be too particular with regard to the administration of these Acts.[101]

Every possible case was seized on by repealers (in the late 70s court reports bulked large in the *Shield*) and although they sometimes defended women whose virtue was dubious, and who might well have

been 'taking them for a ride', they had enough successes to suggest
that the police had a slapdash attitude to evidence and relied greatly on
compliant magistrates. The case of Mary Ann Hart at Woolwich in
1878 illustrates the ambiguity on both sides. The police case rested
entirely on her association with prostitutes; no policeman could
directly attest that she was one but the Inspector in charge was very
confident that she was — though entirely on hearsay evidence. The
defence cast sufficient doubt on the police evidence for the magistrate
to relieve her, but he was in no doubt that the company she kept
might well lead her into prostitution. This was surely a fair assessment of the case; the police could not prove their assertions (which
says something about their diligence as observers) but were probably
correct in assuming that her associations would lead her into
prostitution. Certainly the prosecution may have been premature
and unjustified, but their concern was really with effective control
of the traffic; repealers perhaps made too much of the case as an
example of innocence threatened (it dominated an issue of the *Shield*).
It was hardly an authentic example of legal outrage.[102]

There were better cases. A reformed prostitute was summonsed at
Dover simply on evidence that she had been out late, walking on the
beach.[103] In 1876 in a repeal *cause célèbre* Inspector Anniss was
prosecuted for assault on a respectable shop-girl whose fiancé and
employers stood by her. Miss Murton's case showed the police at their
worst — unsubstantiated innuendo as their chief weapon, though the
fact that the fiancé lived in Littleton's house made the allegation of
conspiracy look credible. The magistrates dismissed the case and a
near riot ensued.[104] Two incidents at Dover reflect poorly on the
quality of the Metropolitan Police. In 1882 Eliza Southey refused to
sign a submission. She was defended by C.J. Tarring, a barrister
member of the NA Committee and Alderman Rees was one of the
magistrates. Between the two of them, the police were pressed savagely
and were forced to admit serving an illegal order on the woman to bluff
her into submission; their identification was suspect and she had no
previous association with brothels or prostitutes. The case was dismissed
and the police criticised for bringing the charge.[105] Elizabeth Burley's
case in 1881 was even more dramatic — chased through the streets by
two CD Policemen, she flung herself into the harbour to escape them,
whereupon they walked away! The repeal movement exerted itself
magnificently. The girl was hurried off to London out of harm's way
(perhaps just as well, as there are suggestions in the NA Minutes that
she was not entirely innocent) and Dover was roused to protest.

Meetings were held, the council dissociated the borough police from the Acts, and eventually the Home Secretary was moved to reprimand and transfer the policemen concerned.[106]

The point of these cases was of course primarily to expose the police in abuses of power — rescue and defence work helped to do this more effectively. This is not to say that concern for the woman was not present, rather that repealers considered regulation to be the worst problem afflicting woman and the chief one to attack. Therefore the police were kept under unremittingly hostile scrutiny: in 1870 the Birmingham repealers Albright and Morgan revealed, probably for the first time, the collusion between the police and hospital authorities at Devonport, after which Inspector Anniss must have become one of the most scrutinised police officers in the kingdom.[107] A female correspondent described to Josephine Butler the steps she had taken to watch the police at work in Canterbury where she had found a particularly flagrant example of police exaggeration:

> The Superintendent told them [the women] a new law had come into operation, *every* girl seen *walking* with a soldier had to be examined, and if she did not submit, she would be imprisoned three or four months with hard labour.[108]

The examining rooms were similarly observed, and complaints collected about painful treatment. Every regulationist assertion that the women approved of the system was countered by evidence that they felt degraded by 'the indescribable compulsory surgical atrocities of the examination room'; petitions were got up and the testimony of the women about their maltreatment became a standard part of most repeal speeches. Certainly the examination was a brusque affair, necessarily so in view of the time allowed for it — in 1877 the Plymouth surgeon examined an average of 70 women each day — and conducted in curious surroundings; morality within the rooms with religious tracts scattered around, immorality without as men waited for the women to emerge.[109] The work of helping the women and scrutinising the operation of the system was not without its hazards: Marshall suffered imprisonment (briefly) and continually complained of harrassment by the police. His employers tried to obtain evidence for a prosecution and instructed him to remain alert in case a chance of charging Inspector Anniss with incitement to breach the peace should present itself. On another occasion Marshall was authorised to employ somebody to be with him when engaged on outdoor work, the intention being to have a reliable witness in case of police insults.[110]

Examples of police misbehaviour were not difficult to uncover (though always hard to prove) as long as a repealer or an agent was there to look after them. But the most spectacular of the scandals thrown up by the Acts came in March 1875 from Aldershot, a town virtually untouched by repeal activity. Mrs Percy, a widow with three children to support, eked out a living as a singer and entertainer in and around the camp. The Metropolitan Police, doubtless regarding such an occupation as but a stone's throw from prostitution, demanded voluntary submissions from her and her 16-year-old daughter, Jenny. When these were refused, the police hounded the mother, making it difficult for her to earn a living and threatening never to let her alone. In despair she poured out her story in a letter to the *Daily Telegraph*, protesting her innocence, and shortly afterwards drowned herself in the Basingstoke Canal.[111] Repealers could recognise a good case when they saw it; Mrs Butler wrote, 'every good cause requires martyrs and this poor woman's death will, I believe, be a means in the hands of Providence of shaking the system more than anything *we* could do'. The case was worked for all it was worth. Bligh was sent to Aldershot to stiffen the Percy family's resolve to tackle the police and defend the deceased's reputation. The children were removed to safety and Jenny Percy herself was lodged with the Butlers. The inquest returned an inconclusive verdict thanks to strenuous efforts by Dr Barr and the police to blacken the character of Mrs and Miss Percy — a jury of publicans said the *Shield* contemptuously — but the press was aroused to good effect. Mrs Butler hired two extra clerks to send letters to every editor in the kingdom — 1,700 of them (the postage alone cost £12) and the results were excellent: *The Echo Daily News Morning Advertiser* all took up the case, though *The Times* confined itself to a brief report of the inquest.[112]

Attempts to prosecute the police foundered — their defence that they had acted within the law was sound, but to Mrs Butler a condemnation in itself: 'this wicked law authorises anything short of murder, and now maybe murder also'. More to the point, the head of the Percy family was an army sergeant and thus subject to official influence. Although Jenny Percy's virginity was attested, the prosecution was dropped, and the 'Percy Fund', opened by the NA at Stansfeld's behest, was applied to the organisation of a great indignation meeting, and then to the support of the Percy children.[113]

Throughout April the agitation prospered with large meetings in provincial towns, culminating in the angry meeting at the Cannon Street Hotel on 4 May 1875 at which Harcourt Johnstone, breaking his usual rule, spoke. Jenny Percy's statement was read out and Shaen, in an inflammatory speech, virtually accused the police of responsibility for a number of other deaths.[114]

The Percy case helped to revive the movement at a critical moment — working-class indignation was genuinely high, indeed efforts were made by popular entertainers to raise a memorial to Mrs Percy at Aldershot, and propaganda circulated widely — a special pamphlet was produced of which 13,000 copies were distributed in the subjected districts.[115] But although the case had a great national impact, it did little to shake local confidence in the Metropolitan Police. Supporters of the Acts were winning victories at repeal meetings at Plymouth in 1877, drawing up petitions of pro-Acts clergy at Portsmouth in 1878, and by 1881 the NA was dissuading the LNA from holding public meetings in the three towns—success was likely only with the best speakers. [116] The local press reported court cases *in extenso* but usually avoided taking sides; a number of papers were unsympathetic, especially the *Western Morning News*, 'one of the most unreasonable and unfair among the newspapers that advocate the Acts', which was attacked by the repeal press for flagrant bias — failing to report large repeal meetings while devoting three and a half columns to a meeting of governors of the Royal Albert Hospital. Against this, the *Devonport Independent* provided fair coverage and was always sceptical about the alleged moral benefits achieved by the Acts.[117] MPs for subjected districts tended to support the Acts — J.D. Lewis and J.H. Puleston, successive MPs for Devonport were leading parliamentary supporters, though even they had at one time given repealers cause for hope; ambiguous phraseology was often the refuge of the MP under attack at elections.[118]

Repealers received some support from local bodies who felt that the Metropolitan Police dramatised the problems faced and improvements achieved for effect, thereby slighting local efforts and reputations. Devonport Borough Council twice defended its town's reputation against Inspector Anniss's claims of dreadful immorality; much was made of these attacks and in 1872 the NA printed 5,000 leaflets giving the council's view of the reliability of the Metropolitan Police.[119] Local police forces were even more angered by claims made for the Acts; the state of the streets was their responsibility and they denied that the Acts had produced any dramatic improvement — in 1882 a

number of Chief Constables and Superintendents were called before
the Commons Select Committee to puncture pro-Acts exaggerations.
Wreford of Plymouth, a particular foe of the Metropolitans also
testified before the Royal Commission and even chaired a meeting of
working men against the Acts.[120] The Metropolitan Police reciprocated
this hostility; Captain Harris alleged that Wreford falsified statistics to
give a better impression of the morality of Plymouth and when asked
why his men did not close down brothels, both he and his successor,
Colonel Pearson, shifted the responsibility to the local police.[121] In
fact, until 1881 the Metropolitan Police did claim to have closed
a number of brothels, but these claims were exposed as false when a
parliamentary return was called for — only one brothel had been
closed as a direct result of their activity.[122] The Chatham Chief
Constable pressed this further in conjunction with the repealer,
Frederic Wheeler; they extracted the names of public houses which
the Metropolitans alleged were brothels, and then discovered that
some were respectable houses — the help of the Licensed Victuallers
Protection Association was thus enlisted. In Portsmouth a number of
sergeants in the local police offered their services as spies against
the Metropolitans — the NA had to turn them down; after all, part
of its case rested on objections to 'spy-police'.[123]

However, this support could not compare with the flood of official
regret from the subjected districts following suspension in April 1883.
A number of clerks to justices were authorised by their benches to
endorse an appeal for the return of the Acts; the Recorder of
Colchester forwarded, with his warm approval, a presentment of the
Grand Jury pointing to increased immorality since suspension;
councils, guardians, justices, clergy, all deplored the loss of the Acts,
and as Campbell-Bannerman shrewdly noted, no two resolutions
were the same, so they were not 'due to organisation, which is so
often traceable in other petitions and resolutions'.[124]

The NA was never so interested in opinion in the garrison towns as
when it had to defend suspension against a barrage of hostile parliamentary questions about local feeling.[125] It sent agents to report
on public feeling in the towns, tried to assemble a deputation of
local repealers to see Harcourt (it was willing to pay expenses of up
to £100 but still encountered a poor response), and asked its old
friends the Chief Constables if they could maintain order without
the Metropolitan Police.[126] In 1884 the regulationist attack concentrated on the increase in disease and Stansfeld issued instructions to
the NA about the collection of evidence to rebut these charges.[127]

A deputation of local repealers was received by Harcourt and asserted against all the evidence that suspension was popular; he was sceptical and received a pro-Acts deputation in a much friendlier manner, professing not to believe that repealers really knew the state of opinion in the towns — against this, the repeal camp could only produce the Chief Constable of Devonport to say, predictably, that his town was never more orderly than now.[128]

Whatever some policemen might say, local authorities in general stood by the Acts — the Chatham Board of Health petitioned annually for their return, and in 1885 its chairman almost carried an amendment in their favour at a repeal meeting conducted by Hugh Price Hughes.[129] Dilke told James Stuart that local authorities were only bothered about the provision of government money and would not pay for the Acts themselves; this explanation for the behaviour of local establishments appealed to repealers — it was noted that Chatham had made do with a smaller police force than other Kent towns and would now have to finance the equivalent of the five withdrawn Metropolitans; economy had been practised at the expense of social morality.[130] Typically, Josephine Butler saw this in a more sinister light: 'In the subjected districts, the municipal spirit was dead, the people had become used to the domination of the War Office.'[131] Yet the debate on conditions in the towns after 1883 in concentrating on respectable opinion, ignored the effect of suspension on the prostitutes themselves. A town missionary writing in 1885 to demonstrate the beneficial moral effects of the Acts, unconsciously showed that suspension had removed one of the props of the prostitute's trade — the illusion of safety for the client. He noted with satisfaction (and quite unaware of the misery revealed) that girls were having to sack children who had acted as servants, they were pawning clothes, selling fruit, could not afford to drink. True they refused his tracts and blamed him for taking away their living, but this seemed a small price to pay for the economic collapse of prostitution.[132]

One way of buttressing opposition to the Acts in the subjected districts, and perhaps disguising its weakness, was to challenge the statistical claims of success. The army and navy medical departments made grandiose claims about reduction of disease, often achieved by comparing different statistical bases, while the Metropolitan Police reports were astonishing documents, moralising about prostitutes, inventing stories about closure of brothels when they were not being closed (nor did the Acts prescribe their closure) and naively boasting the expertise of the CD Police against the supposed unworldliness of the repeal opposition.[133]

The NA always handled the Metropolitan Police, but increasingly turned over the hygienic claims for the Acts to a new body, the National Medical Association (NMA), founded in November 1874. Intended to banish the impression that the medical profession was entirely in favour of the Acts, it was centred on Liverpool and was inspired by Stansfeld's determination to put repeal on a more scientific footing. Mrs Butler was equally keen on the NMA; the LNA provided the services of William Burgess to help with the organisation, and a friend, Dr William Carter, became the honorary secretary. But the undoubted leader of the NMA was another Liverpool doctor, J. Birkbeck Nevins, who devoted himself to the statistical side of the argument, achieving a mastery which sometimes enabled him to defeat the government statisticians. Nevins was a difficult man to work with — for four years during the campaign he would not speak to Mrs Butler — and a poor public speaker who baffled his listeners with medical muddle. He was also inaccurate, much to the NA's displeasure. However, his obituary acknowledged that 'under Dr Nevin's hand, statistics became in a manner living and speaking things'.[134]

To further its work the NMA started a monthly journal, the *Medical Enquirer*, in March 1875. This was a rather dry paper, very exhaustive in its determination to prove the Acts worthless — its articles have Nevins's stamp all over them. Like his pamphlets and tracts, the *Enquirer* did not enjoy much of a sale, and Nevins was constantly obliged to seek subsidies from more prosperous bodies. From March 1878 it only appeared quarterly, and ceased publication in the early 1880s.[135] The NMA was not much of a success — more a vehicle for Nevins's zeal. It recruited more than 120 doctors fairly quickly but failed to develop into an effective national organisation. Its existence was a strength to the repeal cause, and it was able to criticise the medical press's regulationist bias, but the profession as a whole remained unmoved. Indeed NMA members may have been unclear as to its aims — when the NA combed through a pro-Acts petition signed by 174 Liverpool doctors, it found 24 who were members of the NMA.[136] By 1878 it was financially on the rocks, and had to appeal to the NA for help, but this was only offered if the NMA were to abandon its independence. The doctors preferred to soldier on, and managed to borrow large sums from rich friends to do so.[137]

During the sittings of the Commons select committee, Nevins's work was of the greatest importance, both as adviser to Stansfeld and, in public, as an expert witness. However Stansfeld acquired an effective grasp of the statistical case during his four years on the committee, and Nevins's importance diminished. Nevertheless his organisation was of great value in showing that some doctors could see flaws in the Acts.

Preventing the extension of the Acts in any covert form was another priority, given the difficulty of tackling them once in operation. The NA scrutinised parliamentary bills to see if they might offer shelter to regulationists, and savaged those which it thought might. Thus Wheelhouse's Mercantile Marine Hospital Service Bill was condemned because of the facilities for examination which a comprehensive hospital service would provide; his colleague, Captain Pim's efforts to amend the Merchant Shipping Bill for the same purpose were similarly treated.[138] Even the provisions for inspection of factories and the protection of women workers were suspected of misuse if put into the wrong hands.[139] A more obvious danger was that towns might successfully petition to have the Acts applied to them: Newport, Isle of Wight, tried in 1875 whereupon local repealers circularised the whole council against the Acts, and an agent was sent to help. More dangerously, the City of Exeter considered petitioning for the Acts in late 1878; repeal activity was strenuous — four agents converged, the Free Church ministers were roused, the Dean recruited, literature sent to all members of the council and a deputation appeared before it. This very efficient campaign succeeded, the council faltered and the War Office delivered the *coup de grâce* by refusing the application.[140]

But in the towns themselves, repealers had an unimpressive record. The indignation of women subjected to the Acts was scarcely tapped: Rev. Kell at Southampton persuaded 116 prostitutes to petition against police cruelty in 1871, but for the most part there was little response to the angry cries of those like Mary Ann Godden who told the magistrates:

women were now treated as white slaves. She supposed she must submit to the laws of the country; but it was a most indecent law that had been passed during the last four years. Instead of her insulting the officers, they had insulted her by calling her a 'dirty thing'.[141]

Middle-class philanthropy was ill-suited to the potential for civil disobedience. Instead, mediocre meetings with inconclusive results were treated with exaggerated respect and trivial incidents blown up out of all proportion — even the wholly irrelevant issue of the ritualism of a hospital chaplain was thought worth using to try to discredit the Acts by association.[142] As a last resort, repealers simply pretended that poor results were actually good ones. In 1877 F.C. Banks read a paper to the Geneva Congress which was designed to show how well repeal was progressing in the subjected districts. In fact he admitted that five districts were entirely dormant and cited as places where the Acts were strongly opposed Canterbury, where only 5,000 signatures had been collected in six years, and Dover, with 5,453. Vague references to good meetings, strong government influence at work, religious feeling aroused, may well have satisfied a friendly audience, but the admission that, at most, the combined total of signatures from all the towns given against the Acts reached 100,000, serves only to demonstrate that repealers had failed to establish themselves in areas which most mattered.[143]

V

To round off the discussion of repeal organisations (leaving aside the LNA and the denominational bodies for the moment) the regional associations for repeal must be mentioned. The largest two have been encountered already. The NCL covered the six northern counties, and the MCEU the 13 midland ones. Both organisations were well supported and fairly welathy — in their first year of operation they raised £1,082 and £918 respectively.[144] These two were head and shoulders above the other regional bodies — some of which were rather branches of the NA with pretensions to independence.

Scotland had its own National Association from 1873, but although this maintained an office in Edinburgh with a secretary and agent, English repealers criticised the timidity of their Scottish colleagues. Josephine Butler denounced the inability of the Scotsmen to appreciate the significance of women in the movement, and had kind words only for the Edinburgh and Glasgow ladies; while in 1874 the SNA was caught unawares by the general election and had to be given £100 by the NA.[145] Later in the same year, Banks had to go to Edinburgh personally to get the SNA to hold a meeting during the Social Science Congress — and was only able to do so at the cost of excluding ladies from it.[146] The movement never established itself in Scotland — although there were important repealers in Edinburgh, including Professor Calderwood and the Quaker, Eliza Wigham — and in 1882 one of its own members reported that the SNA was dying. When Banks toured Scotland in 1884 he found that it was £60 in debt and had virtually dissolved itself.[147]

In the north-east, Dr Hooppell and Rev. C.S. Collingwood maintained a small but vigorous local association from the start of the campaign right through to final repeal. Based on Sunderland, it held meetings in the towns on the Tyne and Wear and left the country districts to the NCL.[148] In the south-west there had always been active repealers at Bristol, but no electoral work was undertaken until the formation of a Gentlemen's Committee in 1879, when a travelling agent, Rev. E.S. Bayliffe, was appointed.[149] In April 1883 the organisation was expanded and renamed the South-Western Counties' Union, and thus it remained until final repeal; not surprisingly since Samuel Morley was its president, it enjoyed a relatively high income — £376 in its first year, rising to £449 in its second.[150]

Finally to complete the picture, separate Ladies' and Gentlemen's Committees existed in Dublin, Belfast and Cork, but little is known of them and no particular activities are recorded.

Notes

1. *Shield*, 21 Apr. 1883, p. 102.

2. *Shield*, 1 Feb. 1873, pp. 37–9; 22 Mar. 1873, pp. 90–2; 14 June 1873, pp. 193–4.

3. E.g. *Shield*, 5 Feb. 1876, pp. 38–44. The Mayor of Wolverhampton chaired the public meeting at the MCEU's annual conference; he explained that although not a supporter, he was open-minded and felt that he was 'public property' during his year of office.

4. FLB 3802: H.J. Wilson to NCL, EC (circular letter) 13 Nov. 1875; Josephine Butler, *Personal Reminiscences of a Great Crusade* (1896), pp. 178–9.

5. NA, *Annual Report for 1885 and 1886*, pp. 24–5.

6. FLB 3311: Josephine Butler to H.J. Wilson, 29 Oct. 1873.

7. NA EC Minutes, 21 Apr. 1873.

8. NA EC Minutes, 13 July 1874; *Shield*, 24 Oct. 1874, p. 200.

9. FLW Box 82: F.C. Banks to H.J. Wilson, 6 Sept. 1873.

10. FLB 3708: Hudson Scott to H.J. Wilson, 26 July 1875.

11. FLW Box 2: Joseph Edmondson to NCL EC, 29 Feb. 1876.

12. *Shield*, 10 Nov. 1875, pp. 289–91; FLB 3723: H.J. Wilson to NCL EC, 30 Aug. 1875.

13. *Shield*, 7 July 1877, pp. 185–6; FLW Box 2: H.J. Wilson to NCL EC, 6 Apr. 1877.

14. FLW Box 1: H.J. Wilson to NCL EC, 8 Aug. 1882. Between February and July 1882 the NCL obtained 1970 petitions, and another 154 came spontaneously from the North; the rest of the country produced only 665. Put another way, the NCL got 246 petitions per million of population, the rest of the country barely 25 per million.

15. FLB 3277: Joseph Edmondson to H.J. Wilson, 7 June 1873, on the financial arrangements for loaning an NCL agent. His temporary employers kept any monies he might collect.

16. FLW Box 4: *History of the English Repeal Movement*, pp. 6–7 (typescript).

17. See Appendix C for further details on employees and salaries.

18. FLB 24 Jan. 1903: Josephine Butler to G.W. Johnson.

19. E.g. *Shield*, 30 Aug. 1873, p. 281.

20. FLW Box 78: J.E. Ellis to H.J. Wilson, 24 Dec. 1882.

21. NA EC Minutes, 27 Nov. 1882, discussing complaint of J.P. Gledstone.

22. FLB 3285: H.J. Wilson to S.J. Ainge, 18 June 1873; 3288: W.Wastell to H.J. Wilson, 28 June 1873.

23. FLB 3477: Mrs Tanner to H.J. Wilson, 23 May 1875; 3449: H.J. Wilson to Stansfeld, 6 June 1875.

24. Ibid., 3244: Joseph Edmondson to H.J. Wilson, 8 Mar. 1873.

25. *Shield*, 22 Oct. 1870, pp. 263–4.

26. NA EC Minutes, 2 Mar., 9 Mar. 1874.

27. FLB 3249: Josephine Butler to H.J. Wilson, 1 Apr. 1873; 3317: Josephine Butler to 'dear friend', 23 Dec. 1873.

28. FLW Box 82: programme of work, dated 15 Dec. 1872.

29. NA, *Annual Report for 1885 and 1886*, pp. 9–12. Two of Marshall's meetings at Newcastle were said to exceed 4,000.

30. LNA, *Annual Report for 1873*, pp. 6–7; FLB 3313: Josephine Butler to Mrs H.J. Wilson, 12 Nov. 1873.

31. FLB 3195: C.J. Whitehead to H.J. Wilson, 29 Oct. 1872; 3196: Josephine Butler to Miss Priestman, 31 Oct. 1872.

32. FLW Box 82: John Elliott to H.J. Wilson, 19 Feb. 1873. Elliott was also clerk to the Consett Local Board. He asked for £25 p.a. for two day's work per week and was employed.

33. FLB 3250: Josephine Butler to H.J. Wilson, 7 Apr. 1873.

34. NA EC Minutes, 22 Nov. 1880.

35. FLB 3404: Whitwell Wilson to H.J. Wilson, May 1875, objecting to half-educated men addressing public meetings; 3131: C. Herford to H.J. Wilson, 24 Feb. 1872, reporting on agent Hardy: – 'unsuitable for interviewing persons of the upper classes'.

36. Ibid., 3204: H.J. Wilson to John Hardy, 9 Dec. 1872; 3206: H.J. Wilson to Joseph Edmondson, 13 Dec. 1872; 3208: Joseph Edmondson to H.J. Wilson, 14 Dec. 1872; 3280: H.J. Wilson to Joseph Edmondson, 11 June 1873; 3284: H.J. Wilson to NCL EC, 16 June 1873.

37. FLB 3311: Josephine Butler to H.J. Wilson, 29 Oct. 1873; 3269: Josephine Butler to H.J. Wilson, 28 May 1873.

38. NA EC Minutes, 29 June 1874, 6 July 1874, 13 July 1874, 20 July 1874.

39. FLW Box 82: H.J. Wilson to NCL EC, 14 Sept. 1874.

40. FLW Box 2: Items 673–716, 'Correspondence about Burgess', Sept.– Oct. 1876.

41. *Liverpool Daily Courier*, 2 Dec. 1876; *Liverpool Daily Post*, 4 Dec. 1876.

42. NA, *Annual Report for 1874–75*, pp. 16–17.

43. *Shield*, 26 Nov. 1870, pp. 303–9; FLB 3210: George Butler to H.J. Wilson, 24 Dec. 1872.

44. *Shield*, 3 Aug. 1872, p. 1028, criticising *The Times*'s hypocrisy in finding Jacob Bright's speech 'entirely unfit for publication'.

45. *Daily Telegraph*, 18 Mar. 1870, 21 July 1870, critical of the Acts and their defenders; *Daily News* praised by *Shield*, 5 Aug. 1871, for its report on the

deputation to Bruce, attacked by it, 24 Aug. 1872, for its report on the Pontefract election!

46. *Shield*, 18 Nov. 1871, pp. 731–2; it reported the slide towards misrepresentation of the *Spectator*, hitherto favourable to repeal.

47. Benjamin Scott, *A State Iniquity: Its Rise, Extension and Overthrow* (1890), pp. 85, 114–5; Butler, *Personal Reminiscences*, pp. 20–1, 34; J.L. and B. Hammond, *James Stansfeld, a Victorian Champion of Sex Equality* (1932), p. 198.

48. *Shield*, 18 Nov. 1871, pp. 731–2, 17 Jan. 1874, p. 23.

49. Morley was reversing his own attitude, having supported the Acts in the *Fortnightly Review*, Apr. 1870 (Hammond, *James Stansfeld*, p. 134).

50. J.A. and O. Banks, 'The Bradlaugh-Besant Trial and the English Newspapers', *Population Studies*, 8–9 (1954–6), pp. 22–35.

51. NA, *Annual Report for 1880–81*, p. 25.

52. *Shield*, 5 Aug. 1871, p. 602.

53. Josephine Butler, *Recollections of George Butler* (Bristol *c.* 1893), p. 281; *Shield*, 1 Nov. 1874, p. 209.

54. FLB 3839: Josephine Butler to Edith Leopold, *c.* 1875; 3842: Josephine Butler to Mrs H.J. Wilson, 2 Apr. 1875.

55. E.g. *Liverpool Daily Courier*, 24 Dec. 1873, printed an attack on the Church of England petition and gave advance notice that it would not print a reply. Mrs Butler had to protest to another paper.

56. *Northern Echo*, 24 Apr. 1872; *Oxford Times*, 10 May 1873, criticising the Vice-Chancellor for prohibiting the use of a public building for a repeal meeting.

57. *Manchester Examiner*, 18 Mar. 1874.

58. National Library of Wales (Henry Richard MSS) MS 5503B: Josephine Butler to Henry Richard, 6 Nov. 1877 (I owe this reference to Dr D.W. Bebbington); *Shield*, 25 Jan. 1879, pp. 15–16.

59. Besides the earlier articles referred to in chapter 2, see *Westminster Review*, 11 July 1876, for a forceful article opposing regulation.

60. The *Shield* regularly cited *National Reformer* articles of support, e.g. 1 Apr. 1875, pp. 107-8, 8 July 1876, pp. 226-7.

61. FLB Box 78, 643: J.E. Ellis to H.J. Wilson, 28 Mar. 1883; 682: J.E. Ellis to H.J. Wilson, 13 Apr. 1883. Ellis may well have succeeded. The *Pall Mall Gazette* carried a piece critical of the Acts on 13 Apr. 1883 – it pointed out the strength of opposition amongst nonconformists and the working class.

62. FLB 3268: F.C. Banks to H.J. Wilson, defending the *Shield* against Wilson's criticisms; 3741: Josephine Butler to Mrs Tanner, 30 Aug. 1875, agreeing without enthusiasm to support the *Shield* if the rest of the LNA EC wished to; 3876: Josephine Butler to Miss Priestman, 8 Dec. 1875, saying that Mme. Venturi stood in the way of necessary change; 4076: Josephine Butler to 'dear friends', 2 May 1886.

63. FLW Box 78, 887: J.P. Gledstone to H.J. Wilson, 25 Oct. 1883.

64. *Shield*, 1 Nov. 1873, pp. 354–58; NA EC Minutes, 4 Nov. 1872; NA, *Annual Report for 1885–86*, pp. 9–12.

65. See H. Ausubel, *In Hard Times: Reformers Among the Late Victorians* (New York, 1960), pp. 72–8 – this was a common priority among reform movements.

66. FLB 5097: Josephine Butler to friends, 8 July 1871; 3061: Gledstone to Josephine Butler (copy), 24 July 1871.

67. Ibid., 3209: Josephine Butler to H.J. Wilson, 23 Dec. 1872.

68. FLN 54–6: correspondence between F.C. Banks and Godley, Jan. 1874.

69. BL Add. MSS, 44454 (Gladstone Papers) f.41: Josephine Butler to Gladstone, 1 Apr. 1877.

70. FLW Box 5: Stuart to H.J. Wilson, 14 May 1879.

71. FLB 4015: Stuart to H.J. Wilson, 4 Apr. 1884, detailing the assistance given by Mrs and Miss Gladstone in putting pressure on Mr Gladstone.

72. Ibid., 4019: Herbert Gladstone to Josephine Butler, 20 June 1884.

73. D.W.R. Bahlman (ed.), *Diary of Sir Edward Hamilton*, vol. 1 (1972), p. 424; A.B. Cooke and J. Vincent, *The Governing Passion: Cabinet Government and Party Politics in Britain, 1885–86* (Hassocks, 1974), p. 460, Kimberley memo. of Nov. 1895 in Spence Watson MSS.

74. *Nonconformist*, 2 June 1875: a reply from G. Gillett followed on 9 June 1875 pointing out solidarity of Quakers against the Acts.

75. FLW Box 78: J.E. Ellis to H.J. Wilson, 23 Feb. 1883.

76. Sheffield Central Library (Wilson MSS) MD 5890: Joseph Chamberlain to H.J. Wilson, 10 Apr. 1876.

77. *Shield*, 7 Apr. 1877, pp. 91–2; Scott, *A State Iniquity*, pp. 201–10; *Shield*, 23 Mar. 1878, p. 69.

78. *Shield*, 17 Dec. 1870, p. 329; 13 July 1872, pp. 107–8.

79. *Shield*, 25 Nov. 1874, p. 247.

80. FLB 3115: Josephine Butler to her sisters (no date).

81. FLW File IIIA, letter 739: Joseph Chamberlain to H.J. Wilson, 22 May 1883.

82. FLW File I, letter 82; Josephine Butler to H.J. Wilson, 31 July 1874.

83. NA EC Minutes, 25 June 1877. The whole subject of resistance to the Acts in Plymouth and Southampton is discussed in J.R. Walkowitz, ' "We are not beasts of the field": Prostitution and the Campaign against the Contagious Diseases Acts, 1869–1886' (unpublished PhD thesis, Rochester University, 1974), chs. 5–9. The central concern of this valuable thesis is the social context within which the Acts operated.

84. NA EC Minutes, 29 Nov. 1880.

85. *Shield*, 21 Apr. 1877, p. 108.

86. NA EC Minutes, 13 May 1872; 3 June 1872; 2 Sept. 1872.

87. NA EC Minutes, 14 May 1877; 15 Oct. 1877; 19 Mar. 1877.

88. G.H. Dyer, *Sir Wilfrid Lawson* (1878); see also entry in *Dictionary of Quaker Biography* in Friends' Library.

89. *Shield*, 19 May 1877, pp. 137–9 (obituary).

90. FLB 3723: H.J. Wilson to NCL EC, 3 Aug. 1875.

91. NA, *Annual Report 1874–75*, pp. 17-18.

92. NA EC Minutes, 6 Nov. 1876.

93. Ibid., 4 Oct. 1875. The NA EC discussed the SDL weekly as its first item of business from Nov. 1874 to the beginning of 1876. No other item engrossed it to the same extent.

94. Ibid., 17 Jan. 1876; 24 Jan. 1876; 29 May 1876; 13 Nov. 1882; 8 Jan. 1883.

95. Ibid., 18 Mar. 1878.

96. NA EC Minutes, 8 Dec. 1879; 15 Dec. 1879; 1 Nov. 1880; 15 Nov. 1880.

97. *Shield*, 10 Jan. 1874, p. 11; 20 Jan. 1877, pp. 9–10; 2 Mar. 1878, pp. 47–8.

98. See also Walkowitz, ' "We are not beasts of the field" ', pp. 318–9; E.J. Bristow, *Vice and Vigilance: Purity Movements in Britain Since 1700* (Dublin, 1978), pp. 94–9.

99. *Shield*, 16 May 1870, pp. 85, 87; 11 July 1870, p. 155.

100. *Shield*, 14 Oct. 1870, p. 683.

101. PRO HO 45/9322/17273, Captain Harris to H.A. Bruce, 23 Aug. 1872.

102. *Shield*, 14 Dec. 1878, pp. 291–5.

103. Ibid., 25 Oct. 1873, pp. 349–50.

104. *Shield*, 28 Oct. 1876, pp. 325–38; *Devonport Independent*, 7 and 14 Oct. 1876; *National League Journal*, 1 Nov. 1876.

105. *Shield*, 6 May, 1882, pp. 83–5; *Dover Express*, 28 Apr. 1882.

106. *Shield*, 2 Apr. 1881, pp. 68–70; 14 May 1881, pp. 95–6; NA, *Annual Report for 1880–81*, pp. 25–6.

107. Birmingham Reference Library, 562907: *Report of the Deputation to Plymouth* (published by the Birmingham Anti-Contagious Diseases Acts Association for private information only), 1870.

108. FLB 5096: anon. to Josephine Butler, *c.* 1870.

109. *Shield*, 21 July 1877, pp. 201–2; 9 Feb. 1878, pp. 19–20; 16 Feb. 1878, pp. 26–8.

110. NA EC Minutes: 12 and 19 July 1875; 6 and 13 Oct. 1879.

111. Josephine Butler, *Recollections*, pp. 272–77; *Shield*, 22 Mar. 1875, pp. 94–5; 1 Apr. 1875, pp. 97–8.

112. FLB 3839: Josephine Butler to Edith Leupold, *c.* Apr. 1875; *Shield*, 17 Apr. 1875, pp. 109–11, pp. 116–20; *Times*, 21 Mar. 1875.

113. FLB 3888: Henry Bligh to H.J. Wilson, 31 Mar. 1875; 5103: Josephine Butler to Mrs Ford, 20 Apr. 1875; NA EC Minutes, 9 Apr. 1875.

114. *Shield*, 1 June 1875, pp. 133–49.

115. *National League Journal*, 1 Aug. 1875, pp. 4–5; NA, *Annual Report for 1874–75*, pp. 22–3.

116. NA EC Minutes, 10 Oct. 1881; 30 Oct. 1881.

117. *Shield*, 24 Feb. 1877, p. 44; *National League Journal*, 1 Dec. 1883, p. 8; *Devonport Independent*, 8 July 1871, 18 Dec. 1875.

118. *Shield*, 11 Apr. 1874, p. 106.

119. NA EC Minutes, 19 Feb. 1872; *Shield*, 21 Oct. 1882, pp. 200–1; *Western Morning News*, 13 Oct. 1882.

120. *Shield*, 7 Apr. 1877, p. 96.

121. PRO HO 45/9322/17273: Captain Harris to Bruce, 23 Oct. 1871; HO 45/9511/17273A: Captain Harris to Home Office, 15 May 1877, Colonel Pearson to Home Office, Nov. 1882.

122. *Shield*, 18 Nov. 1882, p. 206; NA EC Minutes, 4 Dec. 1882.

123. NA EC Minutes, 2, 16 and 30 Oct. 1882; 31 Oct. 1881.

124. PRO HO 45/9511/17273A: Recorder of Colchester to Home Secretary, 16 Apr. 1884; Clerks of Justices to Home Secretary, 10 June 1884; list of pro-Acts resolutions drawn up by Campbell-Bannerman, 2 May 1884.

125. E.g. *Hansard*, 3rd series (10 May 1883), 279 Col.381 (Talbot); (18 Aug. 1883) 283 Col.1266 (Puleston).

126. NA EC Minutes, 18 June 1883, 16 July 1883, 17 Dec. 1883.

127. Ibid., 25 Feb. 1884.

128. *Shield*, 17 May 1884, pp. 81–90; 21 June 1884, pp. 107–8.

129. Ibid., 16 Feb. 1884, pp. 33–5; 20 June 1885, pp. 91–2.

130. FLW File IIIA letter 736: Stuart to H.J. Wilson, 20 May 1883; *National League Journal*, 1 Sept. 1883, p. 6.

131. *National League Journal*, 1 June 1883, p. 4.

132. Ibid., 1 Jan. 1884, pp. 7–8, reprinting a letter from W. Krause to A.S. Dyer.

133. The *Shield* regularly serialised Captain Harris's reports with pertinent comments, e.g. 8 July 1876, pp. 221–3, 15 July 1876, pp. 229–30, 22 July 1876, pp. 238–9. In 1879 it both reported the Admiralty Solicitor admitting that the purpose of the Acts was not to close brothels (8 Mar. 1879, p. 37) and Captain Harris's claiming to have done just that (12 July 1879, pp. 115–16).

134. FLB 4072: Josephine Butler to a friend, 14 Apr. 1886, on Nevins and Carter; FLW File II letter 533: H.J. Wilson to Josephine Butler, 13 Feb. 1876;

LNA, *Annual Report for 1903*, p. 15; J.B. Post, 'A Foreign Office Survey of Venereal Disease and Prostitution Control, 1864–70', *Medical History*, 22 (1978), pp. 333–4, offers further evidence of Nevins's sometimes casual approach to evidence.

135. *Shield*, 16 Nov. 1874, p. 233; 18 Mar. 1876, p. 91.

136. Ibid., 11 Aug. 1877, pp. 233–4; NA EC Minutes, 1 Feb. 1875.

137. NA EC Minutes, 15 Apr., 29 Apr., 20 May 1878; FLW Box 78: NMA Balance Sheet 1878–79. Subscriptions barely covered the cost of printing the *Medical Enquirer* and the total debt was £372. Donations from E. Backhouse (£150), Stansfeld (£100), Samuel Smith (£50) and others helped to wipe this out.

138. *Shield*, 1 Apr. 1875, pp. 98–9; 29 Apr. 1876, pp. 133–4; 19 May 1877, p. 137.

139. Ibid., 26 Jan. 1878, pp. 11–12; 9 Feb. 1878, pp. 18–19.

140. Ibid., 1 Feb. 1875, p. 31; 1 Mar. 1875, p. 68; 5 Oct. 1878, pp. 250–1; 30 Nov. 1878, pp. 281–2; 28 Dec. 1878, pp. 297–8.

141. *Dover News*, 16 Apr. 1870.

142. *Shield*, 5 July 1873 – a *whole issue* devoted to a meeting at Devonport which was almost won over by a regulationist; 21 Feb. 1874, pp. 62–3.

143. Ibid., 13 Apr. 1878, pp. 91–4.

144. NCL, *Annual Report for 1873*; *Shield*, 31 Jan. 1874, pp. 35–8.

145. FLB 3143: Josephine Butler to H.J. Wilson, received 23 May 1872; NA EC Minutes, 29 Jan. 1874.

146. NA EC Minutes, 7 Sept. 1874 – though the Edinburgh Ladies' Committee had themselves favoured exclusion!

147. NA EC Minutes, 16 Oct. 1882, 14 July 1884.

148. *Shield*, 17 Feb. 1877, pp. 36–7, reporting NE Association's Annual Meeting – income was only £56. The NCL's in the same years was £1,178.

149. FLW Box 5 letter 498: Miss M. Priestman to Mrs C.C. Wilson, 12 Dec. 1879.

150. *National League Journal*, 1 May 1883; *Shield*, 19 Apr. 1884, pp. 63–4; 2 May 1885, p. 60.

6 THE ROLE OF WOMEN IN THE REPEAL MOVEMENT

Although the Ladies' National Association was founded almost accidentally — certainly without any ringing manifesto of the need for women to organise as a sex against the Acts — the mere fact that it operated independently of men, had a profounder effect than many may have realised. Daniel Cooper of the Rescue Society told Josephine Buter:

> At this crisis [the situation in 1869] we heard that the *women* of England were waking up to the consideration of the question. We were rejoiced beyond measure when we saw the announcement of your Ladies' Association in opposition to the Acts . . . We felt on hearing of your Association, that Providence had well chosen the means for the defeat of these wicked Acts. The ladies of England have saved the country from this fearful curse; for I fully believe that through them it has had its death blow. But for the Ladies' Association we should have had no discussion, and the Acts would by this date have probably been extended throughout the country.[1]

The Ladies' Protest at the beginning of 1870 put repeal on the political map, and the LNA shared in the movement's rapid growth. By October, Josephine Butler could boast of having 1,400 members, and the *Shield* was exulting in the LNA as 'the advanced guard of the movement'.[2] At least one advantage of separate organisation from men had been discovered:

> an association of women only . . . is a thing unique in the political history of this country, and your Committee understand that the Government feel some embarrassment as to the manner in which they shall deal with a body composed of such elements.[3]

Thereafter the LNA never contemplated merging with the NA and reminded those who suggested it that 'the members of such an [women's] association are a special power from the very fact of their sex'.[4] Indeed Mrs Butler gloried in the ability of women to manage a movement such

163

as the LNA without male guidance. It was a point of honour that
women should be seen to conduct their own affairs. Thus, when the
Shield incorrectly implied that Stansfeld might have chaired the
LNA's business meeting, she retorted:

> the L.N.A. are in the habit, year by year, of calling together a great
> meeting of women only, and that at such a meeting they would
> consider it a sign of great weakness and poverty of resources among
> women (such as in fact does not exist) if they were to apply to
> a man to act as President . . . but even were these meetings com-
> posed in part of men, the President chosen would always be a
> woman, for on this occasion we deliberately elect to pass our
> Resolutions and make our protests as women, representing an injured
> and outraged portion of our sex.[5]

Of course not all women repealers shared this self-conscious feminism.
Many were timid, and afraid of associating with men in political action
— the Dublin Ladies' Committee was specifically formed for women
unwilling to join a mixed committee; while the Nottingham Ladies'
Committee, unmindful of the struggle to permit women to listen to
debates on the subject, protested to the NA about the presence of
ladies in the Commons gallery during a debate on the Acts — the matter
was referred to the LNA Committee 'with whom the arrangement for
the presence of ladies in the House principally rested'.[6] As late as 1881,
Josephine Butler anticipated that she would lose a number of ladies
from her audience as soon as she mentioned the subject of immoral
legislation.[7]

The other side of the coin was that some male repealers equally disliked working with women, and particularly disliked mixed meetings.
Mundella who was sorely tried by the LNA — 'these women are really
fanatical and scandalous in some of their proceedings' — believed that
meetings of men and women caused scandal and provided the enemy
with ammunition against repealers: 'I believe in meetings in which the
sexes are separated, as many persons of both sexes would come to
such meetings who now absent themselves altogether.'[8] Other northern
repealers shared this view, and Robert Leader forfeited Wilson's friendship because of his newspaper's attacks on women repealers — he disliked 'lady orators' and the idea of women being accepted as public
speakers, though his hostility to the Acts was 'as hearty as ever'.[9] The
issue was resolved at a repeal conference in October 1875 which
unanimously approved mixed meetings.[10]

Simply to have created a women's organisation to agitate on a subject which so many found distasteful was achievement in itself. The more 'respectable' feminist objectives, widening educational and employment opportunities and campaigning for the suffrage, were still in their infancy, yet here were women trespassing upon ground which was anything but proper.[11] They were subjected to tremendous attacks for taking up repeal: the *Saturday Review*, noted for its opposition to feminists, airily chided the Ladies' protest for its alleged ignorance of facts — 'it is a little too much for the ladies to expect us to accept their broad, sweeping, unproved denials of a fact which in innumerable medical journals and in evidence before parliament has been demonstrated'.[12] In the early years, female participation was regularly denounced in parliament by MPs who found the indecency of the subject heightened by it.[13] No debate was complete without a denunciation of the women, sometimes in terms as lurid as those of the *Saturday Review* — 'those dreadful women', 'indecent moenads'.

But the women survived these sorts of attack, and by keeping their nerve and resisting the blandishments of friends and the anger of foes, they matured politically. H.J. Wilson described the first women's meeting in Sheffield:

> C.C.W. [sic — his wife] had to make some announcement, the first time she had lifted up her voice in public and she was terribly nervous. The promoters were astonished at the large number of women who turned up on short notice.[14]

Yet within a year Mrs Wilson had been involved in a violent by-election campaign and subsequently went on to fill her life with philanthropic activity. The LNA was a political nursery in which women learnt to withstand male hostility, and acquired tactical skills to circumvent the most obvious attacks—Josephine Butler urged the deletion of the word 'lament' from an LNA protest: 'We have no time to lament. It brings before me a vision of a number of women sitting down to howl and tear their hair!'[15]

Gradually male hostility to female activism weakened. In 1875 an MP began a speech defending the Acts by praising Mrs Butler's 'character and conduct' which entitled her to 'the highest admiration'; C.H. Hopwood marvelled that this was the first time that an opponent of repeal had 'done justice to the motives of the excellent women in England who have endeavoured to stir up feeling in this matter'.[16] But even in the 1880s a new Speaker tried to exclude women from the gallery during a repeal debate, and Josephine Butler expected to be 'thoroughly abused' for writing to all MPs urging repeal.[17]

When confronted by the Ladies' Protest 'a leading man in the House' is reported as exclaiming:

> We know how to manage any other opposition in the House or in the country, but this is very awkward for us — this revolt of the women. It is quite a new thing; what are we to do with such an opposition as this?[18]

This element of surprise in the mobilisation of women was crucial in launching repeal. Early in 1870 ladies' petitions flooded into parliament: 7,000 from Leeds, 4,000 from York, 6,000 from Bradford, demonstrating the seriousness of the new agitation.[19] However, the contribution of the LNA did not end there; not only did it maintain its independence, it also used it to pursue policies often distinct in their feminine emphasis from those of the rest of the movement.

Thus the moral imperative of the 1870 Protest became the LNA's principal characteristic: the parliamentary campaigners were left to plod through the statistics, demonstrating the defects of the Acts. The women's argument was one of principle, and their aim was broader than repeal alone:

> The ultimate objects of your Society will doubtless extend much beyond the repeal of these Acts of Parliament. Your Association has been called into existence by the shock of this unprincipled legislation, but it will not cease to exist and to work when this legislation is brought to an end.[20]

When repeal was finally achieved in 1886 most of the male associations did in fact dissolve, leaving the LNA to carry on the more difficult fight for equal moral standards.[21] This emphasis on morality later became the orthodoxy for the whole movement; Scott's 'official' history exemplifies it, proceeding from the assumption that *only* a moral campaign could have succeeded. However, in the 1870s the LNA feared that the demand for 'total and unconditional' repeal, though accepted by male repealers, was threatened by their supposed willingness to compromise with a political solution if one could be found. In 1876 it maintained:

> The necessity must never be forgotten for women continuing to

hold their place in the van of the movement. By no other means can the proper view of the subject be kept continually forward, and by no other means can the highest standard of moral purity be held up constantly to view. Further it is only by women that the platform of the contest in which we are engaged can be continually raised to a higher level.[22]

The conflict over Bruce's Bill illustrates the sort of backsliding which the LNA feared from those in parliament. Josephine Butler told Mrs Wilson: '*I and my ladies* will not *in any way* countenance Bruce's Bill, and I am glad *not* to be represented in Parliament at this moment, that I may wash my hands of policy and only hold up *principle*'.[23] The LNA led the opposition to acceptance of the Bill, urging repealers ' 'to prefer, if need be, temporary defeat to compromise – to insist on the recognition of equal rights and responsibilities for both sexes'.[24] Its view prevailed and the movement was induced to return to an uncompromising stance, odious to parliamentary moderates: 'our (so called) *friends* in the House are "disgusted" with our opposition to Bruce's Bill, and lay it upon the absurd fanaticism and suspiciousness of the ladies'.[25]

The LNA was one of the most militant associations during the first four years. It had also adopted a hostile attitude to the Royal Commission, and was the first body to appoint an agent, Samuel Fothergill, 'to bring forward this question at every election, and in some cases to conduct a contest'.[26] After 1874, in common with the rest of the movement, it moderated its tactics – such that it welcomed the Commons select committee in 1879 (in contrast to its intransigence in 1871) and authorised Mrs Butler to testify on its behalf. However this moderation implied no compromise of principle.[27]

Female repealers never tired of referring to their cause as a women's question and this naturally led them to be concerned with the plight of their fellow women, subjected to the Acts. Josephine Butler was eager to make middle-class women aware of the sexist nature of the Acts; she rammed home her message by quoting the bitter complaint of a woman she had met in one of the Kent towns:

It is *men, men, only men*, from the first to the last that we have to do with! To please a man I did wrong, at first, then I was flung about from man to man. Men police lay hands on us. By men we are examined, doctored and messed on with. In the hospital it is a

man again who makes prayers and reads the Bible for us. We are had
up before magistrates who are men, and we never get out of the
hands of men until we die![28]

Although most LNA members viewed the Acts from a distance, and
were unwilling in practice to help victims personally,[29] nevertheless the
LNA (inspired by Josephine Butler) supported work in the subjected
districts to an extent second only to the NA. Agents and LNA workers
often worked there, usually attempting to win over local ladies, but
sometimes attempting large meetings.[30] The LNA twice held its annual
meetings in subjected districts: at Devonport in 1872, and at Woolwich
in 1880; both were reported as successful, and at Devonport a Ladies'
Committee was formed – though, as we have seen, with indifferent
results later.[31]

Yet despite LNA activists' undoubted interest in the operation of
the Acts, one wonders how much they understood of the problems
of those women actually in the police net. It was widely accepted
that middle-class women were not endangered by the Acts –
Josephine Butler quoted working men as saying that 'this law will
not affect the delicate and protected ladies of rank but *our* poor
daughters must be warned speedily of what is threatening them', and
a woman summonsed before the Canterbury magistrates asked: 'Why
should I be examined, and all the girls that are a little better off let
off?'[32]

The LNA's concern (if called upon to choose) was more to defeat
an odious principle than to minister directly to the needs of the Acts'
victims: it approved of rescue work, but in 1878 warned of the danger
of allowing this to divert energies from the main work of repeal; it was
in favour of seeking a Royal Commission on the causes of prostitution,
but again, only after repeal had been carried.[33] Its contempt for the
Acts and their defenders is well illustrated by its reaction to a number
of petitions from prostitutes who supported the Acts – nothing could
be worse than being deluded by material considerations into maintaining the system: 'Your Committee maintains that were these
petitions the spontaneous expressions of the wishes and feelings of
prostitutes, they would constitute the most ghastly and terrible
argument yet adduced against the Acts.'[34] Influenced by its faith
in the virtues of self-help, the LNA (like the rest of the repeal movement) abhorred protective clauses for women in Factory Bills. It
argued that women's labour would thus become expensive and would
be dispensed with – 'these restrictions on grown up women's work

are inevitably pushing women out of work into the street and the gutter — and then they must take to the "best paid industry" — prostitution'. [35] For women already trapped into prostitution, its priority was the removal of the regulation system, not rescue work; for those likely to be sucked in, all it could prescribe was defence of the free labour market. Poverty was correctly recognised as the main cause of prostitution, but the LNA's preoccupation with morality, prevented it from developing responses to this problem.

II

The LNA leadership had to face considerable hostility in the movement's early years from those who agreed with *The Times* that 'the matter of controversy was not such as might be expected to invite the public co-operation of ladies although its discussion is a painful necessity with public men'.[36] They had to be able to withstand allegations that they enjoyed dabbling in filth, and a political thick skin was an undoubted asset. Not surprisingly, women bold enough to commit themselves tended to be accustomed to some form of public activity already.

The LNA's leading figure, Josephine Butler, exemplifies this with her family background of radical philanthropy and an existing interest in social and educational work. The LNA revolved around her charismatic leadership, and her almost mystical ability to inspire her followers was a great asset to the movement. No comparable agitation (temperance, disestablishment — certainly not the suffragists) had a leader able to move an MP to confess: 'I cannot give you any idea of the effect produced except by saying that the influence of the Spirit of God was there.'[37] However there was more to the LNA than simply Mrs Butler; she recognised that administration was not her strong suit, saying: 'It is all very well to have comets flashing about occasionally — but their value is not great in comparison with the steady planets which never err from their orbit.'[38] The LNA's 'steady planets' were a group of ladies who brilliantly complemented Mrs Butler, and, while sharing her background of activism, conformed, far more than she did, to a single 'type'.

Firstly they were nearly all nonconformists (the major difference separating them from Mrs Butler — though she was a rather unorthodox Anglican) and by far the largest group were Quakers whose work for the LNA Mrs Butler frequently acknowledged as crucial in the early years.[39] The most prominent Quaker worker was Mrs Margaret Tanner of Weston-Super-Mare, treasurer of the LNA from 1869 to 1905. She and her sisters, the Misses Priestman, were largely responsible

for the LNA's success in the Bristol area, and shouldered most of the
burden of LNA work when Mrs Butler involved herself in international
work after 1875. Many Wesleyans, Congregationalists and Unitarians
are found in the LNA but of those whose denominations can be
identified, by far the greatest number were Quakers.

The second influence discernible is that of family. Repeal activists
naturally attempted to encourage their families to take a benevolent
view of their actions, and many found it easy to involve relations in
repeal work. The Bright family illustrates this: Jacob Bright was a
parliamentary repeal leader (John Bright's ambivalent attitude
has already been discussed, though he did vote for repeal), his wife
was a founder member of the LNA Executive Committee as was
her mother, Mrs Blackburn of Southport. Also active were Jacob's
sisters, Mrs Samuel Lucas and Mrs Duncan McLaren (whose husband
was another repeal leader in the House) and his niece, Mrs J.P.
Thomasson, and her husband. Other Quaker families were similarly
devoted to repeal: the Clarks of Street, the Priestmans in Bristol and
Bradford, and two sisters who each ran an LNA branch, Mrs Kenway
of Birmingham and Mrs Richardson of York.

Thirdly, LNA leaders had usually been involved, either directly or
through their families, in other radical or philanthropic movements.
Most were active feminists — working for sexual equality and a high
moral standard implied opposition to the idea that a male parliament
could legislate for women. Amongst the most prominent were
Lydia Becker, the suffrage movement's parliamentary agent, Miss
Lucy Wilson and Mrs Wolstenholme-Elmy, both active in the
suffrage and women's education movements. Temperance was
another common interest for many: activists included Miss Tod of
Belfast, Mrs Backhouse of Sunderland, Miss Wigham of Edinburgh
and Mrs Lucas — a great catch as she was president of the British
Women's Temperance Association.[40] A few examples will show how
politically active these women were: Miss Wigham's obituary noted
that 'the Temperance, Peace, Women's Suffrage and every other
philanthropic movement received her assistance by public
addresses, correspondence, or personal labour, while to the poor in
her own town and to all in distress she was a never failing friend'.[41]
Mrs Nichol, also an Edinburgh Quaker (and a member of the Pease
family of Darlington) included among her 'good works and progressive movements' anti-slavery, suffrage, medical education for
women and the RSPCA. Mrs Sheldon Amos devoted herself after
her husband's death to a variety of morality campaigns, suffrage

societies and efforts to help Armenian refugees.

But it was the American abolitionist movement which had the greatest influence on the LNA, especially in its adherence to principle at all costs. Josephine Butler approvingly quoted William Lloyd Garrison's dictum, 'when the necessary revolution in the minds of the people is completed, that in the institutions of the country will follow as the day follows the night'.[42] Garrison's opposition to political compromises, his adherence to principle in the face of adversity, above all his massive sense of conviction endeared him to Harriet Martineau, a prominent English opponent of slavery and later a member of the LNA.[43] Mrs Lucas, Mrs Nichol and Miss Estlin of Clifton were also former abolitionists; Miss Estlin's father had been a famous anti-slavery enthusiast; her obituary noted that 'from him she imbibed the true abolitionist principles which prepared her to take up the cause of women'.[44]

The LNA was run by a small, long-serving executive committee which began in 1870 with a membership of 13 and gradually extended itself until by 1885 it numbered 25. Once elected, members tended to remain until their deaths; in 1900 seven had served continuously since 1870 and 18 since 1880. The main purpose of the EC was to identify prominent women repealers; a list of those willing to serve was presented to the annual meeting and ratified without discussion. This practice encouraged longevity and produced some members who were obviously honorific: thus Harriet Martineau was a member from 1872 until her death in 1876, her place secured by her literary reputation and record of opposition to the Acts; Mrs Nichol remained a member until 1896 though she had been totally blind for the last ten years of her life.

The real work was done by a much smaller group. The executive committee was based in Bristol where the core of its active membership lived: Mrs Tanner, Miss Mary Priestman and the Unitarians, Miss Estlin and Mrs Charles Thomas, Most meetings were held in Bristol with these ladies as the regular attenders — they provided almost half the total attendances at the 72 meetings held between 1875 and 1883, no less than 30 of which were held in Bristol (Mrs Butler attended less than half these meetings).[45] After 1880 the committee met more often in London (of the 22 meetings held there, 17 occurred after 1880) and changes in its composition reflected the LNA's shift towards the capital—for instance members from the north and midlands diminished from eight to six between 1874 and 1885 while the London contingent increased from three to seven.

Josephine Butler's role was a curious one. Officially the honorary secretary, she maintained an office in her Liverpool home for which the LNA paid; from here she directed the LNA agents, and produced a constant stream of ideas, suggestions, directives — in 1872 her postage cost £1 a day. She and Mrs Tanner were given discretionary powers between committee meetings and these she used vigorously — so much so that when she fell ill in 1875, the hard pressed Mrs Tanner had to admit that the LNA was almost paralysed.[46] Yet Josephine Butler was no administrator, so the routine work was dealt with in Bristol — Mrs Tanner paid the bills (though Mrs Butler *was* a good and persistent fund-raiser) while Miss Priestman handled much of the routine correspondence (often with shrewd suggestions from Mrs Butler — who were the best workers in a particular town, why not send annual reports to local papers which are glad to print any news, etc.).[47] After 1875 Mrs Butler was as much the servant of the Federation as of the LNA; indeed she often wrote begging letters to Mrs Tanner on behalf of Stuart, the Federation's treasurer.[48] Yet she remained indispensable — full of energy and ideas — and it was well worth changing the pre-arranged date of the annual meetings to suit her convenience.[49]

The LNA's membership in the years up to 1880 was markedly provincial and especially concentrated in two areas: Bristol and northern England. With the leadership effectively in Bristol, it is not surprising to find an active local committee of which Mrs Thomas was chairman. Indeed ladies were said to be the backbone of the agitation in Bristol and the West, and the Bristol committee was rich — subscriptions totalled £77 in 1875 and £168 in 1876 — and strong (it always returned a list of over 100 members and at its maximum in 1877 provided 15.9 per cent of LNA membership).[50]

Northern membership in the four pre-1880 years surveyed averaged half the total membership, mainly found in large branches such as Leeds, York, Macclesfield or Birkenhead. After 1880 the membership pattern altered: the north ceased to provide such a large proportion (indeed both Lancastria and Yorkshire had reached their peaks in 1874) and London belatedly emerged as a power in the LNA.

In the early 1870s the women of the capital had been little affected by the agitation; in the LNA's first three years, there was no London branch and the inactive London Ladies' Committee preferred affiliation to the NA (possibly to preserve respectability?) until its dissolution in 1872. In 1875 the LNA was reduced to having to ask the NA's assistant secretary, Miss Harrison, to be its London correspondent.[51] However in November 1881 it was decided to

Table 6.1: Regional Distribution of LNA Membership

Year	1870–1		1873–4		1876–7		1879–80		1882–3		1884–5	
Number of subscribers and % of total	subscribers	%	subscribers	%	subscribers	%	subscribers	%	subscribers	%	subscribers	%
Devon and Cornwall	3	0.35	3	0.35	16	1.68	25	2.76	13	1.06	8	0.8
Wessex	33	3.88	41	4.85	47	4.95	45	4.95	49	3.98	40	4.05
Bristol	130	15.25	107	12.7	152	15.9	140	15.4	137	11.17	117	11.75
London	18	2.12	21	2.5	17	1.79	22	2.43	384	31.2	340	34.0
South-east	9	1.05	20	2.38	51	5.33	39	4.3	33	2.68	33	3.32
Central	29	3.4	46	5.45	57	5.95	81	8.95	104	8.45	87	8.75
East Anglia	8	0.94	5	0.59	4	0.43	4	0.42	6	0.48	4	0.4
West Midlands	53	6.2	13	1.54	15	1.57	19	2.1	18	1.46	12	1.21
East Midlands	33	3.88	27	3.2	21	2.2	22	2.43	31	2.52	26	2.62
Peak-Don	2	0.23	14	1.67	59	6.15	52	5.75	25	2.04	21	2.11
Lancastria	233	27.4	147	17.5	152	15.9	79	8.7	107	8.7	56	5.73
Yorkshire	82	9.65	236	28.0	224	23.4	196	21.6	136	11.1	123	12.3
North of England	21	2.47	94	11.2	81	8.45	111	12.25	135	11.0	101	10.11
Scotland	83	9.75	18	2.14	11	1.15	7	0.75	7	0.57	6	0.6
Wales	3	0.35	3	0.35	4	0.43	23	2.54	13	1.06	11	1.11
Ireland	21	2.47	37	4.4	42	4.4	41	4.53	32	2.59	10	1.0
Miscellaneous	91	10.7	10	1.18	2	0.21	–	–	1	0.08	–	–
TOTAL	852		842		957		906		1231		995	
Northern England	338	39.7	491	58.5	516	53.9	438	48.4	403	32.7	301	30.2

Notes: The regions used are those of C.B. Fawcett, adapted by Henry Pelling,
Social Geography of British Elections (London, 1967), 'Northern
England' at bottom comprises the four regions: Lancastria, Yorkshire,
Peak-Don, North of England.
        Percentages do not total 100 because of rounding up.
Source: LNA Annual Reports and subscription lists.

reactivate London by dividing it into district branches. Miss Alicia Bewicke became the London secretary and the coordinator of a remarkable expansion programme — from 22 members (2.43 per cent) in 1880 to 340 (34 per cent) in 1885. By the time of its first annual meeting in 1883, the London branch had set up committees in ten boroughs. Well might Josephine Butler call it 'our youngest and most sturdy child of whom we have reason to be proud' though she felt less at ease with the younger women running it than with the LNA veterans, especially the Quaker women who had been with her since 1869. Miss Bewicke was a particularly trying person to get on with, '*very* excitable and often nearly bringing our cause into discredit by her wild acts and impulses'.[52]

Someone of Miss Bewicke's vigour would have been valuable in the subjected towns where the LNA was pitifully weak. The maximum membership in them was 51 (5.34 per cent) in 1876—7 and, at most, there were LNA correspondents in ten out of the 18 towns, with only Cork having anything approaching a successful branch. Certainly agents and speakers visited the English towns regularly but never succeeded in fostering strong self-sufficient branches.

The LNA membership was relatively wealthy if subscription lists are to be believed; few are for less than 2s 6d, and these are found in branches such as York which made a point of recruiting large numbers. After 1880, the lowest category (2s 6d and under) is maintained at a respectable level only by the adhesion of London, though even there subscriptions had to be a minimum of 2s 6d. Josephine Butler had hoped to recruit working-class women and suggested printing 'a neat little cheap card . . . in the form of a receipt — and the donor's name on it' to encourage them to join.[53] However there is little evidence that they did, other than in exceptional cases where branch secretaries did try to recruit a large membership including poorer subscribers; these exceptions serve only to emphasise the essentially middle-class nature of the LNA. The middle-range categories show increases over the period, though the higher the category the less pronounced it is, until the two highest categories are reached. These declined between 1870 and 1885 causing the LNA's fall in income — the case of the Darlington Quakers illustrates this: in 1872—3 ten people, six of them Peases, gave £59 4s 0d; by 1884—5 the number had dropped to six and the amount to £25 2s 0d.

Membership strength can only approximately be assessed as the only records kept were subscription lists which vary in accuracy and

Table 6.2: LNA Membership — Amounts Subscribed

Year	1870-1	1873-4	1876-7	1879-80	1882-3	1884-5
Under 2s 6d	475 (55.7%)	325 (38.5%)	373 (38.9%)	388 (42.8%)	556 (45.25%)	388 (39.0%)
2s 7d to 5s	127 (14.9%)	193 (22.9%)	239 (24.0%)	226 (25.0%)	277 (22.5%)	254 (25.6%)
5s 1d to 10s	67 (7.86%)	102 (12.3%)	137 (14.4%)	112 (12.4%)	151 (12.25%)	130 (13.05%)
10s 1d to £1	70 (8.25%)	92 (10.9%)	96 (10.0%)	80 (8.85%)	112 (9.1%)	107 (10.75%)
£1 0s 1d to £5	85 (9.96%)	101 (12.0%)	93 (9.7%)	84 (9.3%)	112 (9.1%)	103 (10.35%)
£5.0s 1d to £49	26 (3.15%)	23 (2.73%)	16 (1.67%)	15 (1.66%)	20 (1.62%)	12 (1.21%)
£50 and over	3 (0.35%)	6 (0.71%)	4 (0.43%)	1 (0.11%)	3 (0.24%)	1 (0.11%)
Total membership	852	842	957	906	1231	995
Total subscription income	£992.16.1	£982.13.6	£1160.9.9	£672.19.0	£854.10.4	£523.19.6

Source: LNA Annual Reports and subscription lists.

often include corporate branch subscriptions which conceal the number of individuals. Table 5.2 therefore gives minimum membership figures[54] which show that LNA strength hovered between 850 and 950, rising to 1,231 in 1883 and declining thereafter. This was high in comparison to allied pressure groups; in 1879—80 not one of the LNA's best years, the NA listed 334 individual subscribers, the NCL 184 and the VA 178. A few men subscribed to the LNA (reaching a maximum of 50 (7.1 per cent) in 1874) as the objects and membership clauses of its rules were wide enough to include them, but they made no attempts to influence LNA policy. They were generous donors — T. Thomasson of Bolton regularly gave either £50 or £100 — but never used this economic power to moderate LNA militancy; indeed they may have subscribed to show their support of it.

The typical LNA member during the 1870s was a provincial non-conformist, often a Quaker, with a background of philanthropic or reform activity, a sympathetic family, and often religious connections to sustain her in taking up repeal. In the 1880s the provincial emphasis begins to wane, our typical member may now be a Londoner, or she may come from the south of England where the Annual Reports show that small towns — Grantham, Leominster, Torquay, Ventnor — were acquiring LNA correspondents. This possibly indicates growing respectability, enabling the LNA to break out of its provincial strongholds and establish itself in less likely areas. Above all, in either period she was middle-class, able to afford a high subscription, and unlikely to be found in areas actually subjected to the Acts; as their opponents noticed, LNA members tended to declaim against the Acts only from afar.

III

Even though membership was stable throughout the period, the LNA's income dropped as wealthy subscribers died or otherwise defected. In its early years the LNA had little difficulty in recruiting wealthy donors. Income rose astonishingly from £589 in 1870 to £1,633 in 1873. Virtually all of this came from subscriptions and donations; legacies

Figure 6.1: LNA Income, 1870—85

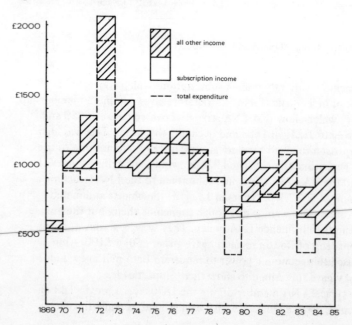

are not found in the accounts until 1884, presumably because the membership was still alive and kicking. It remained at between £900 and £1,100 in the mid-1870s, though was gradually slipping. Until 1879 the LNA committee scarcely ever discussed finance, but thereafter it began to effect economies.[55] Individual subscriptions became more important as the number of large ones diminished, and recruitment campaigns in the early 1880s boosted membership. Understandably the decline was resumed once suspension was carried in 1883, but even in 1885, with an income of £524, the LNA was hardly poor.

Until financial necessity forced innovation upon it, the LNA's organisation is of interest only in so far as its existence proved that women were as capable as men of running a political apparatus. The executive committee had offices and staff in Westminster (shared with the NA and VA) and Liverpool; it employed agents for electoral and agitational work and published considerable amounts of literature. At the beginning of each year annual meetings were held which transacted business, encouraged the membership to zeal during the coming year and directly stimulated activity in the towns where they were held (agents were drafted in to rouse interest in the associated public meetings). This sort of organisation, staffed by professionals on the anti-Corn Law League model, was unremarkable — other repeal bodies operated similarly.

It did, however, demand considerable amounts of money. In the early 1870s this posed no problem and, as Figure 6.2 shows, large amounts were spent on the militant electoral policy. In 1873 when over £1,900 was spent, £1,347 of it was on campaigning; three male agents (Fothergill, Burgess and Bligh) were employed and money was spent freely as part of the general campaign to mobilise opinion against the Acts.

After 1874 the electoral campaign was abandoned and agency work reduced. By 1877 Burgess was the only male agent left, and when he offered to resign the committee accepted, saying that a woman would now be more suitable; Mrs William Goulder was appointed in his place.[56] Her work consisted of holding drawing room meetings to stimulate branches and raise money; the fact that the LNA now had only a woman agent limited its ability to respond to new repeal initiatives. Thus in late 1877 the LNA was unable to respond to an invitation from the MCEU to help in putting pressure on MPs. Women acting on their own were not thought serious and the lack of a male agent was a particular hindrance. Josephine Butler

Figure 6.2: LNA Expenditure, 1870-85

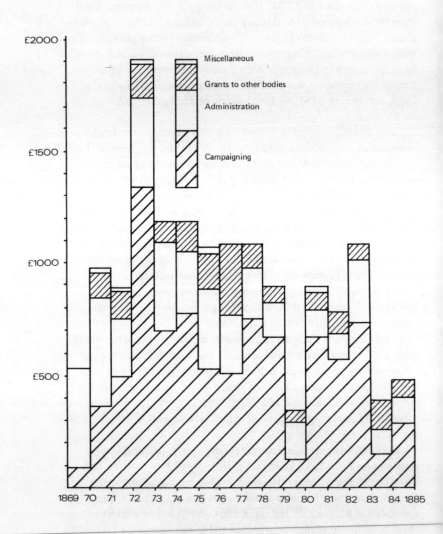

told Martineau: 'Our deputations are generally treated with considerable contempt seeing that we have no votes, as yet. It may be a very
different thing in the future.' She added that however much the LNA
approved the policy of memorialising MPs — the only constitutional
means by which women could influence parliament was by
petitioning.[57] In 1878 the LNA did collect another women's petition,
as in 1871, but again its reception disappointed them, though
petitioning did, of course, have the merit of keeping the branches alive.
Although electoral work dropped off, expenditure remained high
between 1875 and 1878. This was because the LNA resorted to a
policy of working through other associations which they subsidised.
A payment had always been made to the NA for the *Shield*; between
1876—8 and 1881—3 grants were made to the WMNL which also
received free administrative help, as did the NMA and NCL. In 1876
the LNA Annual Report said:

> In fact our Association which was the parent of so many others,
> has for the last year or two practically confined its action in a
> great measure to rendering help, pecuniarily and otherwise, to
> other Societies working in our cause.[58]

By 1878 the accounts were in deficit so the WMNL grant was withdrawn and other small economies made. 1879 saw a slight surplus but
the reserves faced depletion, so when ill health forced Mrs Goulder
to retire at the end of 1879, she was not replaced, and the opportunity
was taken to slash expenditure during 1880 — only £113 was spent
on campaigning. This reduction seems to have had one beneficial effect
— to keep any sort of activity going, voluntary effort had to be relied
on. Two members of the committee, Mrs Steward of Ongar and Miss
Bewicke, began making lecture tours — work hitherto mostly done
by paid agents — with considerable success. Their 1880 tour of the
west country saw Mrs Steward addressing 18 meetings in 22 days and
Miss Bewicke 15.[59]
    Before 1880, members of the LNA were notably inactive; by
contributing to the Association's funds and thereby helping to support
professional agents, the majority could excuse their lack of zeal. The
position of isolated members in small towns, who might not wish
their neighbours to know of their LNA commitment, cannot have
been comfortable. This can be seen in the response to an appeal
made in 1877: branches were invited to submit reports of their
activities for inclusion in the Annual Report, but very few did so. In

1878 only 18 out of 89 towns (20.2 per cent) with branches had any
report to make. A rather desperate call for 'renewal and continued
exertions' was made; these were to include basic activities such as holding
regular committee meetings and women's meetings, petitioning, and
trying to get news into the local press.[60] By 1880, the proportion of
branches sending in reports had declined even further to 16.5 per cent,
but the financial crisis of that year forced the LNA to goad its members
into life. When the state of the funds permitted the employment of
agents again, they were engaged on a short-term basis; every effort was
now made to stimulate branches — Miss Bewicke's work in London
after 1881 caused the Annual Report to call 'the greatly increased
interest in this subject in the metropolis . . . one of the most cheering
experiences of the past year'.[61] Bristol was always reliable; in 1879
it founded outliers at Clifton and Bedminster which soon prospered,
and its members helped to support a local voluntary Lock Hospital;
the Bridport Committee held meetings to put pressure on their MP; the
York branch organised a meeting of 1,000 women in 1879. Gradually
the number of branches submitting reports rose — to 28 (27.4 per cent)
in 1882 and 54 (52 per cent) in 1883. These successes probably em-
boldened the committee, as it decided at the end of 1882 to end the
agency system altogether and rely on voluntary effort with Miss Bewicke
acting as coordinator:

> it has been thought that the time is come when greater and more
> simultaneous work may be done by utilising local interest in the
> cause throughout the country, than is possible by means of an
> organising agency.[62]

Thus financial necessity in the first place had driven the LNA along
the road towards mass involvement, thereby discovering what
Josephine Butler had always known — that amateurs could be as
effective as professionals.[63] The LNA did not succeed in activating all
its members — even in 1883, a year of triumph, almost half the
branches were passive, recipients of whoever or whatever was sent
out from the national offices. The impressive number of branches cannot be taken to imply widespread activity; much depended on the
courage and enthusiasm of the individual secretary or correspondent,
prepared to stand up for her convictions.

Within the repeal movement, the LNA was firmly aligned with the
provincial societies against the London-based NA; its own largely
provincial membership believed that proximity to the parliament

which had passed the Acts *must* be corrupting − only in the provinces
could the movement escape contagion. Mrs Butler put it plainly: 'I
find the gentlemen in London a little slow to move. They cannot I
suppose feel so justly angry, so bitterly grieved as women do about
this.'[64] The split over Bruce's Bill illustrated the gulf between the NA
and LNA, and this gulf persisted into the 1880s. A constant source of
annoyance to the LNA was its obligation to pay part of the *Shield*'s
subsidy without, as it seemed, being able to influence its direction.[65]
The LNA was thus a natural ally for the provincial radicals of the
NCL and MCEU when they challenged the NA in the 1880s.

   This suspicion of the capital was reflected by the LNA's close
connections with the Vigilance Association−Mrs Butler was its
first secretary and six out of the initial committee of ten were LNA
members.[66] Both organisations mistrusted the power of the state
which the VA argued eroded the capacity of the people to defend
themselves.[67] During the 1870s the VA's crusade against state inter-
ference was of great assistance to repealers since one of the things it
was angriest about was the application of compulsion to public
health. Josephine Butler thought it so useful that she considered
making a grant to it by dismissing an agent.[68] In 1873 the Annual
Meetings of the two bodies were held together and she chaired the
VA discussion on the CD Acts.[69] Although its scope was wider, the
VA's view of the Acts was so exactly a reflection of the LNA's that
it was well worth sponsoring as a 'front'.

   In the mid-70s the LNA was a prime mover in the foundation of
two bodies already considered − the WMNL and the NMA − both
originating in Liverpool and initially enjoying the services of the
LNA's agent Burgess. The WMNL was the most regular recipient of
LNA funds and assistance, and when the *National League Journal*
was threatened with closure for financial reasons, the LNA spoke
up strongly in its favour as it contained specifically working-class
material.[70] Local branches saw the importance of enlisting the
support of workers; when the Bristol Trades Council asked to hear
Marshall on the practical application of the Acts, the Clifton ladies
paid his expenses, and the York LNA branch paid the expenses
involved in founding a WMNL branch.[71] In this respect the LNA
membership fully endorsed Josephine Butler's conviction that
working-class support was crucial; and although references to this
alliance are sometimes embarrassingly naive and reveal an un-
conscious class prejudice − tributes to 'fruitful results' obtained by
'the co-operation of cultivated ladies with working men' or cries of

pleasure at receiving soiled petition sheets from workers[72] —none the less the LNA was genuine in its eagerness to demonstrate the support of the working class, and in return, the significance of female involvement was appreciated by the Trade Union movement. In 1873 the *Bee-Hive* congratulated women who opposed 'unjust and eminently unscientific enactments' adding that 'justice is of more consequence than delicacy' in attacking the Acts.[73]

The connection with the NMA is a much more personal one. Dr Carter, one of its founders was an old friends of the Butlers, and he, Nevins and most other medical repealers practised in Liverpool. In a sense they were protegés of Mrs Butler (indeed she claimed as much) and the LNA helped the NMA with money and Burgess's service in recognition of this. The curious thing is that the two bodies were at opposite poles of the movement: 'we — as a body of women — always preferred to lead in anything on the moral side, and step into a secondary place whenever the medical came in.'[74]

IV

To evaluate the LNA's contribution to the repeal movement, one should first try to capture some sense of the courage required and difficulties to be encountered in setting up an organisation for women alone. Simply judging the LNA as one of a number of repeal bodies is to miss one of its principal achievements. At a time when few women dared to lead independent public lives, to participate in a faintly scandalous agitation was to challenge stereotyped attitudes to women's place in society. In 1870 Josephine Butler faced 'the cold looks of friends, the scorn of persons in office and high life, the silence of some from whom we hoped for encouragement, the calumnies of the press'.[75] But in persisting against these odds, she and her colleagues gradually forced men to respect women's rights to engage in such activities. As early as 1872, an MP defended them thus:

> They [the House of Commons] must remember that they were legislating for women who had no opportunity of making them-selves heard except through the disinterested efforts of those of their own sex who had taken up their cause.[76]

J.W. Henley, otherwise a perfect representative of the old-style Tory from the Shires, never ceased to praise the involvement of 'those high-minded glorious women who have so boldly fought this battle in the cause of morality and religion',[77] while Stansfeld chose to announce his public adhesion to repeal at the LNA's 1874 Annual Meeting.

Recognition of their right to campaign was an achievement, but the women of the LNA went further – they campaigned separately. They showed themselves competent to manage an organisation every bit as elaborate as those of their male counterparts; they employed men, they disagreed with men and on occasions won their disputes. The LNA was no submissive front organisation – it held its own ground and insisted on being consulted on policy; Josephine Butler was offended when Stansfeld forgot this: 'I do not *quite* like their not having expressed formally any desire to confer with *us* as an association of women, before taking a decision.'[78] Male repealers came to respect the specifically female contribution: in the 1880s it is common to find them asking the LNA to organise women's meetings as part of coordinated campaigns in particular areas.[79]

Thus the LNA had by the 1880s become an accepted, normal part of the movement – no longer an aberration to be remarked upon, but a legitimate branch of a broad campaign. It moderated its tactics along with the rest of the movement, even in 1879 welcoming a Commons select committee as a means of throwing light on 'the working of an an evil system'.[80] Mrs Butler became a respected figure around the House and her right to campaign no longer questioned – indeed the old battleground of the Ladies' Gallery was completely conquered – LNA members sat throughout the 1883 debates without difficulty and its steward openly showed his sympathy.[81] Large numbers of women could be mobilised: 1,000 attended a public meeting at Nottingham in January 1879, while Miss Craigen, the LNA's last agent, regularly drew audiences of this size in the early 1880s.[82]

The LNA's contribution to the repeal movement can be summed up in two words: credibility and principle. Credibility because until the intervention of women at the beginning of 1870, male repealers had been unable to defeat the apathy, if not hostility, which greeted them. Daniel Cooper, the secretary to the Rescue Society had said despairingly that 'if no other means are found to avail, the women of England must be roused to protest.'[83] But this 'last resort' achieved what he and his fellow workers had failed to: the Ladies' Protest focused attention on the Acts and alerted likely opponents to their existence. It is still rightly regarded as the first blast in the campaign. Principle underlies everything the LNA did. The Acts embodied a differential standard of morality widely regarded as orthodox. The LNA refused to accept this in any way and thus prevented amendment of the Acts; it forced the repeal movement to tackle the question of equality of the sexes rather than simply that of removal of particular and offensive clauses. Josephine Butler insisted that women had to be to the fore in the agitation to keep it directed towards the ultimate goal — to avenge the wrong done to an entire sex:

> It is womanhood which has been wronged for generations, and even our best and truest friends among men are not to be permitted by God, for He will not permit it, to wipe out the wrong. The avenging angel must be one of the sex which has been outraged.[84]

Notes

1. LNA, *Annual Report for 1870*, pp. 4—5.
2. FLB 3048: Josephine Butler to Mrs Buckton, 5 Oct. 1870; *Shield*, 24 Sept. 1870, p. 232.
3. LNA, *Annual Report for 1870*, p. 3.
4. LNA, *Annual Report for 1871*, p. 5.
5. *Shield*, 4 Nov. 1876, p. 347.
6. *Shield*, 28 Dec. 1878, p. 304; NA EC Minutes, 26 Feb. 1883.
7. FLB 3421: Josephine Butler to Mrs H.J. Wilson, 3 Oct. 1881.
8. Sheffield University Library (Mundella-Leader correspondence), 18 Mar. 1874; (Wilson MSS) Box 6: Mundella to H.J. Wilson, 19 Nov. 1875.
9. Ibid., (Wilson MSS) Box 1: H.J. Wilson to R. Leader, 11 Oct. 1875; Leader to Wilson, 2 Nov. 1875; see also FLB 3742: I. Whitwell Wilson to H.J. Wilson, 31 Aug. 1875.
10. *Shield*, 10 Nov. 1875, pp. 289—91.
11. A point which will be developed further in the conclusion.
12. *Saturday Review*, 8 Jan. 1870, p. 46. See also M.M. Bevington, *The Saturday Review 1855—1868* (New York, 1941) ch. 4, p. 118, for a sympathetic discussion of the *Review*'s anti-feminism, stressing it as 'a salutary check on the effusive sentimentality of the time'.
13. *Hansard*, 3rd series (30 May 1870) 201 Cols. 1647—8 (Crawford); (13 Feb. 1872) 209 Col. 345 (Sir James Elphinstone).
14. Sheffield Central Library (Wilson MSS) MD 2479: Wilson's reminiscences, taken down 9 June 1912.
15. FLB: Josephine Butler to repealers (no date).
16. *Hansard*, 3rd series (23 June 1875) 225 Col.369 (Col. Alexander), Col.382 (Hopwood).
17. *Shield*, 22 July 1882, p. 138; FLW Box 78 letter 612: Josephine Butler to H.J. Wilson, Feb. 1883.
18. Josephine Butler, *Personal Reminiscences of a Great Crusade* (1896), p. 20.
19. *Shield*, 14 Mar. 1870, p. 14.
20. LNA, *Annual Report for 1870*, p. 21.
21. See below, chapter 10, pp. 263—4 for the division between libertarians and repressionists in the social purity campaign after 1886.
22. LNA, *Annual Report for 1876*, p. 21.
23. FLB 3130: Josephine Butler to Mrs H.J. Wilson, *c.* Mar. 1872.
24. LNA, *Annual Report for 1872*, p. 8.
25. FLB 3133: Josephine Butler to H.J. Wilson, *c.* 1 June 1872.

26. LNA, *Annual Report for 1872*, p. 13.

27. LNA EC Minutes, 28 Mar. 1879, 16 Feb. 1882.

28. *Shield*, 9 May 1870, p. 79.

29. See below p. 173 and 180 for LNA distribution of membership and levels of activity. Josephine Butler complained to Mrs Wilson of her followers' reluctance to receive 'these poor girls' into their homes (FLB 3442: Josephine Butler to Mrs H.J. Wilson, June 1875).

30. FLW Box 2, letters 762: Josephine Butler to Joseph Edmondson, 5 Mar. 1877, Josephine Butler to H.J. Wilson, 13 Mar. 1877, discussing arrangements for 'some of our veteran ladies to tour subjected towns'.

31. *Shield*, 21 Sept. 1872, pp. 1086–9; 26 Sept. 1872, pp. 1093–5; 7 Feb. 1880, pp. 15–20.

32. *Shield*, 21 Mar. 1870, p. 19; 30 May 1870, p. 14.

33. LNA, *Annual Report for 1878*, pp. 41–6; NA EC Minutes, 22 Jan. 1872.

34. LNA, *Annual Report for 1872*, p. 12.

35. FLB 3327: Josephine Butler to a friend, 4 May 1874; LNA, *Annual Report for 1874*, p. 13.

36. *Times*, 22 July 1871, p. 9 (leading article).

37. E. Moberly Bell, *Josephine Butler, Flame of Fire* (1962), p. 91, quoting Peter Rylands, MP.

38. FLB 3953: Josephine Butler to a friend, 9 Oct. 1882.

39. See Elizabeth Isichei, *Victorian Quakers* (Oxford, 1970), pp. 252–5.

40. Mrs Lucas was active in many social purity and feminist causes, but temperance was her great interest – see her obituary in LNA, *Annual Report for 1889–90*, pp. 13–15; she was the subject of a vulgar hagiography: H.J.B. Heath, *Margaret Bright Lucas, the Life Story of a 'British Woman'* (1890).

41. LNA, *Annual Report for 1899*, pp. 19–20.

42. Butler, *Personal Reminiscences*, p. 307.

43. R.K. Webb, *Harriet Martineau, a Radical Victorian* (1960), pp. 23–4, 151–3.

44. LNA, *Annual Report for 1902*, pp. 15–16.

45. LNA EC Minutes 1875–83. There were 379 separate attendances at these meetings, 183 were the 'Bristol Four'.

46. FLB 3437: Mrs Tanner to H.J. Wilson, 23 May 1875.

47. The Butler MSS at the Fawcett Library contain many letters illustrating Josephine Butler's vigorous direction of LNA policy, full of shrewd, practical advice, e.g. 3190: Josephine Butler to Miss Priestman, 13 Oct. 1872.

48. E.g. FLB 4026: Josephine Butler to Mrs Tanner, 23 Jan. 1885.

49. LNA EC Minutes, 29 Nov. 1881.

50. FLB 3439: Mrs Tanner to H.J. Wilson, 25 May 1875; *Shield*, 20 Jan. 1877, p. 12; LNA, *Annual Reports 1870–86*.

51. NA EC Minutes, 1 Nov. 1875.

52. LNA, *Annual Report for 1881*, p. 20; *National League Journal*, 1 June 1883, pp. 13–16; FLB 3955: Josephine Butler to Mrs Tanner, 30 Oct. 1872; Sheffield Central Library (Wilson MSS) MD 2548: Josephine Butler to Mrs Hind Smith, 7 May 1883.

53. FLB 3050: Josephine Butler to Miss Priestman, 12 Dec. 1870.

54. The possible discrepancy may be assessed by noting that the LNA claimed between 1,100 and 1,200 members in September 1870 while the first reliable subscription list (1870–1) gives a minimum of 852 subscribers.

55. LNA EC Minutes, 28 Mar. 1879 – the LNA owed Mrs Tanner £273 at this stage.

56. LNA EC Minutes, 20 Apr. 1877.

57. FLW Box 5 letter 431: Josephine Butler to R.F. Martineau, 10 Dec. 1877; LNA EC Minutes, 4 Dec. 1877.

58. LNA, *Annual Report for 1876*, p. 21.

59. *Shield*, 10 July 1880, pp. 105–6; LNA, *Annual Report for 1880*, pp. 9–10; LNA, *Annual Report for 1881*, pp. 14–20.

60. LNA, *Annual Report for 1878*, pp. 41–2.

61. LNA, *Annual Report for 1882*, p. 9.

62. LNA, *Annual Report for 1882*, p. 19.

63. See *National League Journal*, 1 Dec. 1881, pp. 14–16, for an article by Miss M. Priestman on 'Ladies' Branch Associations' describing methods to be adopted.

64. FLB Box 3 B6: Josephine Butler to a friend, undated postcard.

65. LNA EC Minutes, 7 Dec. 1878, 24 Jan. 1879: NA EC Minutes, 10 and 17 Feb. 1879.

66. VA, *Annual Report for 1871*.

67. VA, *Annual Report for 1872*, pp. 6–10.

68. FLB 3883: Josephine Butler to 'dear friend', 12 Mar. (1877?).

69. *Shield*, 11 Oct. 1873, p. 336.

70. LNA EC Minutes, 11 Jan. 1877.

71. NA EC Minutes, 16 Apr. 1877; *Shield*, 24 Mar. 1877, p. 73.

72. LNA, *Annual Report for 1876*, p. 15; LNA, *Annual Report for 1878*, p. 18.

73. *Bee-Hive*, 27 Dec. 1873 – it also suggested that the Acts had done more than anything else to convince women of their need for representation.

74. FLB 4072: Josephine Butler to a friend, 13 Apr. 1886.

75. Butler, *Personal Reminiscences*, pp. 213–14.

76. *Hansard*, 3rd series (13 Feb. 1872) 209 Cols.345–6 (A.J. Otway).

77. FLW Box 82 letter 92: J.W. Henley to H.J. Wilson, 1 Oct. 1874.

78. FLB 3992: Josephine Butler to a friend, *c.* May 1883.

79. E.g. LNA EC Minutes, 22 Sept. 1882, 8 Nov. 1882.

80. LNA, *Annual Report for 1879*, p. 19. See above, chapter 3, for the opposite reaction to the 1870–71 Royal Commission.

81. Butler, *Recollections*, pp. 393–4.

82. *Shield*, 25 Jan. 1879, pp. 11–13; LNA, *Annual Report for 1883*, pp. 27–32.

83. In his 'Annual Report for 1869', quoted Benjamin Scott, *A State Iniquity: its Rise, Extension and Overthrow* (1890), p. 96.

84. FLB 3892: Josephine Butler to members of the LNA, 11 Dec. 1877.

7 RELIGION AND THE REPEAL CAMPAIGN

Religion represented a vital, urgent part of life for most middle-class reformers; their political rhetoric was often couched in devotional terms, and their insistence that 'what is morally wrong can never be politically right' owed everything to religious conviction. The Contagious Diseases Acts campaign was emphatically part of the underpinning of politics with religious zeal in the late nineteenth century; Josephine Butler composed countless exhortatory prayers which were eagerly printed by repeal journals. Since they regarded religion as supremely important, repealers strove to demonstrate the full support of religious feeling — failure to have done so would have undermined the claim that theirs was a moral crusade. Stansfeld's first public action as a repealer was to issue an appeal to clergymen and ministers urging denominational support for repeal, and within a few months he was debating how best to approach bishops and trying to recruit Spurgeon, the greatest nonconformist preacher of the age.[1] Both precedent and comparison encouraged this sort of appeal. Had not the anti-slavery movement relied on the support of the godly? Had not the mighty anti-Corn Law League assembled 700 dissenting ministers to buttress its case? And in the 1870s, the Liberation society, the United Kingdom Alliance and other 'semi-moral, semi-political agitations' could fill their platforms with non-conformist spokesmen; nor was the National Church absent when politico-moral issues were debated — High Churchmen joined dissenters in opposing the Bulgarian Atrocities, Evangelicals were the backbone of many moral reform movements.[2] Like these agitations, the repeal movement was much strengthened by religious support. A declaration from a denominational body that the Acts were 'immoral in their tendency, contrary to the law of God, dangerous to the liberty of the subject and do not secure the sanitary and restraining effect for which they were professedly enacted.'[3] was a signal for members to act — a clear indication that the movement was morally untainted, however suspect its area of concern. The greater the number of denominations recruited, the greater the respectability conferred upon the movement — and the more chapels could be used as bases for repeal activity. The NCL concentrated on the denominations in the wake of Stansfeld's call; chapel after chapel received repeal agents and petitioned parliament for repeal; the LNA turned naturally to the chapels when it wished to organise a women's petition.[4]

If chapels were usually receptive to repeal arguments, churches were markedly less so; the Church of England failed to commit itself to repeal, and even more disappointingly, many churchmen believed that the Acts were morally beneficial. Over a third of the signatories to an extensionist memorial in 1868 were Anglican clergy, including three bishops, the masters of eight Oxbridge colleges, seven headmasters and seven rectors of subjected towns.[5] A greater blow, struck directly at the Butlers, came in 1871. George Butler attempted to read a paper on 'The duty of the Church of England in moral questions' to the Church Congress at Nottingham, but was barracked by part of the audience whenever he touched upon social purity. Eventually the chairman, the Bishop of Lincoln, had to ask him to remove these references from the paper so that order might be restored. Josephine Butler persuaded herself that this hostility came from young aristocratic clergy 'put into the Church from motives not the highest' and influenced by 'evil advisers'; but a meeting called by repealers during the Congress was packed with clergy sympathetic to the Acts who made it clear that they resented her presence — especially when she criticised the Church for delaying over repeal as it had delayed supporting anti-slavery.[6]

This diagnosis was entirely correct; the Church was unwilling to take any collective stand over the Acts and indeed could hardly do so given the level of dissension revealed by the Nottingham fracas. An attempt by the NA to convene a meeting of bishops during a synod in 1878 was a fiasco — none at all turned up to meet repeal leaders (including Stansfeld and Johnstone) who had gathered for the purpose.[7] The Convocation of Canterbury had a special committee on social purity which was greatly influenced by regulationist clergy in the subjected districts; its attitude was equivocal, but its failure to pronounce definitely against the Acts ensured it a condemnation from the *Shield*.[8] There was no repeal equivalent to the Church of England Temperance Society, and the Quakers, shocked at the Church's poor response, unfavourably compared it to Anglican activism over the opium traffic.[9] The division amongst churchmen contrasted painfully with nonconformity's opposition to the Acts.

Naturally repeal did attract some Anglican support — and from all sections of the Church. The Butlers were themselves Broad Church; indeed Josephine Butler was spectacularly indifferent to Anglicanism's divisions and talked about a childhood affected by a variety of religious influences which gave her 'the widest ideas of vital Christianity' — her objection was to the Church's stiffness and formality which seemed to prevent it from taking a denominational stand on what was to her a paramount moral issue.[10] She welcomed support from any quarter, whether Broad-Churchmen like Archdeacon Sandford, the first president of the MCEU, Evangelicals like Francis Close, Dean of Carlisle, or Prebendary Fowle of Salisbury, or High-Churchmen — Pusey condemned the Acts as tyrannical and demoralising in 1879.[11] For the Butlers, doctrinal or sectarian differences paled beside the urgent need to secure repeal; indeed George stressed the potential ecumenical benefits of all churches working together against the Acts.[12]

Believing that the National Church had to be with them so that they might demonstrate the true strength of religious feeling, repealers never gave up their efforts to carry it, as an institution, for repeal. They constantly tried to expand their base of support from that of a few distinguished individuals to the clergy in general. Prebendary Fowle secured 1,500 signatures to a clerical memorial in 1873, and when this appeal was repeated in 1883—4, 4,300 clergy signed (28,000 to 30,000 forms were sent out and the NA believed it could have got the number up to 7,000 given time and funds). By 1884 the NA claimed to find less hostility and a more enquiring attitude among the clergy.[13] F.C. Banks was the keenest advocate of a policy directed towards the Church, constantly nagging his committee and never allowing them to forget their commitment to work the clergy vigorously.[14] This persistent belief in the significance of Anglican support contrasts interestingly with the relative indifference shown towards the rather better prospect of attracting Catholics through Manning, who was quite early into the field. He identified himself with repeal in May 1873 and helped in the search for a repeal leader in July 1874; repeal was in the same area as the other moral and social reforms which he supported, and as with temperance, his involvement preceded that of the Anglican episcopate.[15] But little use was made of him — he never became a vice-president of the NA, nor did he speak from repeal platforms. His flock was, of course, far removed from repeal's usual constituency: upper-class 'old' Catholics and slum-dwelling Irish Catholics surrounded middle-class nonconformists socially and aroused antagonisms in equal measure. The influential Wesleyan, Dr William Arthur, an ardent repealer who *was* a vice-president of the NA (from its inception) was an Orangeman who 'waged a life-long war against Popish superstition';[16] as Stansfeld warned Josephine

Butler: 'I rather fear getting Manning; the Protestant feeling against him must be strong now; had we not better leave him in the dark till we get some hold of the Church of England.'[17] Since the latter object was hardly satisfactorily attained, repealers did not dare to arouse Protestant wrath by appealing for Catholic support until 1886, but were beaten to it by the passage of the repeal act.[18]

Manning's support contrasted painfully with the reluctance of Anglican bishops to come forward. William Thomson, Archbishop of York, twice refused to have anything to do with repeal, returning NCL Annual Reports, claiming that they were obscene, and refusing to receive deputations. Mrs Butler was outraged by his behaviour and told Wilson that the NCL did more for the spiritual welfare of the province of York than the Archbishop ever could.[19] She became quite fearless in tackling the higher clergy; an interview with the Archbishop of Canterbury was simply mentioned in passing, and when Exeter seemed threatened by the Acts in 1878, she decided to write a frank letter to the Bishop, not caring whether or not this angered him.[20]

Perseverance never managed to extract from the Church of England an unqualified condemnation of the Acts, but it did help legitimise repeal work and weakened the opposition. Church congresses were attended to carefully: James Stuart and Josephine Buter stirred up opposition to a regulationist in 1874 (revenge for the staged opposition to George Butler in 1871?), and when in 1876 the congress was held at Plymouth, repealers felt obliged to hold a parallel series of meetings.[21] Clergymen were sometimes pusillanimous in their support: Prebendary Leathes of St Paul's agreed to accept a vice-presidency of the NA on condition that he was not asked to subscribe and that publications were sent in sealed envelopes and not frequently![22] Stuart noted the dread of publicity which Anglican clergy seemed to have; he found the Archbishop of Canterbury affable though unwilling to help.[23] Few bishops were willing to follow Moberly of Salisbury or Fraser of Manchester in outright opposition, and amongst the higher clergy the statement of the Dean of Exeter in 1878, attaching 'a higher importance to religious interests than to sanitary expediency' was quite exceptional in its straightforward advocacy of repeal.[24]

In contrast to the hesitancy of the Church of England, the Society of Friends was committed to repeal from the first. The 1870 Yearly Meeting condemned the Acts and urged subordinate meetings to use all efforts to oppose them. As has already been seen, Quaker women were involved in the LNA from its inception, while two Quakers had

convened the 1869 meeting which led to the foundation of the NA.[25]
No denomination was more united in opposition to the Acts; as James
Stuart put it: 'the Friends have always been ahead in most things,
especially in what concerns women';[26] while Mrs Butler found her
closest collaborators among Quakers, and never failed to praise them
for their generous and distinctive contribution to the movement:

> I feel so at home at the *Friends*. Since 1870 for 15 or 16 years I
> have always been asked to their annual meeting, so kindly
> welcomed for my work's sake, though not a Friend . . . They are
> so pugilistic and so obstinate and so gentle and calm. I learned
> much from them in the early years. I delight in them.[27]

The foundation of the Friends' Association for Repeal (FA) on 10
November 1873 was a landmark for the repeal movement. It was
probably a response to a circular which the NA had sent to all
denominations in July 1873 urging them to collaborate more closely
with the movement; the chronicler of the Quaker repeal effort saw it
as the start of 'the appeal to the religious conscience of the nation'.[28]
Since many Quakers were already working for repeal, the new
Association's purpose was chiefly to attract those Quakers unwilling
to join other repeal bodies (the aim was to enrol every adult Quaker)
and to collect money: the *Shield* said that the FA 'will render all the
aid it can to other organisations, and supplement with grants their
pecuniary resources.' and within three days £5,000 had been collected.[29]
The officers were all experienced repealers, and usually supporters of
other agitations as well. Edward Backhouse of Sunderland chaired the
inaugural meeting, and became president; he was also president of
the NCL, a vice-president of the NA, and the largest subscriber to both.
For many years he gave £1,000 per annum to a rescue society; his
other interests included disestablishment, temperance and anti-
slavery — indeed the *Northern Echo* likened him to Garrison (who
died about the same time) in its obituary.[30] The honorary secretaries
were Joseph Edmondson, treasurer of the NCL, Barton Dell of
Bristol, Frederic Wheeler of Rochester one of the few pillars of
opposition in the subjected districts (who later became chairman of
the Executive Committee), and A.J. Naish of Birmingham who was
also an honorary secretary of the MCEU, a former associate of Sturge
in the Complete Suffrage Union and numbered amongst his 'causes'
helping boy chimney sweeps.[31] Common to all these men, and probably
to most Quaker repealers were the peace movement and anti-slavery.[32]

The FA was the first denominational body (the Wesleyans did not follow until February 1874) — appropriately so, given the prominence of Quaker activists. MPs such as Fowler and Jacob Bright handled parliamentary repeal work, and the provincial associations were full of Quakers; indeed it is noteworthy that they did *not* devote themselves exclusively to the FA — confessional politics was not the Quaker way. The MCEU had Naish and Arthur Albright, both wealthy iron-founders; the NCL had Backhouse, Edmondson, George Tatham of Leeds (a teetotaller also committed to a multitude of causes), Priestmans in Bradford, Rowntrees in York. Quaker women were not admitted to the FA despite their prominence elsewhere in the repeal movement; this reflects their 'separate but equal' status, though this was disappearing from the early 1870s, and at the 1880 annual meeting a Women's Committee was set up as an auxiliary to the FA.[33]

F.C. Banks was under no illusions about the FA's primary role — it was to encourage rich Quakers to give more readily by providing them with their own body: 'Mr. Fry told me personally that the Friends' Association was to be an extra backbone to the National'.[34] He seemed to doubt its effectiveness at this, but the success of the first subscription list tells another story. By enlisting the support of prosperous Quaker businessmen, the repeal movement tapped munificent donors and showed the world that it could win over men of substance. Arthur Albright volunteered to tour banks and offices collecting funds; this was a familiar anti-slavery, anti-Corn Law League tactic which, even when it failed to secure funds, showed that repeal was serious, not 'the fancy of a clique'.[35] In the spring of 1874, Barton Dell and Richard Fry toured northern England collecting subscriptions for the FA. They offered to collect what they could for the NA, and within a month had sent in £1,400; in 1874–5 the FA gave the NA £350 directly, and contributed to various special funds.[36]

The FA's own income was handsome: £808 in 1878, £1,160 in 1884 (the NA income then was £1,973). It never had to worry about money. Rather, its problem was one of how to spend its income.[37] There was no need to devote it to Quakers themselves as they were recognised to be virtually unanimous for repeal — the FA therefore turned to other fields. Its close links with the WMNL have already been discussed; together the two bodies worked London in the late 1870s, the FA financing the WMNL's meetings and supporting Lucraft's candidature at Tower Hamlets (the Quaker banker George Gillett was his treasurer).[38] International work also attracted them. Gillett and the Quaker publisher, A.S. Dyer, were prominent in the

campaign to expose the white slave traffic to Brussels. The FA
supported them financially and paid for their work to be publicised.
Similarly they supported work in the subjected districts generously,
and displayed an unsectarian willingness to employ non-Quakers as
speakers: the Baptist, Henry Varley, and the Wesleyan, Hugh Price
Hughes, were both engaged to hold meetings there in the 1880s.[39]
The FA rivalled the NA in its publishing effort. In effect it controlled
two journals — Dyer's *Sentinel* which preached social purity (an
enduring Quaker concern) and the *National League Journal* — and
published through Dyer's firm a wide range of tracts and pamphlets.
Again, there was no particularly Quaker emphasis; in 1879 they
printed 20,000 copies of a speech by the Wesleyan Rowland Rees
and 3,000 copies of a letter from the head of the Temperance Order
of Good Templars.[40] Other churches seem to have been a target for
the FA; in 1874 it paid the NA to send literature to 20,000 clergy
and ministers, while its annual meetings often contained assessments
of the progress in other denominations — progress often assisted by
FA effort.[41]

The Quaker record is impressive; their association was active even
if it did prefer to operate chiefly by financing the work of others; they
were crucial as substantial donors but giving was in no sense a sop to
troubled consciences; as activists, men like Gillett, Dyer or Edmondson
could scarcely be bettered. While it may be conceded that the peculiar
nature of the Society of Friends encouraged competitive philanthropy,[42]
its members' zeal for social purity and humanitarian instincts nevertheless made them outstanding as repealers.

Although Quakers were associated with political dissent they were
not fully part of it. On the great issue of disestablishment they were
relatively unmoved, and their references to nonconformity suggest
that they placed themselves in a separate category.[43] If we turn to the
great dissenting sects, we find another important source of repeal
strength. The Unitarians provided Stansfeld, Shaen and R.F. Martineau;
Congregationalist leaders included Benjamin Scott, Henry Richard and
C.J. (later Sir Charles) Tarring; amongst new dissenters the Wesleyan
Methodists were by far the most important — Percy Bunting, grandson
of the great Jabez, was an activist, as was his sister, Mrs Sheldon Amos,
and Hugh Price Hughes (later to be the leader of the Wesleyan
'Forward Movement') was recruited by Josephine Butler in 1872
when a young minister.[44]

By the mid-1880s there was not a nonconformist denomination
which had failed to declare its opposition to the Acts. A canvass of

nonconformist ministers (similar to the earlier one of Anglican clergy but more successful — the first 7,000 circulars brought back 4,400 signatures)[45] was a great success with 7,800 ministers expressing their support as shown in Table 7.1.

Table 7.1: Nonconformist Ministers for Repeal[46]

		%
Wesleyan Methodist	1,675	21.47
Congregationalist	1,641	21.04
Baptist	1,314	16.85
Primitive Methodist	789	10.12
Free Church of Scotland	640	8.21
United Presbyterians	278	3.56
United Methodist Free Churches	266	3.41
Welsh Calvinists	266	3.41
Unitarians	195	2.50
Irish Presbyterians	188	2.41
Methodist New Connexion	164	2.10
Moravian, Swedenborgian, etc.	146	1.87
English Presbyterians	132	1.69
Bible Christians	106	1.36
	7,800	100.00

The so-called 'nonconformist conscience' has been defined as the 'insistence upon the authority of moral principle in all matters of public policy',[47] and this perfectly summarises the most widely used argument against the Acts. Nonconformists, with their keen sense of the need to bear witness against evil whatever the cost, were natural repealers; Hugh Price Hughes was so convinced of the rightness of the repeal cause that he privately explained away lack of progress in terms of God delaying final victory until the need for equal moral standards was generally realised.[48] It was with exactly this degree of earnestness that repealers strove to underpin their arguments — 'ultimately, nothing is lost by a strict adherence to a sacred principle'[49] was the conclusion drawn by the NA at the end of the campaign. The support of prominent nonconformist ministers was especially valuable for the example which they gave to their congregations: Spurgeon was secured, as was his rival to the leadership of nonconformity, R.W. Dale — though Dale had at one time been an extensionist and claimed only to have dropped the Acts when he ceased to read repeal literature.[50] Wesleyan divines almost unanimously favoured repeal which, given

the nature of the Acts, was perhaps not surprising; but what was
remarkable was the degree to which their connexion organised
officially to secure repeal.[51] Wesleyans had traditionally been at one
remove from the rest of dissent, regarding themselves as inter-
mediaries between the established church and nonconformity:

> Obsessively middle-class and traditionalist, they were not easily
> roused from a half thinking conservatism . . . Unlike the
> Congregationalists, Baptists or certainly the Unitarians, all of
> whom stood well to the left on both counts, Wesleyans were loath
> to join in direct agitation, which they equated with heterodoxy
> and disruption.[52]

Although they were moving towards Liberalism after 1868, a movement which has been called 'one of the most striking phenomena of
our period',[53] Wesleyans were still distinct enough to support Forster
over the Education Act against the massed forces of political nonconformity.[54] Yet, over the CD Acts they displayed opposition more
determined than any other dissenting church except the Quakers.
Indeed it might be argued that the historian who looks for agitations
which enabled Wesleyans to work with other dissenters — thereby
easing their integration into political nonconformity — will find the
campaign against the CD Acts high in the list.

The Wesleyan Methodist Conference condemned the Acts promptly
in 1870, and thereafter in every year until 1886. In February 1874 the
'Wesleyan Society for abolishing the regulation of vice by the state'
was founded at a meeting presided over by the then president of
conference, Rev. G.T. Perks. This was almost an official connexional
society; the president of conference was the *ex officio* head of its
General Committee, and the conference received its report each
year when renewing its protest against the Acts.[55] Why was this
cautious, respectable connexion drawn to commit itself so emphatically
against the Acts?

The most likely explanation is that, uniquely amongst nonconformists,
Wesleyans provided a significant number of soldiers for the army. In
the 1870s less than 4.0 per cent of soldiers were nonconformists
compared to 22—24 per cent Catholics, but when, after 1882, the
figures are further broken down, the vast majority of nonconformists
(5.0 per cent to 0.7 per cent) turn out to be Wesleyans.[56] More than
any other group of dissenters, Wesleyans knew something of conditions
in military towns from the soldiers' point of view; they provided the

first dissenting military chaplain, Dr W.H. Rule, at Aldershot, and under Rule's assistant, C.H. Kelly (who testified against the Acts before the Royal Commission), opened the first Soldiers' Home in 1861.[57] Wesleyan moral and philanthropic work amongst soldiers grew remarkedly from this beginning, but of course had to compete with the earlier and earthier view of the soldier's needs, epitomised by the Acts. Wesleyan chaplains like Rule and Kelly were trying to detach the soldier from the brothel and beerhouse; understandably they regarded the Acts as obstacles in this drive to raise moral standards in the army.

The Wesleyan Society published the *Methodist Protest*, a journal edited by Hugh Price Hughes, and 6,000 copies were distributed monthly through a network of branch secretaries. It was a lively paper, with its emphasis very much on religious protests, and undoubtedly helped to unite the connexion against the Acts. The Society could also boast an impressive array of prominent Wesleyans: ministers like Dr William Arthur, Dr Rule, Dr George Osborn and Dr Punshon, perhaps Wesleyanism's most distinguished preacher; laymen such as Percy Bunting (one of the honorary secretaries), S.D. Waddy MP, and William Mewburn the treasurer who was a rich Banbury merchant — he also acted as joint treasurer of the 'Extension of Methodism Fund' with another member, Sir Francis Lycett. Alderman Rowland Rees of Dover was the Wesleyan repeal hero for his vigorous opposition to the Acts, using his position on the bench to embarrass the police and taking pleasure in describing the results of these clashes;[58] his son, Rev. Allen Rees, was one of the Society's honorary secretaries from June 1878.

But the Society was more successful in mobilising the manse than the financial support of Wesleyanism: in 1877 it found itself £170 in debt; this was in a year when conference congratulated it on its work, when the CD Acts were the only 'political' subject discussed and when its annual meeting was chaired by the president of conference.[59] It was rescued by the City of London Committee, which enjoyed a modest but entirely satisfactory income — its 50 or so city luminaries raised about £110 each year, Samuel Morley usually giving £25; from January 1878 until December 1881 it subsidised publication of the retitled *Protest*, which in theory became non-denominational; there was, however, little change in the contents, as Wesleyans had always been interested in other churches. The City of London Committee was similarly interested in religious opinion — it petitioned the Archbishop of Canterbury in 1877 to no effect — so the two bodies matched well; in any case the City Committee contained many wealthy Wesleyans, such as G.H. (later Sir George) Chubb and the two McArthurs, wealthy merchant MPs.[60] Despite this assistance, the Wesleyan Society was still £140 in debt in 1878, and its position never really improved; in 1884 Banks told Stansfeld indignantly that 'properly worked', the Wesleyans should have been richer than the NA, but in fact owed £50 and the NA had to do much of their routine work in circularising ministers.[61]

Nevertheless, the Wesleyans did at least organise and bear separate witness. Of the other connexions, the United Free Methodists, whose assembly was more willing to debate political issues than most, condemned the Acts in 1870, 1871, 1873, 1879 and 1884; they also sent a deputation to Bruce in December 1872, and when invited to do so, nominated an influential minister, Rev. Thomas Newton, as their representative on the NA committee.[62] The New Connexion, Primitive Methodists and Bible Christians all made occasional protests without ever really contributing any significant strength to the movement. But Methodism as a whole was clearly hostile to the Acts, and when the first Ecumenical Methodist Conference met in 1881, a resolution condemning state regulation of vice was unanimously carried: 'Methodists of all colours, languages, and races united in protesting against official prostitution in every shape and form.'[63]

The behaviour of the Congregational Union, the representative body of the most influential, and socially most prominent dissenting sect, compares rather poorly. Under its influential secretary, Alexander Hannay, the Union's Reference Committee used its considerable powers to obstruct discussion of the Acts for many years.[64] It was not reluctance to tackle political subjects which caused it to hold back – the Union readily pronounced on issues like temperance, education and disestablishment – rather a belief that the subject was unfit for a religious gathering and coarsely handled by the repeal associations. Congregationalism's leading 'political' minister, J. Guinness Rogers, declared himself opposed to the Acts, but deprecated their discussion by the Union, and advised his listeners never to read repeal literature.[65]

Despite this institutional stumbling block, many Congregationalists did oppose the Acts; indeed, as early as April 1873, 885 ministers petitioned Gladstone, and after the Reference Committee turned down an appeal by the NCL in 1874, other means were found for expressing Congregational repeal sentiment.[66] In May 1875 a meeting chaired by Samuel Morley decided to set up a Congregational Committee for repeal,[67] an inactive body, chiefly intended to prove that Congregationalists were opposed to the Acts, despite their Union's silence. Eventually it enrolled 1,900 ministers as members and persuaded all the large county unions to delcare for repeal.[68]

The anomaly of a sect which provided repeal activists such as Benjamin Scott, J.P. Gledstone and Henry Richard (who was the Congregational Committee's delegate to the 1877 Geneva Congress), yet had not declared against the Acts, was a serious concern; the *Nonconformist* chided Congregationalists for their apparent apathy, while the *Protest* ranted against the machinations of the 'omnipotent Committee' which would not be tolerated in Wesleyanism (a sly dig which would not have been lost on Congregationalist readers).[69] Eventually attempts to defeat the Reference Committee's veto succeeded in 1881, though the debate took place only after ladies had left the hall. The Acts were condemned by a large majority, though against serious opposition from a few sincere supporters of their moral effect.[70]

The Congregational Union was the last dissenting body to pronounce officially against the Acts, and its delay had been an embarrassment given the advantages to be derived from the support of a united nonconformist conscience. The Baptist Union had called for repeal in 1871 and again in 1876, though like the Congregationalists, it was far from unanimous, and preferred to avoid a decision if it could:[71] in 1874 and 1879 its General Committee found ways of keeping the issue away from the Union.[72] Nevertheless the Baptists could plausibly be cited by repealers, and prominent ministers such as C.H. Spurgeon or Charles Birrell (cousin by marriage of Josephine Butler and father of Augustine Birrell) were willing to denounce state regulation of vice trenchantly.[73] The only other church to do more than simply pass annual motions was the Free Church of Scotland; its General Assembly petitioned against the Acts regularly from 1872 on, and in 1874 appointed a committee to organise activity within the church — after suspension of the Acts, this committee's scope was widened to a general defence of social purity.[74]

This change was paralleled by a similar one in the objects of the Wesleyan Society which became an official Social Purity Committee of Conference after 1884; the Friends' Association also shifted its emphasis towards the fostering of higher and equal moral standards as the best antidote to regulation, and therefore remained in existence after most of the repeal societies dissolved in 1866.[75]

In short, the repeal campaign in its final years was being assimilated into the growing general movement towards higher moral standards in public life. In the 1870s repealers had pioneered the attack on aristocratic libertinism; by the 1880s reinforcements had arrived: the Association for the Improvement in Public Morals founded by the maverick Marquess Townshend in 1878, the Moral Reform Union founded in 1881 and the National Vigilance Association founded after the Stead revelations in 1885. Repeal connections with all these bodies were strong and thus the movement acquired added respectability by association. It became difficult to accuse repealers of impropriety when they were in such good company. Similarly, religion drew in the timorous and persuaded them that their activism was acceptable: in 1883 and again in 1885 the Friends' Association organised Conventions of Prayer with a wide range of ministers and prominent repealers leading prayers throughout the day and enormous audiences/congregations manifesting a high degree of moral fervour — the emphasis on prayer was a useful one in binding people to the cause.[76] Not all repealers were happy about the emotionalism of this specifically Christian appeal — Josephine Butler was aware of the reservations of Unitarians such as Shaen or agnostics like Mme. Venturi or Mrs Jacob Bright, and even Stansfeld disliked public prayer as a political weapon.[77] However the demonstration of religious support was another matter entirely; he ensured that the presidents of as many nonconformist conferences as possible testified before the select committee about their churches' opposition to the Acts.[78]

Cultivating the support of nonconformity was by then a shrewd political tactic; in 1868 one-seventh of the parliamentary Liberal party were nonconformists, but by 1880 the proportion had risen to a quarter, and increasingly the typical Radical MP was a dissenter.[79] We must now return to the progress of the campaign to see how this change in the nature of Liberalism was to be mobilised for repeal. Stansfeld was convinced of nonconformity's hold over the Liberal party; in December 1882, speaking on the same platform as Dr John Clifford and Hugh Price Hughes he issued this warning:

> When I first entered upon this cause, I appealed to the ministers of all denominations, and I got responses from them. It remains now as it was then, my conviction that upon them and the religious bodies they represent, it will mainly depend whether we win or lose in our time . . . It is their duty, if they are men as well as Christians, to descend into the political arena and to force their convictions on the polling booth and in the constituencies.[80]

Notes

1. *Shield*, 1 Nov. 1874, pp. 221–2; FLB 3340: J. Stansfeld to Josephine Butler, 21 Oct. 1874.

2. G. Kitson Clark, *The Making of Victorian England* (1962), pp. 198–9; R.T. Shannon, *Gladstone and the Bulgarian Agitation, 1876* (1963), pp. 171–6; Brian Harrison, 'State Intervention and Moral Reform in Nineteenth-century England' in P. Hollis (ed.), *Pressure from Without* (1974), p. 294.

3. Methodist Archives, *United Methodist Free Churches: Annual Assembly Minutes*, 1871, p. 77.

4. *Shield*, 25 Nov. 1874, special issue on NCL Annual Meetings; LNA, *Annual Report for 1878*, pp. 17–23.

5. Association for Promoting the Extension of the Contagious Diseases Act, *Third Report on the operation of the Contagious Diseases Acts* (1870), pp. 78–82.

6. Josephine Butler, *Recollections of George Butler* (Bristol *c.* 1893), pp. 239–47; *Shield*, 21 Oct. 1871, pp. 702–5.

7. NA EC Minutes, 12 Aug. 1878.

8. NA EC Minutes, 2 July 1877; *Shield*, 1 Oct. 1881, p. 168.

9. FA, *Annual Report for 1881*; Shannon, *Gladstone*, p. 82, for the Church's division over the Bulgarian atrocities.

10. FLB 3980: Josephine Butler to Bristol friends, probably Jan. 1883.

11. *Shield*, 5 Apr. 1873, p. 111 (Sandford); 20 Jan. 1883, pp. 14–15 (Close); 12 Aug. 1876, pp. 273–4 (Fowle); 12 July 1879, p. 116 (Pusey).

12. *Shield*, 28 Mar. 1870, pp. 30–1.

13. *Shield*, 24 May 1873, pp. 172–5; NA, *Annual Reports for 1883 and 1884*, pp. 25–6.

14. E.g. NA EC Minutes, 28 Jan. 1878, 12 Apr. 1880, 23 Oct. 1882.

15. B.H. Harrison and A.E. Dingle, 'Cardinal Manning as Temperance Reformer', *Historical Journal* 12 (1969), pp. 485–510, discuss Manning's motives for social involvement.

16. *Methodist Recorder*, 14 Mar. 1901 (obituary).

17. FLB 3340: Stansfeld to Josephine Butler, 21 Oct. 1874.

18. NA, *Annual Report for 1885. and 1886*, p. 16.

19. FLB 3209: Josephine Butler to H.J. Wilson, 23 Dec. 1872; 3007: fragment by Josephine Butler, *c.* 1874.

20. FLB: Josephine Butler to Miss Priestman, 25 Oct. 1878.

21. FLW Box 82 letter 82: Josephine Butler to H.J. Wilson, 31 July 1874; *Shield*, 21 Oct. 1876, pp. 313–16.

22. NA EC Minutes, 17 Dec. 1877.

23. FLW Box 5 letter 444: James Stuart to H.J. Wilson, 2 Apr. 1878.

24. *Shield*, 14 Dec. 1878, p. 290. See also Desmond Bowen, *The Idea of the Victorian Church* (Montreal, 1968) ch. 6, for the episcopacy's generally sluggish attitude to reform; and Edward Bristow, *Vice and Vigilance: Purity Movements in Britain Since 1700* (Dublin, 1978), pp. 76–7, 100–2, for the Church's willingness to listen to the more conventional Ellice Hopkins denouncing male sexual misconduct. Unlike George Butler, she *was* given a hearing.

25. M. Gregory, *The Crowning Crime of Christendom* (1896), pp. 7–8.

26. James Stuart, *Reminiscences* (1911), p. 227.

27. FLB: Josephine Butler to Miss Forsaith, 13 Mar. 1898.

28. NA EC Minutes, 14 and 21 July 1873; Gregory, *The Growing Crime*, p. 8.

29. *Shield*, 29 Nov. 1873, pp. 385–6; Friends' Library, *Minutes of the Friends' Association*, 15 Nov. 1873.

30. *Shield*, 31 May 1879, pp. 89–90; *Northern Echo*, 24 May 1879.

31. *Birmingham Post*, 31 Mar. 1889.

32. See Elizabeth Isichei, *Victorian Quakers* (Oxford, 1970), p. 106.

33. FA, *Annual Report for 1880*; *Shield*, 29 May 1880, p. 84; Isichei, *Victorian Quakers*, pp. 107–9, 253.

34. Fawcett Library, *Letter Book of the N.A. 1883–86*: F.C. Banks to J. Stansfeld, 22 May 1884.

35. FLW Box 82 letter 50: Josephine Butler to H.J. Wilson, 22 Oct. 1873.

36. NA EC Minutes, 9 Mar., 13 Apr. 1874; NA, *Annual Report for 1874–75*, p. 10.

37. *Shield*, 8 Mar. 1879, pp. 39–40; 7 June 1884, pp. 100–2.

38. *Shield*, 9 June 1877, pp. 155–6; FA, *Annual Report for 1879*.

39. FA, *Annual Report for 1884*.

40. FA, *Annual Report for 1879*.

41. Ibid.; NA, *Annual Report for 1874–75*, p. 16.

42. Isichei, *Victorian Quakers*, pp. 215–19, 238.

43. Ibid., p. 200.

44. John Kent, 'Hugh Price Hughes and the Nonconformist Conscience' in G.V. Bennett and J.D. Walsh (eds.), *Essays in Modern English Church History* (1966), p. 181.

45. NA, *Annual Reports for 1883 and 1884*, pp. 26–7.

46. NA, *Annual Reports for 1885 and 1886*, p. 16.

47. H. Lovell Cocks, *The Nonconformist Conscience* (1943), p. 35.

48. Methodist Archive, Hugh Price Hughes to Dr G. Osborn, 1 Mar. 1881.

49. NA, *Annual Reports for 1885 and 1886*, p. 19.

50. Benjamin Scott, *A State Iniquity: Its Rise, Extension and Overthrow* (1890), p. 193 (Dale committed himself to repeal at an MCEU conference, 8 Dec. 1874); FLW Box 78 letter 659: J.E. Ellis to H.J. Wilson, 6 Apr. 1883.

51. If the NA figures are to be believed, virtually every Wesleyan minister must have signed the nonconformist petition; 1,675 were claimed, while the number of active ministers (excluding probationers and supernumaries) was 1,510 in 1881 and still only 1,588 in 1891 – C. Cook and B. Keith (eds.), *British Historical Facts 1830–1900* (1975), p. 227.

52. Stephen Koss, *Nonconformity in Modern British Politics* (1975), p. 19.

53. John F. Glaser, 'Nonconformity and Liberalism, 1868–1885. A Study in English Party History' (unpublished PhD thesis, Harvard University, 1948), p. 276; see also pp. 102–3, 115–17.

54. Koss, *Nonconformity*, pp. 25–6.

55. Methodist Archive, *Minutes of the Wesleyan Methodist Conference* (1870), XVIII, p. 154; (1874), XIX, p. 199; *Shield*, 14 Feb. 1874, pp. 50–1.

56. H.J. Hanham, 'Religion and Nationality in the Mid-Victorian Army', in M.R.D. Foot (ed.), *War and Society* (1973), pp. 163–4.

57. O.S. Watkins, *Soldiers and Preachers Too* (1906); C.H. Kelly, *Memories* (1910).

58. *Protest*, 16 Oct. 1878, p. 95.

59. *Methodist Protest*, 16 Oct. 1877, pp. 87–9; *Shield*, 26 July 1877, pp. 213–14, 25 Aug. 1877, p. 228.

60. *Methodist Protest*, 16 Nov. 1877, pp. 100–2; *Protest*, 15 Jan. 1878, p. 3, 'it will still be our *raison d'etre* to represent distinctively – although not exclusively – the religious and Christian aspects of the great movement'.

61. *Protest*, 16 Oct. 1878, p. 90; *Letter Book of the N.A. 1883–86*, F.C. Banks to J. Stansfeld, 22 May 1884.

62. Methodist Archive, *U.M.F.C. Annual Assembly Minutes, 1870–1886*; *Shield*, 7 Dec. 1872, pp. 1175–6; NA EC Minutes, 9 Nov. 1874, 12 Jan. 1885.

63. *Protest*, 28 Oct. 1881, p. 86.

64. Glaser, 'Nonconformity and Liberalism', pp. 101, 228, 243–4; NA EC Minutes, 27 Oct. 1873: the Congregational Reference Committee refused to put an NA memorial before the Union. At the same meeting a very favourable response from the Primitive Methodist General Committee was reported!

65. *National League Journal*, 1 Dec. 1881, p. 9.

66. *Shield*, 12 Apr. 1873, p. 120, 15 Nov. 1874, p. 203; Glaser, 'Nonconformity and Liberalism', p. 243.

67. *Shield*, 1 June 1875, pp. 149–50.

68. Scott, *A State Iniquity*, pp. 200–1; *Shield*, 20 Jan. 1877, pp. 14–15, 30 Nov. 1878, p. 287.

69. *Nonconformist*, 23 Jan. 1878; *Protest*, 20 Nov. 1879, p. 99.

70. *Nonconformist and Independent*, 19 May 1881; *Protest*, 20 June 1881, pp. 65–9.

71. *Shield*, 7 Oct. 1871, p. 681; 28 Oct. 1876, pp. 339–40; *Methodist Protest*, 16 Oct. 1876, p. 82.

72. *Shield*, 16 Nov. 1874, pp. 234–45; 17 May 1879, p. 79.

73. For Birrell (1811–1880) see Butler, *Recollections*, pp. 222–3 and her obituary of him in the *Protest*, 20 Jan. 1881, p. 5.

74. *Shield*, 1 July 1874, p. 152; 19 July 1884, p. 125.

75. Methodist Archive, *Minutes of the Wesleyan Methodist Conference*, 1884, p. 276, 1885, p. 263; Friends' Association *Annual Report for 1885*.

76. *Shield*, 17 Feb. 1883, pp. 33–8, 21 Feb. 1885, pp. 22–5; Butler, *Recollections*, pp. 394–5.

77. FLB 3980: Josephine Butler to Bristol friends, *c.* Jan. 1885.

78. NA EC Minutes, 21 Nov. 1881; *Shield*, 8 July 1882, special issue on religious evidence before the select committee.

79. Glaser, 'Nonconformity and Liberalism', pp. 423–6; T.W. Heyck, 'British Radicals and Radicalism, 1874–1895: A Social Analysis', in R.J. Bezucha (ed.), *Modern European Social History* (1972), p. 34.

80. *Shield*, 23 Dec. 1882, p. 223.

8 THE LIBERAL STRATEGY

I

By 1879 the repeal movement was stagnating: its parliamentary
strategy was no more than the annual repetition of forlorn repeal bills,
and in the country Josephine Butler pessimistically noted a falling off
in activity — though with the excuse that 'bad times like the present,
are always unfavourable to social movements for reform, and our cuase
is no exception to this rule'.[1] Paradoxically it was the government
which came to the rescue. When C.H. Hopwood got up to move the
first attack of the session (against the army estimates on 17 March)
the government replied by promising a select committee to look
into the Acts' operation. When the committee was appointed on 11
June 1879 both Stansfeld and Johnstone were members, and so felt
debarred from going on with the annual repeal bill which was withdrawn at the end of July.[2]

Repeal organisations were not dismayed; the NCL conceded that
the committee was weighted in favour of the Acts, yet because it
would publicise the campaign, it must be 'heartily accepted with all
the responsibilities it involved in regard to the production of evidence
against the Acts'. The LNA, which had been the body most hostile
to the Royal Commission in 1870, welcomed the committee, while
the *Protest* talked about 'one of the most important and significant
signs of progress' and called the appointment of the committee
'another fatal blow to the fabric of iniquity'.[3] One can easily understand the welcome, for the select committee was a godsend to the
movement: its MPs were spared the embarrassment of another futile
defeat, and could instead begin to attack the Acts in a fashion they
found congenial; repealers in the country could focus their activities
on the committee as an alternative to the annual bill, and it had the
advantage of not being an inevitable anti-climax and disappointment.

Stansfeld and Johnstone insisted upon having skilled assistance for
their work on the select committee, and after an unsuccessful approach
to Joseph Edmondson, it was agreed that the NA would allow Banks
to undertake the administrative work. To supervise the evidence they
wanted someone legally qualified, and as their 1870—1 choice, Douglas
Kingsford, was not available, they retained another barrister, S.W.
Casserley, for his work.[4] He proved to be an excellent chief of staff:

organising the evidence of repeal witnesses, ensuring that they worked
from prepared briefs on which they were rehearsed before testifying, and
conferring regularly with Stansfeld and Banks to plan the repeal case.[5]
Careful preparation meant that the officials could occasionally be
tripped up, despite all the facilities at their disposal – certainly the
Army Medical Department suffered at Stansfeld's hands.[6] Yet repeal
successes were achieved with trivial resources: a three guinea subscription to a medical library which enabled the NA to borrow seven books
at a time; J.H. Lynn poring over statistics, and laboriously indexing
evidence as it was given to the committee; Nevins supplying hygienic
refutations of official arguments.[7] The NA devoted itself to this work,
raised a special fund of £2,000 to defray the additional expenses, and
put its entire staff behind Stansfeld and Johnstone; it delighted in
quoting its enemies' angry references to its strength, while privately
aware of how much it was stretched to keep up with the mountain of
evidence amassed by the committee.[8] It was all the more galling that
this 'laborious and tedious work' was little appreciated by some
provincial repealers who wearied of the committee's seemingly interminable deliberations and included the NA in their condemnation
of the whole thing. Banks knew better – the NA exhausted itself to
work the select committee effectively.[7]

The repeal press was convinced of the committee's importance.
All the journals reported and commented upon its progress, and the
Shield in particular serialised every scrap of evidence – including that
of regulationists (it defended this practice, saying that it believed in
fair play, and that this testimony condemned itself).[10] Week after
week whole issues were devoted to transcripts of evidence, as if there
was little else to report – which, on the domestic front, was indeed
the case. Furthermore, this obsessive attention demonstrated to
repealers the ability of their advocates on the committee – something
more effective than an annual test of strength was proceeding, as
Stansfeld (and after January 1881 Hopwood) interrogated official
witnesses using their forensic skills to emphasise favourable evidence
and denigrate unfavourable. The publicity afforded was so valuable
that Stansfeld walked out in protest when the committee went into
camera to discuss an individual case affecting the police – his
object was to expose precisely those facts which other members
found delicate.[11]

The committee was weighted against repeal: when first appointed
only five out of the fifteen members were repealers, and this proportion
was approximately maintained throughout its existence. However, the

Protest made the point that this was the first parliamentary enquiry *per se* to include repealers; and the difference was noted from the first, as Stansfeld extracted from the Director-General of the Army Medical Department the admission that he did not know the provisions of the Acts.[12] Besides Stansfeld and Johnstone, the most prominent repeal members were Hopwood (from January 1881), William Fowler (from July 1880), and Thomas Burt, the miners' MP. All these MPs disqualified themselves from speaking in public on the subject while the committee was sitting – this created organisational difficulties, though in a way the enforced separation emphasised their indispensability and raised their stock in the movement.[13]

Against Stansfeld and his small group there stood an equally determined group of regulationists led by George Cavendish-Bentinck, Judge Advocate General in Disraeli's government; from July 1880 he was joined by his Liberal successor, George Osborne Morgan. Both men supported the Acts enthusiastically and defended them with vigour, yet – this apart – they had nothing in common: Cavendish-Bentinck was an aristocratic fool whose appointment to office by Disraeli was treated as a perverse joke. He was a silly late-night obstructionist who liked to tilt at Gladstone, though he was usually mauled for his pains. Repealers regarded him as a rake, and his behaviour seems to support this – he lost his balance when discussing the Acts, and his defence of them coarsened into brutal sarcasms which horrified many.[14] Mundella's observation gets his measure: 'a little, mean drunken aristocrat, without the slightest capacity for business. He is notorious in the House of Commons for his muddled speeches, and unsteady gait after dinner'.[15]

Osborne Morgan was a striking contrast – an able lawyer, and a radical with a record of support for nonconformist causes – his own speciality was the Burials Bill which he carried in 1880; but on the CD Acts he was implacable and in the 1870s had recorded five votes in their favour. This clear commitment discredits Gladstone's assertion of Morgan's impartiality, and still more so Morgan's grotesque claim that he had joined the committee with an open mind.[16] Repealers assailed him for his partisanship, and surmised that he had misled the government into believing he was impartial.[17] Once on the committee (and he replaced a repealer, Shaw Lefevre) he was assiduous in attendance (58 out of a possible 61 sittings). Cavendish-Bentinck was equally meticulous (66 out of 70). As Judge-Advocates, the two men represented the official military interest and could rely on those MPs with service connections – as repealers never failed to point out in their analyses of the background and connections of members of the select committee — all designed to prove self-interest as motivation.[18] The only representative of a subjected district, Sir Henry Drummond Wolff, MP for Portsmouth, supported the Acts.

The select committee made agonisingly slow progress: it sat nine times in 1879 to hear the official medical evidence supporting the Acts — a fairly weak case was put up, and the *Shield* felt confident that repealers could do better when their turn came.[19] But although Nevins testified for three days in March 1880, the general election put an end to the committee, and delays in reappointing it meant that it met formally only to recommend its continuance in the next session (it was later put about that the delay was deliberate — the military departments needing time to respond to Nevins's attack).[20] Twenty-five sittings were held in 1881 to hear more evidence on the medical aspects, and a further 31 in 1882 to take evidence on the moral and social efforts of the Acts. In both these years the committee was working as effectively as it could, but the great lapse of time inevitably caused some exasperation and by 1881 had revived demands for a repeal motion in parliament.

The 1880 general election was an important step forward for the repeal movement, even if it did disrupt the select committee's work. Repealers had been preparing unobtrusively for some years, and by 1879 had a fairly extensive constituency organisation throughout the north and midlands; by-elections had been watched carefully and on occasions the repeal movement had intervened (as at Oldham in 1877) but the ruthlessness of the earlier campaign was absent.[21] The LNA, which had harried MPs at the end of the Gladstone parliament, decided not to bother petitioning members of the expiring parliament, and remarked mildly:

> much pains have been taken, however, by the Electoral Repeal Associations to ensure in every locality where we have fellow workers that the questions shall be brought before the individual candidates for parliament.[22]

When a branch of the NA was founded at Kings Lynn in October 1879 (the Wesleyan superintendant in the chair) its objects typified the moderate approach to electoral work which had become the rule:

> to secure good deputations to wait upon members of Parliament and candidates for Parliamentary election . . . also to present well

signed memorials to them, and to request gentlemen from time to time to write to them personal letters.[23]

In November 1879 the NA published a manifesto, 'The Coming Struggle' in anticipation of the expected election — it enjoined repealers to approach MPs and candidates individually, and it specifically acknowledged the existence of more powerful claims to attention, 'questions of foreign policy, agricultural and commercial distress etc.'.[24] The NA spread the word effectively — even before parliament was dissolved on 24 March 1880 it had sent out 12,800 communications, and had 200,000 leaflets waiting for distribution; ten female clerks had been hired, and Banks had prepared marked-up lists of candidates. The whole operation was elaborate and thorough.[25]

Another contrast with the 1874 election was the attitude displayed to party politics. Repealers had only to look at parliamentary votes to see that their hope lay with the Liberals, and they had long been working within the Liberal party, nudging it towards acceptance of repeal.[26] Naturally they liked to continue the fiction that theirs was not a party question — indeed Wilson observed that Conservatives could find no better way of splitting the Liberal party (which had brought in the Acts) than to undertake their repeal;[27] but this was not to be taken seriously. On 20 March the *Shield* told its readers: 'on this particular occasion, not to let the cause of repeal affect their conduct at the poll'; on 3 April it went further:

> having regard to the tremendous importance of the moral and political questions involved in the actual contest between Liberal and Conservative rule, it would be unwise to insist upon making our subject a test question during the elections.[28]

This was effectively a call to vote against 'Beaconsfieldism', and apart from the WMNL, repeal organisations identified loyally with this policy: the NA sent out masses of literature and its agents toured the southern counties; the NCL circularised 5,000 selected voters, and its two agents toured the north; the LNA recommended memorials to candidates so that none could claim ignorance after the election.[29] No threats were issued.

This approach avoided any danger of 'spoiling' the Liberal vote — the lessons of 1874 had been well learnt, and the new political realism extended to eschewing inflated claims of electoral influence. It was enough that the Liberal victory added greatly to repeal strength in parliament.[30] William Shaen estimated that it now contained 179 repealers, 232 supporters of the Acts and 241 MPs whose views were unknown.[31] 153 known regulationists had gone, but only 41 repealers had retired or been defeated, and new MPs not committed to the Acts by earlier votes given in haste were regarded hopefully.[32] The NCL boasted of returning 57 repealers from the north, while only 20 regulationists were elected (a reduction of 21),[33] and parliamentary leadership was strengthened by the return of William Fowler and the election of two committed repealers, Charles McLaren and J.P. Thomasson. All five repealers on the select committee were re-elected, but five of their Tory opponents were defeated.

Repeal strategy in the election had been strikingly vindicated; instead of trying to coerce the Liberal party, repealers had supported it loyally and modestly. They had reason to believe that they had acquired political credit upon which they might eventually hope to draw. Other groups were of course in the same queue for reward, so repeal success would, to some extent, depend on its ability to push itself forward, and on the ability of regulationists to continue to hold their position. In this sense, though it probably did not realise it, the LNA was correct to argue that 'whatever our gains in the House, public opinion will ultimately decide the question'.[34]

The Liberal party was now an important target — and a practicable one given Liberalism's growing identification with moral reform since Gladstone's return to active and popular politics in 1876. Though the NA still insisted that it was not a partisan body, it agreed to advertise in a Liberal Directory in 1881,[35] while provincial repealers positively gloried in their Liberalism. They recognised that their brand of provincial, dissenting radicalism was increasingly important within the party, and wished to use their advantage to press repeal's claims. R.F. Martineau and the MCEU successfully championed the policy of appealing to provincial Liberalism, and persuading local associations to include repeal in their programmes.[36] If this emphasis conflicted with London's nervousness of partisanship, then as good Birmingham NLF men they were perfectly willing to take on the capital. They had always disliked the NA's pretensions within the movement — indeed the MCEU tried to evade payment for the *Shield* because the NA insisted on its right to collect funds in the midlands[37] — and Martineau was eager to capture central direction of the campaign from feeble metropolitan hands.

H.J. Wilson heartily agreed with this aim; ever the man of business he regularly found fault with the NA: 'It is a very unhappy thing

that the movement is so weak in having no well-administered headquarters', he moaned to Stansfeld in 1875.[38] In the 1880s he led the
provincial attack on London's alleged sluggishness, criticising its
bureaucratisation and timid methods, and finding the *Shield* boring —
full of foreign news which did not interest him. The disloyalty
towards the NA was often remarkable — perhaps the provincial defeat
over petitions still rankled; the NCL had to spend £127 to collect
2,000 petitions in 1882 (excluding salaries and Mrs Wilson's free help),
and the MCEU flatly refused to collect petitions in the midlands, and
made the NA do it.[39] Provincial repealers had scant regard for the NA:
they had advanced in the provinces, whereas it remained static in the
capital, supported by a diminishing group of activists with no
specifically Liberal credentials.

Table 8.1: Most Active Members of the NA Executive Committee,
1883[40] (those who attended more than 16 meetings — maximum 38)

J.H. Levy	36	arch-individualist and bulwark of the VA; Professor at Birkbeck College
Miss L. Wilson	32	edited the VA's *Journal* from 1880; disliked by Mrs Butler
W. Shaen	31	chairman of NA
R. Hampson	25	
Mrs R.R. Glover	22	
G. Gillett	22	Quaker banker and secretary of FA
Mme. E. Venturi	20	editor of *Shield*; Stansfeld's sister-in-law; ally of Miss L. Wilson
M.E. Marsden	17	

The average attendance at an NA committee meeting in 1883 was 10·78,
in 1872 it had been 14·54; fewer meetings were held (38 against 48)
and fewer people attended regularly. The impression is of an organisation
active enough but beginning to turn in on itself.

The provincials, in contrast, were recruiting effectively in the early
1880s; one such example is J.E. Ellis the Nottinghamshire colliery
owner, a Quaker radical who became active in 1882, and thereafter was
among the most energetic of northern repealers. Religious, family and
friendship influences all conspired to draw him in: also a repealer was
his brother-in-law, Joshua Rowntree of Scarborough, with whom he
shared many other interests; Edmondson knew him and suggested
giving him office in the repeal movement to attach him more closely;
James Stuart was a great friend and Henry Wilson became one during

their political work together in the 1880s.[41] All these men had their
special interests: Ellis, the new man, acted as an unofficial whip,
chasing up MPs; Stuart was the diplomat amongst them, a good
political 'fixer', always inclined to seek compromises, but with
excellent connexions in the government; Edmondson was the
ideologist; Martineau the anti-NA conspirator; Wilson the coordinator
of the radical campaign.

Their aim was to capture the Liberal party. Immediately after the
1880 election Wilson suggested a memorial to prominent Liberals —
but so arranged as to disguise its repeal origins.[42] However this posed
problems for the regular leadership: a generation gap separated
Stansfeld from the radicals, and in any case, his strength was his
prominence in Westminster politics; while Josephine Butler's style
of inspirational leadership was worlds removed from their tactics.
In practice these leaders were respected for their contributions, and
went unchallenged (though sometimes resented); but there was a real
desire to circumvent, if not replace, the NA, for it utterly failed to
recognise the difference between the obsolete militancy of a 'hard'
electoral policy (which it revived in June 1880)[43] and the provincials'
faith in the Liberal party. When Johnstone made way for Dodson (a
defeated minister) and received his coveted peerage, the NA sent
agents to Scarborough to challenge the candidates. This provoked the
wrath of Johnstone and the Rowntrees, who were recommending
Dodson in the name of Liberal unity, and outrage from Henry Wilson
at his territory being invaded by the unsubtle Londoners: 'All this is to
be taken in connection with the frequent, if not continual cause of
complaint we have had of the over-bearing and unconciliatory attitude
of the National Association.'[44]

R.F. Martineau's first assault on the NA came in July 1880 at a
conference called to determine the repeal movement's post-election
policy. Warmly supported by Wilson, he proposed that uniformity of
action should be secured by means of sovereign delegate conferences —
the problem which provincial repealers encountered was the ability
of NA branches in the London area to outvote the larger provincial
bodies at the existing informal conferences. However, this proposal
was killed by Stansfeld, who wanted to avoid any restrictions on the
leadership's powers, and a milder resolution was substituted.[45]

By this time, Stansfeld was the parliamentary leader in all but name;
it was to him that the repeal organisations turned for instructions,
and he mapped out the parliamentary campaign subject to Johnstone's
approval.[46] When the latter went to the Lords in July 1880 (as Lord

Derwent) Stansfeld assumed the full leadership, though he was careful to require complete freedom of action; this was agreed to at another conference in August.[47]

Stansfeld was available as leader because of his exclusion from Gladstone's recently formed Cabinet. This was not particularly surprising; for six years he had neglected the front bench for repeal work — a luxury which only an indispensable ex-minister could afford — and Stansfeld was not that. He had been an efficient head at the Local Government Board from 1871 to 1874, but one who had favoured the Poor Law interest at the expense of Simon's medical side; Kimberley, a shrewd observer, thought him a limited politician.[48] Other than his administrative ability, his chief claim to inclusion had been his position as a leading provincial radical; but this claim was weakened during the Disraeli years by the emergence of a new generation of men whose claims on the Liberal party were far stronger by 1880. To put it bluntly, Gladstone accommodated Chamberlain by dropping Stansfeld.[49] This was a serious blow to an ambitious leading politician. He still had hopes of office and Edward Hamilton had expected him to receive a Cabinet post;[50] but all Gladstone offered was the chairmanship of Ways and Means, and this invitation to political oblivion was courteously declined.[51] In private, Stansfeld expressed his indignation: 'I don't intend to let W.E.G. [sic] snuff me out, but I shall be heard of again bye and bye I hope.'[52]

This exclusion is of course the basis of Stansfeld's reputation today; the required sacrifice which makes him a tragic historical figure, who preferred principle to career; but at the time it hit him hard, and his parliamentary performance noticeably deteriorated.[53] As far as repeal was concerned, a brave face was shown, but like Johnstone, Stansfeld used his new position as parliamentary leader to excuse himself from 'outside' work.[54]

Even while nominally under Johnstone, Stansfeld had proved himself an excellent leader. As a leading House of Commons man he commanded attention and dispelled the belief that repeal could not attract serious non-crank politicians. Mrs Butler recognised the value of this contribution: 'I am glad he is able to give the impression that he is not a weak monomaniac! for he will be all the stronger as a champion of our cause',[55] and for F.C. Banks, Stansfeld's public support in the autumn of 1874 was the most cheering event of that otherwise dispiriting year.[56] His status gave him the added advantage of being able to settle quarrels within the movement from 'on high': in the month of this first public speech against the Acts, he is to be found gently pressing Mrs Butler (addressed in letters as 'Josephine') into sinking her differences with Mundella and welcoming the former Royal Commissioner into the movement.[57] His political grasp was most important; before 1874 repealers had certainly lacked this flair for uniting different styles of activist.

But as soon as Stansfeld became involved, a new sense of purpose appeared – he immediately suggested a conference of repeal associations to thrash out the question of petitions against memorials.[58] Indeed, conferences were his preferred method of disciplining his followers. They enabled him to explain his intentions and rally support with comprehensive speeches from the platform. Even the most fractious repealer could hardly fault Stansfeld's willingness to consult the movement; he was positively keen to do so – thus a conference of repeal associations in 1881 was called 'by Mr. Stansfeld's express desire' to discuss tactics,[59] and he was willing to bend before a weighty demand, in this case for a repeal bill. But in general, freely conceded conferences were a superb means of controlling the movement's impulsive tendencies. On one subject alone did Stansfeld insist on differing from the bulk of repealers: he believed in elaborating a coherent socio-medical policy and in fully discussing the question of treatment for venereal disease. The usual repeal view was that no palliatives could be considered before repeal was carried, and that separate facilities were wholly to be condemned; Stansfeld argued that thus to bury one's head in the sand was to offer regulationists a splendid opportunity to brand repealers as anti-medical purists. He was not this (though many repealers were) and always refused to adopt an extremist position on the provision of separate facilities; repeal MPs were always powerfully induced towards moderate positions on medical issues, by their over-riding need to persuade the House of Commons.[60]

However, he fully agreed with provincial radicals on the need to woo the Liberal party; indeed, among his achievements, directing his movement towards cooperation with his party stands high. As early as January 1876 he advised repealers against trying to cover the whole country with an electoral organisation; the constituencies disliked outside pressure (he could have added that when applied it had not worked) so it was better to ensure that all urban seats had committees of electors ready to raise the question, as they saw fit, at the next election.[61] Not only was this a repudiation of the pre-1874 strategy, it was also an invitation to repealers to form committees in precisely those urban seats which the Liberals needed to win back in order to regain a majority. In the years of Tory rule, no one worked harder than Stansfeld to make repeal acceptable to the Liberal party and provide it with claims for recompense whenever the Liberals should return.

After 1880, though still vital in both the Commons and the select committee, Stansfeld's position in the movement came to be questioned, though never challenged. He was still the only 'great name' but no longer the repository of political awareness — H.J. Wilson and his colleagues were now more representative of provincial Liberalism than he. In a sense he was being left behind in the early 1880s and probably knew it — Stuart said that Stansfeld was obsessed with Gladstone's perfidy in dropping him: 'that is Stansfeld's mania . . . it is a full delusion, he did not work for the party from 1874 to 1880 and could not expect Gladstone to do anything else for him'.[62] Stansfeld's 'growing feeling of resentment and distaste' towards Gladstone was suggestive of his unhappiness in the 1880 parliament — passed over, neglected and committed to a cause which alienated him from the front bench to which he aspired, his position was unenviable.[63] Personal grief played its part. His wife was dying and the necessity of attending to her distracted him; W.S. Caine suggested that he let the 1882 repeal bill debate fizzle out so that he might get away to her, and Josephine Butler found him in 1882 too often paralysed by worry and ill health, readier to declare his intentions than to act on them.[64] All these considerations meant that by the end of 1882 he was unwilling to do anything for repeal outside the House of Commons and told a repeal audience that they had no option but to rely on his judgement.[65]

II

By comparison, H.J. Wilson and his colleagues were positively full of bounce, and as the select committee dragged on, increasingly impatient. Martineau continued to try to get around London's dominance (no sooner was Stansfeld confirmed in the leadership than Martineau was calling a conference of officers together — in Birmingham, not London)[66] but the problem remained of what to do while waiting for the committee to report.

1881 was a depressing year. The *Shield*'s pages were enlivened only by foreign news — and there were spectacular successes to be reported in Brussels and in Paris, where the municipality impotently tried to abolish the *Police des Moeurs* (hailed as a great victory by Hugh Price Hughes).[67] The domestic scene was dreary — further serialisation of evidence before the select committee, and a return to the discontinued practice of printing reports of all meetings; the *Shield* was desperately short of interesting material with which to fill its pages. Morale declined to such an extent that Banks was told to stop a revision of the list of NA General Committee members; though intended as a tidying-up to exclude the dead and infirm, the process was giving an alarmingly large number of people an excuse to withdraw from the committee.[68] Similarly, large numbers of likely MPs were declining the honour of vice-presidency.[69] Parliamentary activity was limited to Hopwood asking a series of questions on the operation of the Acts — the propriety of doctors serving as magistrates and so forth. Disastrous attacks were also made on the military estimates — the *Shield* disingenuously explained them away by suggesting that MPs did not understand the nature of the motions.[70]

When Stansfeld called a repeal conference at the end of October, he was just in time to forestall another attempt by Martineau to impose provincial-led unity. He had issued two circulars; one pessimistically analysed the state of the movement, and urged it to 'become a Party' in order to get out of its trough; the other proposed an elaborate federal structure, the main object of which would be the removal of the NA from the centre of the movement.[71] This scheme was not proceeded with: Stansfeld's conference was too open to be a suitable forum for constitutional discussion — as the NA committee realised with relief.[72] By way of compensation, he made a notably pugnacious speech, admitting that the select committee was making slow progress and criticising the government for putting Osborne Morgan on it. Best of all, he promised to introduce a repeal bill in the next session.[73]

When the Bill came on late in July 1882 it made no impact.[74] There was little time available, especially after an unsuccessful piece of Irish obstructionism aimed at clearing the galleries, and Stansfeld could not make a full speech. Instead he more or less apologised for bringing the Bill in given the government's difficulties (with the Arrears Bill?) and concentrated on attacking one or two fallacies; for instance that all repealers were opposed to treatment for VD. Childers replied for the government in a conciliatory vein, promising to consider both the committee's report and the evidence on which it was based. The Bill was defeated without a division. Under the circumstances the *Shield*'s comments were moderate: Stansfeld had obliged the government to acknowledge its responsibility to act on the committee's report, and for the moment nothing more could be done.[75] Not everyone took it so calmly. H.J. Wilson thought repeal was so far away that the NCL should employ agents again, and he asked leading radicals how the campaign might be revived. Carvell Williams replied that Stansfeld had been inadequately supported, but that the House simply had not been interested; repealers would have to make theirs a party question and force it on MPs.[76]

This was not the whole story. He shrewdly added that private measures tended to go to the wall in the face of government business. Indeed the erosion of the private member's rights *vis-a-vis* government demands for parliamentary time was a feature of the period, and necessitated a change in tactics.[77] Just as the UKA switched from the Permissive Bill to the Local Option resolution, so too did the repeal movement alter the thrust of its attack. A resolution was not a new idea: Whitbread had suggested using it in 1874, but the NA had rejected the idea; Stansfeld had considered it in 1876 — but more to inform public opinion than to circumvent obstruction.[78] By 1878 the press of government business crowding repeal out was obvious (and deliberate, thought the *Shield*),[79] and the attractions of a resolution — easier to introduce and harder to talk out — were making it desirable simply on procedural grounds.[80] For this reason, Stansfeld decided that the next repeal debate would be centred on a resolution — though later he chose to argue that as a wider, more 'principled' measure it was in itself preferable to a straight repeal Bill.[81] In a political sense too, a resolution had a possible advantage — it might attract the votes of MPs like Childers who disliked regulation but would defend existing legislation; and, judging by later remarks, many supporters of the Acts did not believe the government would act on a mere resolution. The *Shield* thought otherwise: 'The carrying of the resolution would take the life out of the Acts, and leave it to the Government to see that they were decently interred.'[82]

The issue was now to hand, for the select committee finally reported at the beginning of August 1882. It had dragged on for too long, contributing to the slump in morale in 1881, but it was now clear that the careful management of the repeal case had ensured an exceptionally good run of evidence — especially when compared to earlier enquiries (see Table 8.2).

To have produced more witnesses than the official side was a feat in itself, but to have beaten them in the provision of clerical witnesses was outstanding (though admittedly all but one of the repeal clergy were nonconformist ministers representing their denominations). The moral case was reinforced by town missionaries, Cooper of the Rescue Society and Mrs Butler herself; in sharp contrast to her appearance before the Royal Commission, she submitted to the discipline of the

Table 8.2: Attitudes of Witnesses to Regulation before the 1879—82
Select Committee[83]

	Before the 1879—82 SC			Before all the enquiries		
	For	Against	Neutral	For	Against	Neutral
Doctors (military)	4	—	—	27	1	3
Doctors (official)	5	—	—	27	1	1
Doctors (civilian)	1	5	—	20	14	20
Policemen	9	5	—	22	6	1
Military men (officers)	—	—	—	6	1	1
Civil servants	—	—	—	6	—	—
Clergy	7	12	—	16	18	—
Matrons/nurses	1	—	—	5	2	—
Miscellaneous	8	15	—	21	29	1
	35	37	0	150	72	27

NA's managers and learnt by heart the details in her evidence.[84] But
although the moral emphasis of the objections to the Acts is thus
clear, more practical objections were not neglected: Casserley had
persuaded the local police at Plymouth and Devonport to testify
against their metropolitan rivals, which they did, making 'good,
telling witnesses';[85] and the Chief Constable of Glasgow had been
summonsed to explain how his force achieved the moral and police
benefits claimed for the Acts, without them.[86] The medical evidence
was also favourable — Nevins was able, and the NA believed that it
had managed to prove the military statistics quite unreliable — much
of the credit for this going to Stansfeld for his cross-examination of
Surgeon-General Lawson.[87] This was the only breakthrough in all the
evidence given before the committee; otherwise both sides stuck to
the positions they had been holding for over ten years and simply
tried to drown their opposition with evidence.

Not surprisingly, the two groups on the committee chose to submit
separate reports — the mistake of the Royal Commission was not to
be repeated. The majority report, drafted by the chairman,
O'Shaughnessy, a Home Ruler, was a complete endorsement, indeed
almost a eulogy of the Acts; it found no fault and only regretted the
impossibility of extension. Stansfeld drafted the minority report
which six members signed. This was an unambiguous condemnation
of the Acts which found them deficient on every conceivable ground.
This report was the better argued from the evidence; the regulationist
one was an uncritical resumé of the evidence of those responsible for

operating the Acts, whereas the repealers showed a greater interest in probing the true state of affairs in the subjected towns. All this was pointed out by the repeal press, with an eye to Childers's promise that the government would consider the evidence as well as the reports: the *Shield* even analysed the marginal references in both reports to show how much fairer were those in Stansfeld's.[88] The minority report was reprinted in great numbers and made the basis of the winter campaign in 1882—3; as the *Shield* put it:

> Repealers have reason to thank God that all skirmishing under false colours is ended, and ended also is the long truce forced upon us by the insidious tactics of our opponents. The Majority Report is a declaration of war.[89]

But not all repealers followed the *Shield* in the conclusion it drew: 'Not only is the government not for us; it is against us, and it would be worse than folly not to take full account of this fact in the coming struggle.' It was all very well to grumble about the government's lack of faith, but to identify it as the target for attack as the *Shield* was doing,[90] seemed to be the prelude to resuming the irreconcilable tactics of ten years before. This might be acceptable to the twin dictators of NA policy (as Wilson saw them) — Mme Venturi and Miss Lucy Wilson — but it was not the strategy desired by provincial repealers. Wilson had consulted the much respected J.H. Raper of the UKA who had urged the need for better organisation to oblige MPs to commit themselves to repeal — efficient working would ensure no omissions.[91] To bring this about, the exasperated provincials were once more plotting the subversion of the NA's leadership; they were determined to create an organisation which *would* concern itself with the Liberal party, and not perpetrate gaffes such as scheduling a repeal conference at a time when it would clash with a meeting of the NLF — as the NA did in 1881.[92]

At the end of August, Wilson began the process with a circular to northern activists in which he was startlingly offensive to the NA and urged the adoption of UKA/Liberation Society methods in the protracted struggle he now envisaged. The NA was simply not up to this, so a new delegate body would have to be set up, preferably centred on Birmingham rather than London, incorporating the NA if it was willing, but proceeding without it if not.[93] Wilson had already taken the precaution of sounding out other bodies such as the FA and the WMNL; the MCEU made the arrangements for a conference and one of its vice-chairmen, a vigorous barrister named Jesse Herbert (praised by Martineau as 'desperately in earnest') began secretly lining up support for the provincial strategy.[94] Josephine Butler was enthusiastic. She wanted to retain the support of the NA if possible (Shaen was thought especially valuable) but if not, personal considerations should no longer stand in the way: 'the languid or perfunctory workers will either receive new life, and run in step with us, or they *must* be left behind.[95] Her ally, James Stuart, agreed with this, but ever the conciliator, suggested ways of selling the new scheme to Stansfeld and the NA, with the need to carry Shaen again seen as a priority.[96] Actually, the intended victims failed to see the threat: Stansfeld adopted an independent stance, encouraged Wilson's attack and urged the NA to comply with provincial demands;[97] while the NA committee, unaware of Wilson's lobbying, failed to meet at all in August or September and when it met again in early October, lamely agreed to the MCEU-organised conference.[98] The provincials held the NA in contempt. One wing, represented by Stuart, wanted to capture and reinforce it before weakness caused its disappearance; the other, represented by Edmondson, would let it die if 'a more vigorous heir' could be found. But all agreed with him that 'our real want is less machinery *more work*'.[99]

The MCEU issued a circular on 23 October convening the conference; again it argued that the movement was near to collapse and needed a new central delegate body to pull it round, and Jesse Herbert annexed a scheme of government for a 'Parliamentary Committee'.[100] Shaen immediately protested to Martineau in the strongest terms, and the NA issued a counter circular alleging deception by the MCEU, a petulant thing which Herbert rightly criticised as indicating that the NA seemed more concerned to defend its leadership than to advance the cause.[101]

The conference on 7 November 1882 was the most acrimonious ever held; so much so that no report was published in the repeal press, and only a manuscript account prepared for Wilson survives.[102] It was well attended — 25 organisations were represented (10 of which were LNA affiliates) and there were 59 delegates, of whom 27 were women. Debate raged for two hours with the NA refusing to concede the need for a new body and the militants apparently drawing back from an open break. Eventually a compromise was reached: the NA would sponsor the new body as *its* Parliamentary Committee, and the provincials ambiguously agreed to cooperate with it. Only those willing to work energetically would be allowed onto the committee. The tone of the provincial assault is conveyed by a manifesto issued by the MCEU to coincide with the conference; this was a moralistic call to arms demanding a brazen attitude to conventional prudence: 'That which the supporters of the Acts say is too horrible to be discussed, must surely be too horrible to be endured?'[103] Given their impatience for constructive action, the provincials regretted their agreement to the compromise before the ink was dry. Ellis talked of the NA's 'dog in the manger' attitude and admitted that sympathy for a feeble old guard had prevented many from doing what they knew to be right.[104]

Wilson soon overcame any scruples about fair dealing. As the NA sedately set about forming its Parliamentary Committee (the Executive Committee waited a week before considering the matter at its next ordinary meeting) he set about undermining their efforts. Reporting to the NCL Executive Committee he announced that two committees were to be set up, one by the provincials, one by the NA. He recommended having nothing to do with the latter.[105] This was straining the compromise to breaking point; another coordinating committee was the last thing the conference had intended, but Wilson was a determined man. Ellis and the MCEU accepted this scheme with little hesitation and all began pre-empting the NA's market by capturing various repeal societies for their committee. Only Stuart remained eager to avoid a clash, professing to see signs of a change of heart in the NA; Wilson, however, was now happily and energetically heading for such a clash.[106]

His committee met for the first time on 29 November. It adopted the title 'Political Committee' to distinguish it from the NA's 'Parliamentary Committee' and limited its activity to the north and midlands. The intention was to implement the conference's demand for vigorous action, but without reference to the NA.[107] Wilson naturally became the secretary. He recognised that he would not be acceptable generally as chairman, and Stuart was secured for that post. He was thereby tied to the provincial cause, even though he could not rid himself of the desire to reconcile the two sides. The conspiracy was successfully kept from the Londoners until two days before the meeting, when George Gillett of the FA sent a hurt letter to Wilson protesting against this separatist move, a betrayal, as he saw it, of the conference's decision. But even on the day of the meeting, Banks was so much in the dark that he sent Wilson a chatty note with the latest parliamentary news, little realising what Wilson's meeting (which he had heard about 'by merest accident') was up to.[108] After a decent interval, Wilson formally notified him of the Political

Committee's existence, and the NCL and MCEU declined to be associated with the Parliamentary Committee.[109]

They missed nothing. The NA's committee was late in the field and never succeeded in establishing its *raison d'être*. It could not co-ordinate because the Political Committee made a better job of this, and soon lapsed into being a mere subcommittee. Wilson's committee, as he later gladly admitted, was a new development 'of Liberal politicians who felt impelled to press on the Liberal Government their desire to bring about the repeal of the C.D. Acts'.[110] In this way, repeal was following in the steps of the Liberation Society by addressing itself directly to the Liberals — in March the nonconformist MPs had begun to meet regularly to concert action on religious issues.[111] An important tactical shift had thus been made, largely due to Wilson's zeal, and although it was later played down by repealers — 'some difference of opinion' was how the *Shield* recalled it in 1898 — the change was a significant one of principle, and as it turned out, of practice also.[112]

III

The Political Committee united Liberal repealers in a concerted effort to swing the party organisation against the Acts. Wilson immediately circularised his members, urging them to attend the National Liberal Federation's meeting at Ashton on 19 December, and here they scored an important success.[113] Stuart was chosen to second a vote of confidence in the government, and used his speech to warn them that their record on moral progress failed to match up to that on social and political progress; he blamed the evil influence of officials, but remained confident that the government 'could wipe away this source of future disintegration of the Liberal party'.[114] Benjamin Scott thought the choice of Stuart to second the vote showed government support for repeal.[115] This was obviously incorrect, but it would be nearer the truth to say that it showed the drift of NLF thinking.

Wilson and Ellis were hard at work reinforcing this — ' "in and out" of the House of Commons stirring people up' as Josephine Butler gratefully recorded.[116] Ellis spent much time working on individuals such as the Whig MP, Cecil Foljambe: 'this matter of Repeal is one of personal fag', he told Wilson adding that no Association could use personal contacts in the way a few prominent Liberals could.[117] Wilson too was getting at the same group, circularising Liberal office holders with a memorial to Gladstone, and spurred on by J.H. Bell, the influential editor of the *Northern Echo*, approaching the

NLF leadership to get repeal accepted as part of the programme — this would enable them to renew their approach to Gladstone in the cause of Liberal unity as well as party morality.[118] Stansfeld had already warned the Liberal leadership that it risked the disintegration of the party by refusing repeal, and the great Christian Convention in January 1883 underlined the nonconformist repugnance for the Acts; the message was clear.[119]

It was also getting across. Stuart dined Chamberlain and Dilke in Trinity and both declared their commitment to repeal; Chamberlain positively gushed.[120] Ellis, Stuart, Martineau and Wilson kept up the pressure in the first months of 1883 with an avalanche of personal letters to Liberal MPs, designed to support Hopwood who had secured time to move a resolution on 27 February. The NA was also active with its well tried methods; its office strained to keep up with the mountain of correspondence and petitions; Banks imaginatively urged repealers to present their petitions through hostile or lukewarm MPs, and not to overburden friendly ones.[121] Large scale constituency pressure was drummed up to support Hopwood. An MP told Josephine Butler that 'the amount of pressure from the country [was] unprecedented in the history of any agitation', and in the lobby she 'saw members with both pockets projecting, full of private letters. One man is said to have had 500 private letters in one day from constituents, and in despair (!) he determined to vote for repeal.'[122] The tide was turning: at the LNA Annual Meeting in February three hitherto inactive MPs sat on the platform; and at the Newcastle by-election earlier in the month the three candidates vied with each other to declare their opposition to the Acts — John Morley was elected, and when he was introduced on the evening of 27 February he immediately went and sat next to Hopwood and asked what he could do.[123]

Unfortunately there was nothing he could do. Despite intensive lobbying of MPs a few days before (Ellis had by now succeeded in getting at young Whig MPs such as Grey and Elliott through Cecil Foljambe) and a virtual siege of the lobby on the night — Cardinal Manning was there to influence the Irish MPs and the Westminster Palace Hotel housed an all day women's prayer meeting — the resolution was crowded out by other business, and Hopwood could only promise indignantly to renew the effort.[124]

A group of MPs immediately balloted for time to introduce a motion, all intending that it should be for repeal.[125] Fortunately Stansfeld was successful, and 20 April was fixed as the date. The offensive was renewed — a meeting of friendly MPs discussed how best to support Stansfeld, and 60 MPs (representing 200 pledged repealers) memorialised Gladstone on 11 April asking him to receive a deputation. On the following day, 12 April, the General Committee of the NLF unanimously pressed for immediate repeal,[126] and then on 13 April the *Pall Mall Gazette* topped this off with a powerful leader pointing out that the Acts had not been such a success and wondering 'whether the game is worth the candle'. Better to have done with 'the scandal of the agitation'. The Cabinet cracked and agreed at its meeting on 14 April to make the subject an open question; and Hamilton used precisely the *Gazette*'s phrase when noting the decision in his diary two days later.[127]

Naturally Wilson made much of the NLF result to pressure Liberal MPs; all received a circular, and Stuart drew the resolution to Hartington's attention.[128] Repeal was now regarded as a Liberal policy. To his own followers in the north, Wilson sent a circular analysing the attitude to repeal of every northern MP, urging pressure on the undecided,[129] and at Scarborough, W.S. Caine warned his running mate, Dodson, that he would lose his seat if he failed to vote for repeal.[130]

But despite their efforts, repealers like Caine, Ellis or even Stansfeld were pessimistic about their chances on 20 April; this time, however, careful preparation did pay off, and the debate vindicated Stansfeld's style of parliamentary leadership.[131] His speech was a lucid exposition of his minority report — any MP who had managed to avoid the recent deluge of repeal propaganda could have innocently supposed that he was listening to the author of a widely supported majority report. Stansfeld demolished his opponents' arguments: hygiene, efficiency, alleged moral improvement, better public order, the government's statistics, all were analysed and dismissed. He dealt at length (and, he insisted, reluctantly) with the failure of the Acts to eliminate VD. This was a crucial point — he had to persuade MPs that the Acts were statistically proved not to be worth defending. There is no doubt that he succeeded.

The opposition was bungled and no match. Osborne Morgan led with the standard public health defence of the system, insisting on its popularity in the subjected towns and the efficacy of official reclamation work. A side-sweep at repealers who disapproved of treatment for VD was immediately rebutted by Stansfeld. This rehash was no reply to an up-to-date challenge to the Acts, but Cavendish-Bentinck was worse; his speech was a mixture of boorish attacks on his opponents and unsupported assertions about the benefits of the Acts. O'Shaughnessy, the chairman of the select committee tried to defend his report, but his analysis of the statistics confused matters without shaking Stansfeld's case.

Only two members of the government spoke. Hartington announced the Cabinet's decision not to defend the Acts, but to let parliament decide. He admitted that most members of the Cabinet supported repeal; only the other service minister, Northbrook, and the Home Secretary, Harcourt, followed him in defending the Acts. Childers represented the other ministerial view; he had opposed compulsory examinations since 1875, but as he favoured retaining certain parts of the Acts, he had supported the compromise embodied in Bruce's Bill. He could not vote for a repeal Bill, but would support the resolution. Among the other MPs who spoke were a significant group of new members including Thorold Rogers and George Russell who seemed offended by the bland acceptance of the Acts hitherto shown by their older colleagues and predecessors. The repeal case had the best of a worthwhile debate, and when the division was taken the resolution was carried by the handsome majority of 72 (182: 110) in this, the first ever parliamentary vote for repeal.[132]

The press immediately acknowledged the importance of the vote: *The Times* regretted it, and paid Stansfeld a very backhanded tribute about his lack of worldliness, but had to concede that the resolution was 'the death-blow of the Acts'; the *Echo*'s record as the only consistent supporter of repeal amongst metropolitan papers permitted it to talk of Stansfeld's vindication against 'the opposition or the indifference of the Go-with-the-Stream Press' and the *Pall Mall Gazette* agreed that this was a triumph of morality over expediency.[133] But repealers found difficulty in appreciating the magnitude of their success; naturally their papers exulted, but discussion in private was altogether more cautious. Josephine Butler learnt that the three ministers who favoured the Acts had been given the job of framing the government's response; naturally she suspected this 'lovely trio' of wishing to devise a compromise.[134] She suggested a test of any measure: does it take cognizance of the needs of an immoral man who may have future relations with the woman in question? If so, it would fail.[135]

The government's decision was to withdraw the police and suspend examination while considering further permanent arrangements. Hartington announced this on 4 May and justified it by saying that the House would hardly vote money for a system of which it had just voted its disapproval. Regulationist MPs were furious and Hartington, who had once declared that the Acts would continue to be implemented until a repeal Bill was carried, only just managed to evade a reasonable charge of inconsistency.[136] When further pressed by Puleston on 7 May, he grew bolder and announced that the Acts conferred permissive powers on the government which the House could remove by denying it supply.[137]

Nearly two months elapsed before the government produced its measure, and during this lull a serious split developed amongst repealers. Everyone knew that the government was in a quandary; Hamilton noted that the conflict between the Acts and resolution gave rise to a curious constitutional position, and the press accused the government of having abdicated responsibility for implementing the law.[138] The *Shield* reacted badly to the uncertainty, one moment reviling the government, the next making pathetic appeals to it; whereas the Political Committee was much more conscious of the need to await the government's decision and then work to modify and improve it — a view urged on them by Dilke and Chamberlain and warmly espoused by Stuart.[139] Stansfeld endorsed a 'wait and see' policy when addressing that usually militant audience, the LNA Annual Meeting on 10 May.[140]

Only the NA stood out nervously against this tendency, issuing on 28 May a manifesto full of militant statements about positive legislation not being their concern, and special treatment for VD sufferers offending repeal principles.[141] It provoked a storm: Stansfeld thought it premature; Wilson disliked its negative emphasis; the NCL was interested in the promotion of social purity and refused to sign. Many other societies wanted amendments before they would endorse it; even Josephine Butler's attitude was muted and realistic — she told an LNA conference that abolition of separate Lock Hospitals was a long-term aim which should not be pressed for the moment.[142] Stansfeld hurriedly summoned a private conference to extract a vote of confidence and impose some unity on the movement.[143]

The reaction to the government's Detention in Hospitals Bill, published on 5 July, showed that this unity was illusory. The Bill repealed the Acts, but included greater powers of detention in the hospitals (which would be retained) especially if combined with parts of the Criminal Law Amendment Bill, then in the Lords. Its curious title suggests the regret felt by the service ministers at the loss of the Acts, but it did dismantle the examination system. Stansfeld thought the Bill reasonable as long as clause 5 (permitting transfers from prison to hospital) was deleted, and the Political Committee, meeting on 9 July, agreed to endorse it subject to amendment.[144] The provincial repealers were acutely aware of the need to get the government moving somehow; Stansfeld did not believe that this Bill stood much chance of getting the necessary time, but he wanted to encourage the government to act, and not leave the repeal Bill to a private member, with all the added difficulties which that involved. The London activists, principally Levy, Mme Venturi and Miss Lucy Wilson, thought differently, and at the NA EC's next meeting they bullied their colleagues into taking up a hostile attitude to the Bill; the *Shield* then came out with acid criticisms of it, and a call to mobilise.[145]

Stansfeld and the Political Committee were aghast; Wilson talked of 'deplorable action', Herbert wondered how they were to persuade MPs to take them seriously if their policy vacillated like this, Ellis revealed depths of loathing for the Londoners and happily reported that even Stuart was 'disgusted and provoked' and would now be willing to strike firmly against the NA − unlike his tenderness in December 1882. Stansfeld was the hardest hit. Nursing his dying wife, he found that his sister-in-law and oldest friends had turned against him.[146]

While the NA was recovering from the attack, and trying to mend its fences, the government Bill was quietly dropped; it had received no support from the divided repeal movement, while the other side was busy attacking it for haste in abandoning the Acts. One opportunity was thus lost, but on the other hand as long as the Liberal government remained in office, the repealers were in no danger. Government immobilism now favoured them, and regulationists faced the same weight of ministerial inertia as had delayed repealers for so long. Conservatives used repeal tactics: debates on the estimates, questions about local expressions of regret over suspension (just as repealers had asked questions about individual cases of abuse), but none of this had any effect. Hartington brushed off the attempts of the Fourth Party (both Wolff and Gorst represented dock-yard towns) to embarrass the government, and grew firmer in his resistance to them. In 1884 he told Puleston: 'the effects of these Acts on the health of the Army were, owing to the extremely partial character of their operation, very slight, and also extremely fluctuating'.[147] Stansfeld could hardly have put it better.

As loyal Liberals, the provincials were in a dilemma as to how much pressure to apply. Stansfeld reasserted control at a conference held at Birmingham in October and the NA reluctantly came into line behind him.[148] Moderation was now the keynote − Stuart wrote to Chamberlain 'as a Liberal' to urge the government to drop clause 5, suggesting that they were being 'led a foolish dance by the pro-Acts officials'.[149] Furthermore, the movement was increasingly seen as a

Liberal auxiliary; for instance, the Political Committee was included in Schnadhorst's circular to associations which might wish to put up resolutions to the NLF.[150]

In private, Stansfeld was well aware of the government's problems and the general political situation. He warned the NA that 'the Liberal party will look very much askance upon anyone seeking to attack the Government on the eve of a Reform Bill'.[151] In public he was willing to make fighting speeches, arguing that he would hold the government to its duty, and in February 1884 the Political Committee decided that he would have to bring in another resolution even at the risk of defeat.[152] Maintaining morale was still necessary, and in fact there was a substantial falling off in activity (measured by NA turnover – the smallest since its foundation) when the resolution failed to materialise.[153] The dilemma remained: how to use repeal strength to convince the government that it should act, without endangering it? A deputation to Harcourt in May 1884 was rudely received, and told that the government would not reintroduce its bill.[154] A memorial to Gladstone in June was more kindly received, and Herbert Gladstone replied tactfully, pointing out that pressure of business prevented any chance of carrying repeal and any attempt would only assist Tory obstructionists. Time was on the repealers' side now that 'the sting of the Acts' had gone.[155] Indeed, when the effects of suspension were discussed during the Estimates debate in July, the debate was raised by regulationists and the repeal contribution was slight.[156] But the NA found the lack of action exasperating and in October 1884 broke its silence with a circular to Liberal office holders threatening repeal as a test question at the next election if nothing was done. Wilson exploded against a policy 'unwise and impracticable', but this was a line increasingly difficult to hold once the Reform Act was out of the way.[157] Dr Ewing Whittle of Liverpool expressed rank and file impatience at the MCEU Annual Meeting in January 1885:

> in the great crisis of 1880, the whole Liberal party was appealed to to sink all crotchets, and to give their undivided support to a Liberal government. Those who had been called 'crotcheteers' – a name I am not ashamed to own – did throw themselves in with the Liberal party. What was the consequence? A great Liberal victory. What thanks did we get for it? Sneers and scorn and contempt by all the purely party men. Personally . . . I resent it. Now let us in the next General Election sink to crotchets.[158]

However when the NA began abandoning the pro-Liberal policy, setting up electoral committees and trumpeting the need to be uncompromising (quoting Cobden in support) — the leading provincials had had enough. After a plot to 'capture' the NA had been foiled, Stuart, the Butlers and the Wilsons finally severed their connections with it.[159]

The sudden reappearance of a hostile Tory ministry in June 1885 cancelled any damage done by the schism—it reminded repealers of the dangers posed as long as the Acts remained on the statute book — and the Tories were not going to repeal them. At the November election, an overtly non-partisan attitude concealed an inevitable bias towards the Liberals — in July, of 225 candidates known to favour repeal, only 15 had been Tories — and the idea of repeal becoming a test question was quietly dropped.[160] In a crisis, repealers had to agree that their best chance lay with the success of the Liberal party, and they were well rewarded: 261 repealers wre returned of whom 221 were Liberals.[161] The parliamentary leadership was reinforced by H.J. Wilson's election for Holmfirth.

Repeal MPs in the new parliament immediately formed a caucus and prepared to move a new resolution: appropriately it was Wilson who secured a date, though it was lost when the Liberals returned to office in February.[162] However, this gave repealers the opportunity to wield their party influence: Stansfeld let it be known that his substantial group would not brook further delay, and under the circumstances the government felt obliged to defer to radical sentiment. Campbell-Bannerman, the Secretary for War, circularised his colleagues on 12 March advising cooperation,[163] and when on 16 March Stansfeld moved a resolution that the Acts ought to be repealed, it was with the knowledge that he had government support. The debate was surprisingly easy — an amendment to continue making payments to hospitals was divided on the defeated 245: 181 with government tellers (Gladstone himself intervened to help); the resolution was carried without a division.[164]

Translating it into a repeal Bill was now urgent as the Commons was becoming more and more preoccupied with the Home Rule Bill. Stansfeld badly wanted the government to make a fitting end to the campaign by taking on the Bill itself; only thus could time be guaranteed. When Arnold Morley dithered, he and Stuart appealed directly to Gladstone who agreed to give government facilities.[165] On 25 March the Bill had an unopposed second reading; on 26 March Stansfeld was invited to take Chamberlain's place in the Cabinet as President of the Local Government Board, his old office. This, he told his sister, was 'a kind of *amende honorable* implied rather than expressed', though he had no illusions about the government's prospects.[166] Stuart took charge of the bill which got through the Commons on 2 April after some momentarily worrying obstruction by Cavendish-Bentinck, and the Lords bowed to public opinion. The Royal Assent was given on 15 April, and Stansfeld telegraphed the good news to Mrs Butler, then in Naples. After a 16-year struggle she exulted: '*that* abomination is dead and *buried*'.[167]

Notes

1. FLB 3899: Josephine Butler to BCGF EC, 11 Jan. 1879.
2. *Hansard*, 3rd series (11 June 1879) Col. 1695; *Shield*, 26 July 1879, p. 120.
3. NCL, *6th Report for 1879 and 1880*, p. 7; *Protest*, 17 Apr. 1879, pp. 39–40.
4. NA EC Minutes, 24 and 31 Mar., 5 and 12 May 1879.
5. E.g. NA EC Minutes, 16 June 1879, 28 Feb. 1881, 30 Jan. 1882.
6. NA EC Minutes, 4 Apr. 1881.
7. NA EC Minutes, 28 Feb. 1881, 17 July 1882.
8. NA, *General Report for 1880 and 1881*, pp. 40–1.
9. *Letter book of the N.A., 1883–1886*, F.C. Banks to J. Stansfeld, 22 May 1884.
10. *Shield*, 15 Oct. 1881, pp. 181–97.
11. NA EC Minutes, 5 June 1882.
12. *Protest*, 17 July 1879, pp. 79–80.
13. FLW Box 5 letter 499: Josephine Butler to Mrs H.J. Wilson, 29 Dec. 1879, searching for substitute speakers for MPs.
14. H.W. Lucy, *A Diary of Two Parliaments, the Disraeli Parliament, 1874–1880* (1885), p. 298; Paul Smith, *Disraelian Conservatism and Social Reform* (1967), p. 197 suggests that Disraeli appointed Bentinck to stop him becoming a backbench dissident.
15. Sheffield University Library (Mundella-Leader correspondence) 12 Mar. 1874.
16. *Hansard*, 3rd series (27 Apr. 1883) 278 Col.1275 (Gladstone); (7 May 1883) 279 Col.65 (Morgan).
17. *Shield*, 1 Nov. 1881, pp. 199–208 (Stansfeld attacking Morgan at a conference on 25 Oct. 1881). For Morgan, see *D.N.B. Supplement*, p. 1064.
18. See Rev. J.P. Gledstone, *Observations on the Recent Select Committee of the House of Commons* (1882), p. 2; *National League Journal*, 1 Dec. 1882, p. 9.
19. *Shield*, 11 Oct. 1879, pp. 156–9.
20. *Shield*, 7 Apr. 1883, p. 90.
21. NCL, *5th Report for 1877 and 1878* discusses all by-elections in its area and claims a gain of two.
22. LNA, *Annual Report for 1879*, pp. 18–19.
23. *Shield*, 8 Nov. 1879, p. 171.
24. NA EC Minutes, 3 Nov. 1879; *Protest*, 20 Nov. 1879, pp. 117–19.
25. NA EC Minutes, 10 Nov. 1879, 22 Mar. 1880.
26. E.g. FLB 3818: George Tatham to H.J. Wilson, 6 Dec. 1875 – on getting repeal inserted into the Liberal programme.

27. *Shield*, 21 Feb. 1880, pp. 22–6 (Wilson was speaking at the MCEU Annual Meeting in Derby).

28. *Shield*, 20 Mar. 1880, p. 37, 3 Apr. 1880, p. 45.

29. NA, *General Report for 1880 and 1881*, pp. 23–4; NCL, *6th Report for 1879 and 1880*; LNA, *Annual Report for 1880*, pp. 8–9.

30. *Protest*, 20 Apr. 1880, pp. 39–40 admits that repeal had been overshadowed by 'the all-absorbing question of Foreign Policy'.

31. *Shield*, 24 July 1880, pp. 111–16.

32. *Shield*, 17 Apr. 1880, pp. 53–6.

33. NCL, *6th Report for 1879 and 1880*.

34. LNA, *Annual Report for 1880*, p. 16; see H.J. Hanham, *Elections and Party Management: Politics in the Time of Disraeli and Gladstone* (1959), p. 124 and D.A. Hamer, *The Politics of Electoral Pressure: A Study in the History of Victorian Reform Agitations* (Hassocks, 1977), pp. 150–1 for the Liberation Society's similar strategy.

35. NA EC Minutes, 25 Apr. 1881.

36. E.g. *Shield*, 11 Feb. 1882, p. 26 for report of the King's Norton Liberal Association commending repeal to their MPs, one of whom, the regulationist G.W. Hastings, was present.

37. NA EC Minutes, 22 Oct. 1877.

38. FLB 3449: H.J. Wilson to J. Stansfeld, 6 June 1875.

39. FLW Box 1 letter 887: H.J. Wilson to NCL EC, 13 Dec. 1883; *Letter Book of the N.A. 1883–1886*, F.C. Banks to J. Stansfeld, 22 May 1884.

40. Abstracted from NA EC Minutes; see chapter 3 (p. 72, above) for equivalent figures for 1872 (a comparable year in terms of activity).

41. A. Tilney Bassett, *The Life of the Rt. Hon. John Edward Ellis MP* (1914), p. 41; Elizabeth Isichei, *Victorian Quakers* (Oxford, 1970), p. 206; FLW Box 78 letter 365: Joseph Edmondson to H.J. Wilson, 10 Oct. 1882; J. Stuart, *Reminiscences* (1911), pp. 227–8.

42. NA EC Minutes, 12 Apr. 1880.

43. NA EC Minutes, 28 June 1880; *Shield*, 26 June 1880, pp. 94–5.

44. NA EC Minutes, 26 July 1880; *Shield*, 7 Aug. 1880, p. 118, 21 Aug. 1880, pp. 130–1; FLW Box 2 letter 814d: Circular, H.J. Wilson to NCL EC, 28 July 1880; 814f: H.J. Wilson to NCL EC, 11 Aug. 1880.

45. *Shield*, 24 July 1880, pp. 111–16; FLW Box 2 letter 814b: Circular, H.J. Wilson to NCL EC, 28 June 1880.

46. E.g. NA EC Minutes, 24 Feb. 1879 – Stansfeld informs the NA of the session's parliamentary activities.

47. *Shield*, 28 Aug. 1880, pp. 133–37; NA EC Minutes, 23 Aug. 1880.

48. R.J. Lambert, *Sir John Simon 1816–1904, and English Social Administration* (1963), pp. 520–1, an unflattering picture of Stansfeld with a devastating opinion by Lowe; Ethel Drus (ed.) 'A Journal of Events During the Gladstone Ministry, 1868–1874, by John, first Earl of Kimberley' *Camden Miscellany*, 21 (1958), p. 21 (4 Mar. 1871), p. 43 (3 Dec. 1873).

49. BL Add. MSS 44463 (Gladstone Papers) f.224: Gladstone to J. Stansfeld, 27 Apr. 1880 (cancelled) referring to the 'representative principle' which Gladstone cannot set aside.

50. Josephine Butler, *Recollections of George Butler* (Bristol *c.* 1893), p. 338; D.W.R. Bahlman (ed.), *The Diary of Sir Edward Hamilton*, vol. 1 (Oxford, 1972), p. 2.

51. BL Add. MSS 44463 (Gladstone Papers) f.195: Gladstone to Stansfeld, 25 Apr. 1880; f.281: Stansfeld to Gladstone, 29 Apr. 1880.

52. Stansfeld MSS (in family hands): Stansfeld to Mrs W.A. Case (sister), 31 May 1880.

53. The classic statement of Stansfeld's sacrifice is Sir Robert Ensor, *England 1870–1914* (1936), p. 171; see also J.L. and B. Hammond, *James Stansfeld, A Victorian Champion of Sex Equality* (1932), pp. 218–19. Obituaries in *The Times* and the *Standard*, 18 Feb. 1898, stress the adverse effect on Stansfeld.

54. *Shield*, 1 May 1880, p. 61, 7 Aug. 1880, pp. 117–18; for Johnstone's refusal see NA EC Minutes, 27 July 1874.

55. FLB 3828: Josephine Butler to H.J. Wilson, 19 Dec. 1875.

56. *Shield*, 24 Oct. 1874, p. 194.

57. FLB 3341: J. Stansfeld to Josephine Butler, 23 Oct. 1874.

58. NA EC Minutes, 7 Sept. 1874.

59. *Shield*, 15 Oct. 1881, p. 187.

60. NA EC Minutes, 5 and 12 July 1875, Stansfeld and Johnstone preventing the NA from issuing a hasty anti-medical manifesto; see also Hammonds, *James Stansfeld*, pp. 202–5.

61. *Shield*, 5 Feb. 1876, pp. 38–44. He was addressing the MCEU Annual Meeting at Wolverhampton, 18 Jan. 1876.

62. FLW Box 78 letter 620: J.E. Ellis to H.J. Wilson, 22 Feb. 1883 (reporting a conversation with Stuart).

63. A. Jones, *The Politics of Reform: 1884* (Cambridge, 1972), pp. 260–1; see also p. 15.

64. FLB 3935: W.S. Caine to anon., 27 Aug. 1882; 3952: Josephine Butler to R.F. Martineau, 2 Oct. 1882.

65. *Shield*, 23 Dec. 1882, p. 223.

66. FLW Box 2 letter 615a: H.J. Wilson to NCL EC, 15 Sept. 1880.

67. Methodist Archives MSS: Hugh Price Hughes to Dr G. Osborn, 1 Mar. 1881.

68. NA EC Minutes, 17 Jan. 1881.

69. Ibid., 3 Jan. 1881, seven including J.F.B. Firth and Ashton Dilke; 17 Jan. 1881, ten including G.O. Trevelyan; 24 Jan. 1881, three including S. Whitbread.

70. *Shield*, 20 Aug. 1881, p. 168; *Hansard*, 3rd series (4 Aug. 1881) 263 Col.908: Labouchere moving reduction of the army estimates – defeated 80:13.

71. FLW Box 78 letters 315 and 316: two printed circulars from R.F. Martineau, 11 Oct. 1881.

72. NA EC Minutes, 17 Oct. 1881; a particularly large meeting (16 members) to discuss the Birmingham circulars.

73. *Protest*, 25 Nov. 1881, pp. 98–102; *Shield*, 1 Nov. 1881, pp. 199–206.

74. *Hansard*, 3rd series (19 July 1882) 272 Col.1079ff.

75. *Shield*, 22 July 1882, pp. 137–8.

76. FLW Box 1 letter 844g:H.J. Wilson to NCL EC, 9 Aug. 1882; FLB 3942: J.P. Gledstone to H.J. Wilson, 11 Sept. 1882, reporting Carvell Williams's views.

77. Edward Bristow, 'The Liberty and Property Defence League and Individualism', *Historical Journal*, 18 (1975), p. 768, discusses the scope for destroying constructive legislation which 'shrinking opportunities available to private members' bills' offered the LPDL.

78. NA EC Minutes, 2 Mar. 1874; *Shield*, 16 Dec. 1876, pp. 365–72.

79. NA EC Minutes, 15 July 1878; *Shield*, 20 July 1878, p. 201.

80. *Shield*, 3 Mar. 1883, p. 41, argues that resolutions are the only viable means of pursuing an agitation in the House of Commons.

81. NA EC Minutes, 27 Nov. 1882; FLB 4005: J. Stansfeld to Emile de Lavelaye, 5 Sept. 1883.

82. *Shield*, 17 Feb. 1883, p. 29.

83. *Report of the Select Committee on the Contagious Diseases Acts (1866–*

1869), *PP* 1882 (340), ix. Thre were also four earlier interim reports summarising evidence only.

84. FLB 3925: Josephine Butler to George Butler, 4 May 1882.

85. NA EC Minutes, 27 Feb. 1882.

86. *PP*, 1881 (851), viii, QQ7478–90, 7611–647, Appendix 21, Tables 1–5.

87. NA EC Minutes, 4 Apr. 1881.

88. *Shield*, 21 Oct. 1882, pp. 198–9.

89. *Shield*, 12 Aug. 1882, pp. 155–6.

90. See also *Shield*, 16 Sept. 1882, pp. 175–6.

91. FLB 3939: H.J. Wilson to J.H. Raper, 1 Sept. 1882; 3943: J.H. Raper to H.J. Wilson, 12 Sept. 1882.

92. NA EC Minutes, 10 Oct. 1881: H.J. Wilson protested about this, but without effect.

93. FLB 3938: H.J. Wilson to NCL EC, 31 Aug. 1882.

94. FLB 3948: R.F. Martineau to H.J. Wilson, 28 Sept. 1882; 3951: Jesse Herbert to H.J. Wilson, 1 Oct. 1882.

95. FLB 3952: Josephine Butler to R.F. Martineau, 2 Oct. 1882.

96. FLW Box 78 letter 372: James Stuart to H.J. Wilson, 12 Oct. 1882.

97. FLW Box 78 letter 368: J. Stansfeld to H.J. Wilson, 9 Oct. 1882; NA EC Minutes, 21 Aug. 1882.

98. NA EC Minutes, 9 Oct. 1882: it thereby postponed a conference of its own.

99. FLW Box 78 letters 382 and 383: James Stuart to H.J. Wilson, 17 and 20 Oct. 1882; letter 386: Joseph Edmondson to H.J. Wilson, 23 Oct. 1882.

100. FLW Box 78 letter 388: circular issued 23 Oct. 1882; letter 391: scheme of government.

101. FLW Box 78 letter 394: Shaen to R.F. Martineau, 26 Oct. 1882; letter 425: Jesse Herbert to H.J. Wilson, 2 Nov. 1882; NA EC Minutes, 30 Oct. 1882.

102. FLB 3077: MS Report of Conference at Birmingha, 7 Nov. 1882.

103. *Protest*, 23 Dec. 1882, pp. 114–16.

104. FLW Box 78 letter 430: J.E. Ellis to H.J. Wilson, 8 Nov. 1882.

105. FLW Box 1 letter 846: H.J. Wilson to NCL EC, 8 Nov. 1882.

106. FLW Box 78 letters 431–43: record Wilson's effective lobbying during November 1882.

107. FLW Box 78 letter 472: H.J. Wilson to NCL EC, 6 Dec. 1882 reporting the meeting.

108. FLW Box 78 letter 462: G. Gillett to H.J. Wilson, 27 Nov. 1882; FLB 3974: Banks to H.J. Wilson, 29 Nov. 1882.

109. NA EC Minutes, 11 Dec. 1882.

110. FLW Box 4: typescript 'History of the English Repeal Movement', 1915.

111. J.F. Glaser, 'Nonconformity and Liberalism, 1868–1885. A Study in English Party History' (unpublished PhD thesis, Harvard University, 1948), p. 508.

112. *Shield*, Nov. 1898, p. 167 – the article also misdates the dispute to 1881.

113. FLW Box 78 letter 480: H.J. Wilson to Political Committee, 8 Dec. 1882; letters 505–30: replies indicating approval; the Leeds repealer, Ald. George Tatham, attended specially.

114. *Shield*, 6 Jan. 1883, pp. 5–6.

115. Benjamin Scott, *A State Iniquity: Its Rise, Extension and Overthrow* (1890), p. 218; see also p. 122 for his tribute to the effectiveness of the Political Committee.

116. FLW Box 78 letter 491a: Josephine Butler to Mrs H.J. Wilson, 19 Dec.

1882.
117. Ibid., letter 573: J.E. Ellis to H.J. Wilson, 1 Feb. 1883.
118. Ibid., letter 568: H.J. Wilson to Liberal office holders, Jan. 1883; letter 545: J.H. Bell to H.J. Wilson, 3 Jan. 1883.
119. *Shield*, 23 Dec. 1882, p. 223, reporting Stansfeld's speech to a repeal conference on 14 Dec. 1882.
120. FLW Box 78 letter 592: Stuart to J.E. Ellis, 10 Feb. 1883.
121. NA EC Minutes, 21 Feb. 1883; *Shield*, 7 Apr. 1883, p. 90.
122. Liverpool University Library (Butler MSS) MS 8.4(3) B1: Josephine Butler to A.S. Butler, 3 Mar. 1883.
123. Ibid.; *Shield*, 17 Feb. 1883, p. 29, 3 Mar. 1883, p. 48.
124. FLW Box 78 letter 623: J.E. Ellis to H.J. Wilson, 23 Feb. 1883; Liverpool University Library (Butler MSS), MS 8.4(3) B1: Josephine Butler to A.S. Butler.
125. See *Shield*, 17 Mar. 1883, p. 84 for a discussion of the propriety of this tactic.
126. *Shield*, 21 Apr. 1883, pp. 92–4; NA EC Minutes, 9 Apr. 1883; Ellis proposed the motion, Spence Watson seconded.
127. BL Add. MSS 44644 (Gladstone Papers) f.28 Cabinet minutes, 14 Apr. 1883; D.W.R. Bahlman (ed.), *The Diary of Sir Edward Hamilton* (Oxford, 1972), p. 423 (entry for 16 Apr. 1883).
128. FLW Box 78 letter 676: Stuart to H.J. Wilson, 11 Apr. 1883; letter 679: circular to Liberal MPs.
129. Sheffield Central Library (Wilson MSS) MD 2549: H.J. Wilson to NCL members, Apr. 1883.
130. FLW Box 78 letter 699: W.S. Caine to Joshua Rowntree, 18 Apr. 1883.
131. *Hansard*, 3rd series (20 Apr. 1883) 278 Col.749ff.
132. See above, chapter 5, for Gladstone's regard for the tone of the debate and surprise at the size of the majority.
133. *Times*, 21 Apr. 1883, p. 11; *Echo*, 21 Apr. 1883; *Pall Mall Gazette*, 21 Apr. 1883.
134. Sheffield Central Library (Wilson MSS) MD 2548: Josephine Butler to Mrs Hind Smith, Apr. 1883.
135. FLB 3995: circular dated 1 May 1883.
136. *Hansard*, 3rd series (4 May 1883) 278 Col.1865ff.
137. Ibid., (7 May 1883) 279 Col.52ff. He thus belatedly confirmed the repeal case for attacking the estimates over the years (see *Shield*, 29 June 1872, p. 987).
138. Bahlman, *Diary of Sir Edward Hamilton*, p. 433 (entry for 8 May 1883); *Newcastle Daily Journal*, 8 May 1883.
139. FLW Box 78 letter 736: Stuart to H.J. Wilson, 20 May 1883; letter 739: Chamberlain to H.J. Wilson, 22 May 1883.
140. *Shield*, 19 May 1883, pp. 154–7.
141. NA EC Minutes, 28 May 1883 (the manifesto was principally the work of J.H. Levy and Miss Lucy Wilson); *Shield*, 2 June 1883, p. 165.
142. FLW Box 1 letter 861: H.J. Wilson to NCL EC, 11 June 1883; NA EC Minutes, 18 and 25 June 1883; *Shield*, 2 June 1883, pp. 168–72.
143. NA EC Minutes, 4 June 1883; LNA, *Annual Report for 1883*, pp. 19–27.
144. NA EC Minutes, 9 July 1883; FLW Box 1 letter 866: H.J. Wilson to NCL EC, 10 July 1883.
145. NA EC Minutes, 16 July 1883; *Shield*, 21 July, pp. 200–1, 204–5; FLW Box 1 letter 828: Miss I.M.S. Tod to H.J. Wilson, 24 July 1883, a fascinating eye-witness account of the meeting.
146. FLW Box 1 letters 793–856: Wilson's correspondence about the NA's

action.

147. *Hansard*, 3rd series (28 July 1884), 291 Col. 687.

148. *Shield*, 3 Nov. 1883, pp. 258–61; NA EC Minutes, 15 and 29 Oct. 1883.

149. FLW Box 79 letter 960: Stuart to Chamberlain, 5 Nov. 1883.

150. Ibid., letter 974: Stuart to H.J. Wilson, 2 Dec. 1883.

151. NA EC Minutes, 4 Feb. 1884.

152. *Shield*, 16 Feb. 1884, pp. 25–31; Liverpool University Library (Butler MSS) MS 8.4(2): Josephine Butler to A.S. Butler, 10 Feb. 1884.

153. NA EC Minutes, 16 Feb. 1885.

154. NA, *Annual Report for 1883–84*, p. 22; see also J.L. and B. Hammond, *James Stansfeld*, pp. 242–4.

155. FLB 4019: Herbert Gladstone to Josephine Butler, 20 June 1884.

156. *Hansard*, 3rd series (28 July 1884) 291 Col.671ff.

157. NA EC Minutes, 13 and 27 Oct. 1884; *Shield*, 6 Sept. 1884, pp. 145–6.

158. *Shield*, 7 Feb. 1885, p. 13.

159. *Shield*, 15 Nov. 1884, pp. 173–5; NA EC Minutes, 18 and 27 Apr., 4 May 1885.

160. For the enormous amount of work done by the NA during the campaign, see *Annual Report for 1885–86*, pp. 8–14 and *Shield*, 12 Dec. 1885, pp. 157–61.

161. LNA, *Annual Report for 1885*, p. 17.

162. Sheffield Central Library (Wilson MSS) MD 2615: a set of letters from Wilson to his family describing his first weeks in parliament and the steps the repeal group were taking to force themselves forward. Predictably, Wilson expressed his admiration for the discipline of the Irish party.

163. J.A. Spender, *Life of Sir Henry Campbell-Bannerman G.C.B.*, vol. I (1923), p. 105.

164. *Shield* 20 Mar. 1886, pp. 37–46; FLW Box 1 letter 966: H.J. Wilson to Mrs H.J. Wilson, 17 Mar. 1886; FLB 4071: Mrs Tanner to Josephine Butler, 17 Mar. 1886.

165. J. Stuart, *Reminiscences* (1911), p. 221; see also Hammonds, *James Stansfeld*, p. 258; A.B. Cooke and J. Vincent, *The Governing Passion: Cabinet Government and Party Politics in Britain, 1885–86* (Hassocks, 1974), p. 16.

166. BL Add. MSS 44496 (Gladstone Papers) f.44: Stansfeld to Gladstone, 26 Mar. 1886; Stansfeld MSS (in family hands): Stansfeld to Mrs W.A. Case, 30 Mar. 1886.

167. Liverpool University Library (Butler MSS) MS 8.4(3) B1: Josephine Butler to her children, Easter Sunday, 1886.

9 POLITICAL CONNECTIONS AND ALLIANCES IN THE REPEAL CAMPAIGN

I

> So long as the Tories are in power we shall not carry our point, but when the day for a Liberal government to be returned comes, we shall be on the winning side.[1]

Thus wrote J.P. Gledstone in 1876 and we have seen how enthusiastically provincial repealers pursued a policy of collaboration with the Liberal party. By no means all Conservatives, however, supported the Acts: Henley, Russell Gurney and Sir Robert Fowler were notable opponents, and a Conservative repealer reminded the *Shield* that the Acts had all been carried by Liberal governments.[2] But appeals to the Tories were never really on, and Mrs Butler was surely correct in doubting their willingness 'to make political capital of our question . . . they are too much attached to the Acts in general'.[3] By 1878 the *Shield* was unmoved to hear that some Conservatives were trying to get their candidate at the Reading by-election to oppose the Acts; a Liberal would be a better supporter of Johnstone's bill.[4]

Conservative repealers were never of much importance as a proportion of their party, whereas the proportion of Liberals who were repealers increased over the five major divisions on the Acts from 15.9 per cent to 40.5 per cent. On the opposite side, Liberal supporters of the Acts declined in number and importance within the party, until by 1883 they were as weak within it as Conservative repealers were within theirs. Conservative supporters of the Acts were already stronger than Liberals by 1873, and in this year and in the two divisions of the Disraeli parliament, over half the party voted for the Acts. Within the Liberal party, MPs who described themselves as being on the 'left' largely went for repeal. (See Tables 9.1 and 9.2.)

After the confusion of the 1870 vote there was never any doubt about their allegiance: furthermore, since there was no consistency in *Dod*'s labels (see Table 9.2), radicals such as Trevelyan, Rylands and P.A. Taylor have to be omitted because they were content to describe themselves as Liberals. By 1883 to be a Liberal meant that an MP might well be a repealer; to be an advanced Liberal or a radical meant

234

Table 9.1: Party Votes in the Five Major Repeal Divisions on the CD Acts

24 May 1870	— Repeal Bill; debate adjourned 229:88	(Division List 84)
21 May 1873	— Repeal Bill; put off 6 months 251:128	(Division List 87)
23 June 1875	— Repeal Bill; put off 3 months 308:126	(Division List 152)
19 July 1876	— Repeal Bill; put off 2 months 224:102	(Division List 189)
20 April 1883	— Repeal resolution *carried* 182:110	(Division List 68)

	Repealers						Non-repealers					
	Con.		Lib.		Total		Con.		Lib.		Total	
1870	30	10.7%	60	15.9%	90	13.7%	83	29.8%	148	39%	231	35%
1873	16	5.7%	114	30.2%	130	19.8%	146	52.5%	107	28.2%	253	38.6%
1875	20	5.7%	108	36%	128	19.7%	236	67%	74	24.6%	310	47.5%
1876	11	3.1%	93	31%	104	15.9%	183	52%	43	14.3%	226	34.8%
1883	16	6.7%	168	40.5%	184	28.2%	85	35.6%	27	6.5%	112	17.4%

Notes: All totals include tellers.
Party totals are expressed as percentages of party strength at the beginning of each parliament, Home Rulers being counted as Liberals. (Source: T. Lloyd, *General Election of 1880*, pp. 5, 134.) Repeal and non-repeal totals are expressed as percentages of the size of the House of Commons (658 in 1868, 652 in 1874 and 1880).

Table 9.2: Votes of MPs in CD Acts Divisions Who Described Themselves as 'Advanced Liberal' or 'Radical'

	1870		1873		1875		1876		1883	
	R	NR	R	NR	R	NR	R	NR	R	NR
Advanced Liberal	7	5	10	—	11	—	10	—	15	1
Radical	4	3	5	—	7	—	9	—	9	—

Notes: Descriptions from *Dod's Parliamentary Companion* (1870–85).
R: repeal; NR: non-repeal.

that he probably would be.

If we examine the regional breakdown of three divisions (disregarding the confused 1870 division and the government-whipped 1875 vote), we find repeal strength chiefly in English borough constituencies which provided at least half the vote in each of the three. (See Tables 9.3 and 9.4.)

Elsewhere, substantial support was found in Scotland, rather less in Wales and Ireland. Regulationists came overwhelmingly from England. Wales and Scotland soon declined, and by 1883 Ireland was the only 'fringe' to provide a reasonable number of supporters of the Acts. County conservatives were the largest single group, but they never attained the same significance as did borough Liberals on the other side.

The predominance of borough Liberals was predictable — this was where the radicals were found, and this is where the gains were made in 1880 which made repeal possible in 1883. Another factor suggests itself: this is nonconformity's political base. After 1880, of 90 nonconformist MPs, 78 sat for boroughs, mostly in England,[5] and their increase at that election can be directly related to gains in the boroughs. The support of borough members gave repeal a useful propaganda advantage over the enemy. The borough electorate was so much greater than that in the counties that defeats could be explained away as resulting from defects in the representative system. It was argued that the size of the electorate on each side demonstrated the strength of popular support for repeal. Thus (to take the most extreme example) success in 1883 could be made to look this impressive:[6]

Table 9.3: The Divisions of 1873, 1876 and 1883 Distinguishing Regional Patterns (The percentages for Liberals are of total repealers, those for Conservatives are of total non-repealers.)

| | 21 May 1873 | | | | 19 July 1876 | | | | 20 April 1883 | | | |
| | Repeal | | Non-repeal | | Repeal | | Non-repeal | | Repeal | | Non-repeal | |
	L	C	L	C	L	C	L	C	L	C	L	C
England	86 (61.5%)	17	73 (45.5%)	120	63 (60.5%)	8	20 (65%)	146	112 (61%)	12	14 (65%)	73
Wales	4 (2.8%)	0	11 (1.9%)	5	4 (3.8%)	0	4 (4.4%)	10	14 (7.6%)	0	5 (0.8%)	1
Scotland	22 (15.7%)	1	10 (1.5%)	4	21 (20.2%)	2	3 (3.5%)	8	26 (14.1%)	0	1 (0.8%)	1
Ireland	9 (6.3%)	1	14 (7.2%)	19	5 (4.8%)	1	15 (6.6%)	15	16 (8.7%)	3	9 (5.3%)	6
University	0	0	1	5	0	0	1	4	0	1	0	2
Totals	121	19	109	153	93	11	43	183	168	16	29	83
	140		263*		104		226		184		112	

Notes: All divisions include tellers, that for 1873 includes pairs also.
*This total includes one unclassifiable vote as the *Shield* used a defective division list.
Source: *Shield*, 7 June 1873, p. 188; 29 July 1876, p. 246; 1 May 1883, p. 137.

	Repealers	Non-repealers
Liberal borough electorate	1,016,371	20,637
All other Liberal electorates	518,941	107,370
Conservative electorate	139,013	538,115
	1,674,325	666,122

Such tables were even more cheering when a defeat had to be explained away. This ruse had an impressive radical pedigree. In 1849 the defeat of Cobden's arbitration motion was mitigated by noting that MPs in its favour represented four million inhabitants, those against only three million.[7]

Table 9.4: The Divisions of 1873, 1876 and 1883 Distinguishing English Boroughs and Counties (The percentages for Liberals are of total repealers, those for Conservatives are of total non-repealers.)

	Liberal Repealers		Conservative Non-repealers	
	All England	English Boroughs	All England	English Counties
1873	86 61.5%	76 54.5%	120 45.5%	78 29.6%
1876	63 60.5%	57 55%	146 65%	79 35%
1883	112 61%	93 50.5%	73 65%	43 38.4%

Source: *Shield*, 7 June 1873, p. 188; 29 July 1876, p. 246; 1 May 1883, p. 137.

Two parliamentary preconditions for the unexpected repeal success in 1883 can be identified. Given the almost complete party identification on the issue, the Liberal victory in 1880 was crucial in providing the requisite Liberal majority — of the 147 MPs voting in 1883 who had been elected since the previous division in 1876, 101 were repealers. This is where pressure from within the party had counted; Stuart later described how Cambridge Liberals had organised a women's petition, a resolution to Gladstone from the Liberal 200, letters to doubtful MPs from leading Liberals and memorials from clergy, nonconformist ministers and JPs.[8] Secondly the proportion of Conservatives prepared to continue defending the Acts had slumped to 35.6 per cent (of a party which had already suffered a 17.4 per cent loss at the 1880 election). The 1883 division was the smallest of the five major ones surveyed; only 292 MPs voted, so with 9 pairs and 4 tellers a total of 314 members expressed an opinion.[9] Of the 344 who were absent, the *Shield* knew the opinions of 226, and these divided firmly in favour of the Acts — 159 were supporters (97 of them Conservatives) and only 67 repealers. Had they voted in any numbers, the majority would have been threatened, but the force behind the Acts had withered. Repealers naturally attributed this to popular pressure persuading MPs to abstain, but it may equally well have been weariness at the prospect of having to face the untiring pressure of a zealously conducted agitation.

This strategy was far from unique; the repeal movement was but a part of a network of interrelated agitations for moral and social improvement which were increasingly exerting pressure on and through the Liberal party. And by the 1880s they had every expectation of being listened to; as Wilson noted grimly in December 1882:

the backbone of the Liberal party is more and more teetotal and philanthropic in its sympathies. If this ministry is going to ignore these truths, and think that the Nonconformists and Radicals and Teetotallers who won the Elections in 1880 will be satisfied with killing the Egyptians, and attending to Electric Lighting and Bankruptcy Bills, I am afraid they will ere long be repeating the history of 1873—74.[10]

The methods employed by repealers were common to all reform movements: the subscription-based popular organisation with its bureaucracy, public meetings, publications, parliamentary campaign and demonstration of working-class support, were all to be found in the campaign for disestablishment, temperance, repeal of the Vaccination Acts and international arbitration — to name only the most prominent.[11] The only difference of method between the repeal movement and the rest is that repealers did not regard the May Meetings, centred on Exeter Hall, as necessarily the apex of their year — but they did advertise in the 'May Meeting Guide', and indeed received a reduction in price because of the proprietor's sympathy.[12] Common membership also bound reform movements together; none of its prominent activists was exclusively committed to repeal — Baxter Langley, William Shaen and Henry Wilson have all been observed embracing a wide variety of causes, and catholicity of agitational taste was the basis of this sort of political life.[13] This is not to suggest that everybody supported everything. Osborne Morgan was a bitter enemy

both of repeal and women's suffrage, yet in every other respect he
was a model reformer: he was for disestablishment and the Permissive
Bill, his maiden speech had been for the abolition of University
Tests, he carried the Burials Acts in 1880 (after trying for ten
successive sessions), as Judge Advocate he abolished flogging in the
army in 1881, and he worked to improve the material conditions of
women — helping women's education and pushing the Married
Women's Property Act through in 1882.[14] Obviously one or two
lapses are permissible before a reformer ceases to figure in the list
of 'all purpose radicals'.

All these movements shared a common pedigree — they venerated
the memory of the anti-slavery and anti-Corn Law agitations; both
successful, both models for reformers of how pressure should be
applied. Even more directly their success released experienced men
for other work — Isichei observes that 'Victorian agitations tended to be
each others' heirs, and the success of the League freed energies for
the Peace Movement'.[15] The anti-Corn Law League showed reformers
how to organise, and its leaders were seen as exemplars of disinterested
statesmanship; however, as W.S. Jevons observed about the UKA,
reformers drew a simplistic moral from the League's success — namely,
that any sufficiently determined agitation would inevitably secure its
ends. They forgot that the League's objective had differed completely from theirs, and had been politically altogether more
promising.[16] Not all reformers were so crude. Edmondson, discussing
tactics in the aftermath of the 1883 resolution, urged repealers to
offer the government 'a golden bridge over which to retreat with
honour' and cited anti-slavery and the League as precedents.[17]

The anti-slavery campaign as the epitome of disinterested human-
itarianism was an earlier and even more potent inspiration than the
League. Morality vanquishing expediency was exactly the point for
most reformers: Henry Wilson likened the Bulgarian atrocities
agitation to anti-slavery, while repealers so admired American
abolitionism that they appropriated the term for themselves — an
early work on the movement was entitled *The New Abolitionists* and
the BCGF's eventual title was International Abolitionist Federation.[18]
In 1870 the *Shield* praised George Thompson, 'the advocate of human
freedom', for speaking at a repeal meeting, while, for Mrs Butler,
William Lloyd Garrison represented the cause of humanity — during
an English tour in 1877 he stayed in her house and was introduced
to her children in the hope that they might be imbued with his fixity
of principle — and she made the comparison explicit by talking of 'the

active persecution and ignoble treatment to which the modern reformers like the abolitionists in America, were at times subjected'.[19] Garrison's declared opposition to the Acts and his pronounced moral suasion attitudes commended themselves to repealers; Mrs Butler's recovery from serious illness in 1875 was aided by having a 'fat book' on the anti-slavery campaign read out – the thought of the two causes, both combating suffering, helped to revive her.[20]

One attitude which the anti-CD Acts campaign illustrates supremely well is the hostility and reserve towards London displayed by provincial reformers. This, however, was nothing out of the ordinary: W.S. Caine said that he was not much impressed by the NA 'but then *all* London Societies are badly managed', and ingrained suspicion of the metropolis compounded with bureaucratic difficulties – 'friction between the local branch and the central organisation' – caused rancour and wasted effort in many a reform movement.[21]

The violence of the repeal movement's early approaches to parliament is also to be found elsewhere: enthusiastic petitioning, deluges of propaganda (usually aimed more at comforting the faithful than at converting anyone), assaults on MPs in their constituencies, above all a refusal to be in any way discouraged in adversity – this was the style of popular radicalism. In 1873 the *Herald of Peace* showed that it had the measure of the enemy:

> What we have most to apprehend . . . is not so much hostility as indifference . . . The only way to remedy this is to galvanise members by a stream of electricity from without, and to awaken their sympathies by proving that the subject is one which is near to the hearts of a large body of their constituents.[22]

The provincial reformer wanted an MP willing to load himself up with a portmanteau of worthy causes. Such men could be found, though they were always a minority in the House and were labelled 'faddists' or 'crotcheteers'. Those unwilling to rise to the required standard were penalised (usually by electoral pressure). Backhouse would not support Isaac Lowthian Bell, 'a miserable whig', because of his refusal to support disestablishment, repeal of the CD Acts, repeal of the 25th clause and the Permissive Bill.[23] Mundella expressed his contempt for MPs who ran away before the division on the Permissive Bill to avoid antagonising one side or the other by their vote.[24] Turnouts for reform divisions were low: the number voting in the five major divisions on repeal averaged 350 (53.7 per cent of the House);

the Permissive Bill's average between 1868 and 1875 was only 338 (51.1 per cent); the successful vote on arbitration in 1873 was carried in an extremely small house of 190 (28.8 per cent).

Fear, however, is not the only explanation. Most reformers outside parliament shrank from accepting (if, indeed they realised) that the House of Commons operated totally different political conventions to theirs. Chapel-type oratory and moral fervour were all very well in the north, but they appeared ridiculous at Westminster, and those who refused to adapt to the norms of the parliamentary club diminished their credibility within it.[25] Most MPs were simply not interested in reformers' preoccupations; they would discuss reform 'fads' only when compelled to do so. Mundella believed that 'the natural repugnance of the majority to enquire into such a disagreeable business induces Parliament to maintain the [C.D.] Acts in the belief that they are promoting order, decency and morality'.[26]

Reformers in parliament were often given a rough time. A sympathetic hearing was given only to those willing to defer and adapt to the traditions of the House. One such was Edward Miall whose 'prudent and judicious conduct' even though he was a 'radical parson turned politician' earned him the praise of an experienced commentator:

> Mr. Miall . . . was well aware that the House of Commons was not a public meeting, and that to speak there effectively on such a subject was altogether a very different matter from writing in the columns of the *Nonconformist* or addressing an audience of willing listeners at Crosby Hall; and therefore, not withstanding the expressed disapprobation of some of his too zealous followers . . . he bided his time, never attempted to bully the House, nor obtruded himself and his opinions upon it when it was unwilling to learn.[27]

Only in the 1880s, when the parliamentary Liberal party was increasingly composed of such men, did reformers secure some measure of acceptance — thus when Stuart entered parliament in 1884, Edward Hamilton thought he would do well, despite his 'nasty crotchets'.[28]

Reformers could be appallingly naive: George Gillett, 'a representative religious philanthropist' was said by Ellis to be 'a very good fellow but not the faintest political instincts', he 'eyes politicians, MPs and such people as me rather dubiously'.[29]

Gillett was an unworldly dreamer, better at planning a purity crusade than a campaigning strategy; F.W. Newman was positively eccentric in his obsessive support of every reform cause — he described himself as 'anti-everything', loved a struggle and preferred to be on the weaker side.[30] Even if they avoided crankiness, reformers could display shockingly poor judgement. Josephine Butler's fixation with repeal was such that she could not help promoting it to first place in the political scene given the slightest encouragement. After browbeating Bruce in 1871, she wrote of 'a new era coming' when 'Irish land bills and the like will not henceforth be the engrossing matter for parliaments to deal with'.[31]

Tactical crudity was the corollary to this obsessiveness; 'all or nothing' demands were common. Thus the UKA might well have thought itself fortunate to have a prominent Manchester Tory, W.R. Callendar, as a vice-president; but he was nonetheless indignantly rebuked by the Alliance's secretary when he conciliated the Manchester Licensed Victuallers by seeking and obtaining their endorsement in 1874.[32] For many reformers sheer hard work, zeal and persistence took the place of realistic consideration of the problems involved; an anti-vaccinationist declared in 1877 that his movement had to 'get into a towering passion: it was not enough to have a good cause. No reform movement has ever been gained by argument alone.'[33] Why bother thinking about tactics when morality was so obviously on one's side? Thus many a cause was spoilt by the tedious repetition of internally directed propaganda, often marred by exaggeration.[34] All this suggests that reformers were as much concerned to demonstrate their own virtuous activity as actually to win their struggle. The moral uplift of doing that which was right, possibly even the satisfactions of office holding, could become ends in themselves. In the repeal movement a more realistic attitude was emerging in the 1880s. Wilson remained contemptuous of Londoners, but his radicalism became saner, more directed; when it was thought that Stansfeld might get back into office in 1882, Wilson viewed the prospect without concern — people should do things other than repeal, besides which it would be good to have a friend on the front bench.[35] But London repealers did not share this more worldly attitude, and their stubborn refusal to compromise with political reality showed them to be still firmly located in the half-world of self-validating, self-satisfying reform activity; as J.E. Ellis said in 1883 when vexed by the NA: 'There is an element in this Repeal agitation which does not want to die out.'[35]

II

Feminism is a good place to start tracing the repeal movement's connections with other causes. The Acts were all about morality and
sexuality, and those concerned to repeal them could reasonably be
supposed to be in favour of improving the status of women generally.
In the LNA the movement had a female auxiliary of real importance
in the general feminist front, but what of male repealers? Were they
committed to the women's cause?

Stansfeld certainly was. When he retired in 1895 the *Review of
Reviews* called him women's 'foremost champion' and added that
he 'held a watching brief on behalf of women, and whether he was in
office or out of it made no difference in the assiduity with which he
served the cause of his fair clients'.[37] Besides championing repeal
and consistently supporting female suffrage, Stansfeld had appointed
the first woman Poor Law Inspector in 1873 and had played a leading
part in the campaign for women's medical education.[38] The leaders
of the women's movement presented him with a memorial of their
gratitude upon his retirement, and after his death a fund was raised
to set up the Stansfeld Trust which employed a scrutineer to check
legislation from the feminist viewpoint. Wilson too supported
women's suffrage, though as a sound party man he worried about
the effect which too narrow an extension of the franchise would have
on the Liberal vote. Despite his wife's suffragist enthusiasm, he was
on the point of voting against it in 1892, until the brutality of anti-
suffrage arguments recalled him to the women's cause.[39]

The *Shield* argued from the first that the repeal movement could
only help the suffrage campaign, and many supporters believed that
the Acts had been passed so easily because women lacked the vote.[40]
Josephine Butler was a convinced suffragist who argued that the vote
would spell the end of the Acts — and she cited regulationists who
also believed this.[41] In the early 1880s she drew women's attention
to the municipal vote which, in the subjected districts, could
be used 'to purify the governing bodies of men tainted with the evil
system around them'.[42] By then, however, the two movements are
often found acting in tandem; LNA branches were carrying motions
in favour of both repeal and women's suffrage, and when in 1884
the *Shield* published an article rhetorically asking 'ought repealers
to be in favour of women's suffrage', the answer was of course 'yes'.[44]

In parliament, regulationists were the mainstay of the anti-
suffrage vote; 65.5 per cent of MPs opposed to the Women's
Disabilities Bill in 1870 also voted against repeal Bills; by 1876 the

proportion had risen to 70 per cent. In 1883, Hugh Mason failed to carry a women's suffrage resolution by a much smaller margin (132:116) than was usual, and as with the 1883 repeal resolution, the big change lay in the absence of a large number of anti-suffrage regulationists — their proportion of the total anti-suffrage vote slumped to 25 per cent and turnout was well down. This parallel change in the fortunes of repeal and suffrage after 1880 is noteworthy — though, unlike repealers, the suffragists suffered a shattering defeat in the following year. Repealers provided between 40 per cent and 52 per cent of suffrage votes and maintained their proportion consistently.[44] In general the leaders of the two sides in each case lined up consistently: prominent repealers such as Stansfeld and Jacob Bright were enthusiastic suffragists; their leading opponents, Puleston, Osborne Morgan, Cavendish-Bentinck opposed votes for women. Leading anti-suffragists such as E.P. Bouverie, A.J.B. Beresford-Hope and J.H. Scourfield also supported the Acts.

Anti-military feeling was strong in the repeal movement; as early as July 1870 Baxter Langley was delightedly reporting in the *Herald for Peace*:

> how completely the agitation against the C.D. Acts is taking the form of an anti-military movement. Wherever I go my Peace arguments are enthusiastically cheered . . . there is this healthy sentiment amongst working-men and middle-class politicians.[45]

Repealers regarded the existence of a standing army as an inducement to vice, and were glad to join the peace movement's attack on militarism. The two agitations were seen as going hand in hand and supporters believed that success in one would mightily reinforce the other.[46] Edmund Jones, when a delegate of the Liverpool Workmen's Peace Association to the Paris Peace Congress in 1875, declared:

> Probably there would never have been a Contagious Diseases Act in this country but for the standing army which has furnished an excuse to men who desired one, that provision must be made for our soldiers to keep them healthy, even at the expense of the wives and daughters of England.[47]

Mundella included the monstrous expense and 'horrible' moral consequences of it in a general condemnation of the whole idea of a professional army, but repealers had a more specific objection when they condemned those army regulations which prevented most soldiers from marrying.[48] This encouragement of the market in vice was the nub of their argument against the armed forces — or rather the army, for the existence of a 'standing' navy was never attacked. However, the military interest's power to obstruct repeal incurred a dispropor- tionate amount of odium. One repealer was so angered by this that he wanted to make military men ineligible to sit in the House of Commons, and the *Shield* regularly enumerated and berated the strength of the military there.[49] Mundella, in 1872, described the House as 'full of soldiers and sailors and others who regard the C.D. Acts as models of good legislation'.[50]

Since they faced a common enemy, there was every reason for the peace and repeal movements to work together, which they often did: Josephine Butler addressed meetings of the Peace Society and supplied them with speakers, and in turn the 'Captains' of the Peace Society at York are to be found helping the NCL to advertise a meeting addressed by Stansfeld in 1879.[51] Furthermore, the two movements shared a concern for higher standards of citizenship, both were interested in the soldier as a moral being and a citizen, and this identification can only have helped the repeal cause given that the Peace Society was much more of a 'respectable' body, well regarded by the press.

Its parliamentary leaders — Henry Richard, Thomas Burt, Sir Alfred Illingworth, Sir Wilfrid Lawson, Sir Joseph Whitwell Pease, Peter Rylands, Henry Labouchere, Samuel Whitbread — all voted for repeal; in seven divisions spread over three parliaments a constant majority of anti-military voters were repealers — in all cases over 60 per cent. The presence of government tellers defending the military side in each case did not deter them from voting against military expenditure or adventures.[52]

Repealers believed that the army was closely linked with the aristocracy, and audiences loved to hear the two denounced together, for the immorality of the upper classes was another stock-in-trade of every repeal speaker — and very much tied to their hostility to parliament and metropolitan sophistication.[53] A constant feature in Josephine Butler's writings is the comparison of upper-class ignorance or hostility with lower-class commitment: 'No peeresses there, but the humblest people' was her description of a Salvation Army meeting; indeed peeresses approached her for advice on reclamation work.[54] When an Oxford clerical don praised the efforts of humble repeal workers, she exulted: 'what a cause ours is for bridging over religious and class prejudice!'[55]

Others shared her dislike for the upper classes. Edmund Jones inveighed against 'aristocratic licentious men' who seek 'to drag into the meshes our wives, sisters and daughters, and to endeavour to keep them fit for their vile purposes at the public expense';[56] and the *Shield* often discovered cases of officers' immorality being accepted while that of their men was punished.[57] The repeal campaign was fighting against a style of aristocratic libertinism which, by the 1870s and 1880s, was being successfully evicted from the upper reaches of society. In 1878 Josephine Butler welcomed the conversion to repeal of Lord Townshend as 'evidence that our principles are beginning slowly to permeate upwards' — furthermore, he founded the 'Association for the Improvement of Public Morals' precisely to influence those people (i.e. the upper class) who would not join existing repeal bodies.[58] However, as long as aristocratic debauchery remained a whipping-post for the movement, it provided a further link with the other radical agitations.

The repeal campaign's attitude to the state and interventionism was uncomplicated. Whereas other moral reform agitations with similar 'individualist-minded' memberships either needed the assistance of the state to achieve their aims (for instance temperance) or its cooperation to carry out their work effectively, as with the RSPCA, all repealers desired was that the state should cease its interference in areas more properly the concern of moral agencies.[59] They had no need to evolve justifications for calling in the state, indeed they could and did indulge in exaggerated criticism of the execution of the Acts, likening closed courts to the Star Chamber and suggesting that the Acts presaged the decline of municipal government.[60] Indeed repealers were suspicious of any legislation which might facilitate extension — they scrutinised a Sanitation Bill in 1874 lest it might enable local authorities to bring in regulation unobtrusively, and were roused to protest against the Factory Bill in 1877 because of the restrictions it placed on women's work.[61]

Many repealers objected to the Acts as reinforcing an expanding state which sapped the citizen's constitutional rights; Johnstone vigorously opposed state intervention, while J.W. Henley was one of the purest individualists in the House — opposing the Plimsoll agitation he suggested that the increase in the number of wrecks was related to the increase in legislation.[62] F.W. Newman's opposition to the Acts was grounded in his hatred of the state and desire to revitalise local institutions: as he put it, 'if law be centralized, it always lingers far beyond men's needs'.[63] For these men the Vigilance Association for the Defence of Personal Rights (VA), which grew out of the repeal movement in 1871, was an umbrella for their individualism and connected repeal with other anti-state agitations.[64] Initially dominated by Mrs Butler and Miss Becker, by 1880 the VA was in the hands of London repealers, J.H. Levy and Miss Lucy Wilson. It argued against a range of 'interfering' legislation and opposed compulsion in public health as weakening the resolve of the people to defend themselves.[65]

The VA and the repeal movement agreed that officials were to blame for the stealthy extension of state control, an interesting anticipation of a modern hypothesis. In 1874 the *Shield* caught a civil servant advocating extension of the Acts and the examination of merchant seamen, and two years later Wilson claimed that 'the official heads of the great spending departments' were implicated in spreading libels about Stansfeld.[66] But these titbits apart, repealers had no hard evidence to reply on. However, their assertion that the real enemy was not the government but its officials was probably well founded, and in the 1880s there was much speculation on the best means of circumventing the pernicious influence of civil servants and getting directly at ministers such as Hartington.[67]

The Metropolitan Police as agents of central authority were naturally regarded with great hostility; any evidence of their un-reliability was taken up with enthusiasm.[68] Indeed this hostility was quite unreasonably generalised into an attack on the behaviour of members of provincial forces — it is not clear what purpose was served by revealing police abuse outside the subjected districts.[69] Certainly repealers dreaded a European-style police tyranny over moral behaviour, but their chief practical concern was to prevent the centralisation of police forces. The 1877 Prisons Act, criticised by the VA as 'an alarming advance upon the path of centralisation and personal government', seemed a disturbing augury in this respect;[70] and an amendment by Rylands against transferring control of prisons to the government was well supported by repeal MPs who constituted 50 per cent of his minority.[71] Thereafter, the danger of a centralised police obsessed Josephine Butler whose correspondence is full of it, and in 1879 she published *Government by Police* which emphasised her belief in the virtues of local control.[72]

Fear of the state drew repealers closer to those inclined to shift the blame for the nation's woes onto the shoulders of 'meddling doctors'. At its most extreme this attitude is exemplified by the speaker at the VA's 1881 Annual Meeting who declared: 'we never had these small-pox panics before the establishment of the Medical Department of the Privy Council, but since it has been created, whenever a few cases occurred in the metropolis, the public mind was worked up into a state of panic about it'.[73] Certainly, the medical profession chose to associate itself closely with officialdom in order to help establish preventive medicine firmly; not surprisingly, their struggle provoked a libertarian backlash which paid too little attention to the purity of the doctors' motives.[74]

In one sense the doctors helped to create the grounds for opposition by exaggerating the results to be obtained by employing compulsion. Their failure was more evident in relation to the CD Acts than the Vaccination Acts, but in both cases the shattering of early, grandiose medical claims produced a fatal loss of confidence.[75] Further they tried to insist that they possessed a monopoly of knowledge, and that medical opinions, resting on expertise not available to the layman, should not be questioned.[76] Naturally this attitude provoked indignant opposition — Josephine Butler exploded after reading a letter in *The Times* from F.C. Skey:

> I am astounded at the audacity of his declaration 'Our profession *and our profession alone has a right to dictate* . . .' in the matter of the Contagious Diseases Acts! This kind of assertion, which I fear expresses the opinion of some of these aristocratic doctors is calculated to make the medical profession (as a friend expresses it) 'stink in the nostrils of the moral and religious people of England'.[77]

Obviously this sort of claim if proved even marginally doubtful would justifiably cause those opposed to medical pretensions to redouble their efforts; in 1876 the *Shield* talked about 'freedom from medical tyranny' being 'of more importance than any sanitary theory' and, as usual, self interest was cited as the motive for medical defence of the Acts (though with little justification when applied to the entire profession).[78] The doctors defended themselves clumsily, declining the opportunity of debates on repeal platforms (fair enough given the partial treatment usually meted out, but politically maladroit), and refusing to let repealers attack the Acts at BMA conferences.[79] Even more objectionably, the Social Science Association, the medical profession's loyal ally, succeeded in preventing repealers from presenting papers after they had won three successive victories in 1869, 1870 and 1871 — the Association's chairman for most of the period was G.W. Hastings, a regulationist Royal Commissioner and, although a lawyer, a member of the BMA.[80] Nevertheless the NA took social science congresses seriously and each year mounted a major propaganda effort to coincide with them; winning the attention of progressives was thought a worthwhile aim despite all the rebuffs visited on the movement.[81]

Dislike of what the *Pall Mall Gazette* sneeringly called 'the claims of medical experts to settle moral and legal questions without right of appeal' led the NA towards cooperation with the VA in a general onslaught on medical empire building.[82] Together they opposed additional powers for doctors in the Factory Bill of 1878, and in 1883 they objected to the compulsory notification of infectious diseases.[83] As to anti-vivisection, another movement assaulting medical pretensions, Stansfeld chaired the first meeting of the Victoria Street Society in December 1875, though once it was safely under way, he dropped into the background.[84]

The clearest parallels and similarities in attitudes to medicine are with the anti-vaccination campaign. Repealers were careful not to entangle themselves with the other movement — no point in fighting someone else's battle.[85] However, given the common enemy and inter-related memberships (the Hume-Rotherys, leading opponents of vaccination in the 1870s were repealers as was P.A. Taylor, their parliamentary champion in the 1880s), it is reasonable to expect the two movements to be treading the same path. After 1880, they do so to an uncanny degree: under its chairman, William Tebb, the London Society for the Abolition of Compulsory Vaccination pursued the same tactics as the repeal campaign in its latter stages — it directed its activities towards parliament, established its command of the statistical argument, began to discredit the assertions of the medical establishment and win doctors to its cause, and cultivated the working class (probably more successfully than did repealers).[86] In parliament, repealers were strongly identified with opposition to vaccination; they made up 58.5 per cent of the vote for the second reading of Pease's Penalties Bill in 1878 and 53 per cent of Taylor's majority on first reading of an anti-compulsion Bill in 1883.[87] These two movements successfully challenged the medical profession as part of a general (though by no means justified) reaction against its attempts to educate public opinion. They had no particular secret for success: hard work enabled them to puncture foolishly inflated medical claims; supple tactics enabled them to take advantage of this success.

Where the anti-vaccinationists had much in common with the

repealers, the temperance movement was admired more for what it was. After all, the UKA's aim was to persuade parliament to put restrictions on the drink traffic, while it could be argued that the repeal movement was, without in any way approving of it, trying to remove regulations on 'the traffic in vice'. *The Times* exploited the inconsistency in 1872: 'We hope the extreme solicitude for "civil liberty" will commend itself to those who are thinking of preventing their fellow countrymen from buying a glass of beer.'[88] However, the moral basis of the temperance case overcame such problems, and of the three leading repealers, H.J. Wilson was a devoted UKA man. Stansfeld, as a brewer, might have had difficulties, but he emphasised that his brewery refused to engage in the tied house trade, and indeed, made the supply of good beer to private residences sound positively philanthropic. He had no trouble from teetotallers, and his obituary in the *Morning Advertiser* was cool — the trade's organ regarded him politically as a suspect brewer.[89] Mrs Butler was no teetotaller, but she was enthusiastic about temperance methods: 'the idea of combatting sexual vice in the same vigorous and extensive manner in which drunkenness is combatted is one which everyone of us should strenuously support.'[90]

It was the excellence of temperance organisation, especially that of the UKA, which impressed repealers. Mrs Butler thought very highly of J.H. Raper, the UKA's parliamentary agent, who was advising Wilson on tactics by the 1880s; and much effort was put into trying to enlist the support of temperance societies.[91] This policy enjoyed some success. Josephine Butler worked effectively on the Good Templars, and other organisations declared their support.[92] That the UKA's tactical advice was sought is interesting, for, as W.S. Jevons argued in 1876, its refusal to accept anything less than its total demands made it 'the worst existing obstacle to temperance reform in the kingdom'; when Jevons's article was pointed out to the NA Executive Committee, it was received very coolly.[93] The Alliance did retreat slightly from its irreconcilable position when it adopted the local option resolution.[94] and the repeal movement followed it in this in the 1880s. It might be argued that Wilson and his provincial colleagues reassessed their tactics as part of a general appreciation of the need to tackle parliament more subtly, and in particular, through the Liberal party. In such a reassessment, the mighty UKA, strongest of all moral reform organisations naturally took the load.

In parliament the leading temperance radicals such as Lawson, Burt and W.S. Caine were repealers; the brewers' champions, Watney and Wheelhouse supported the Acts. Once again, J.W. Henley's determination to defend individual liberty at whatever cost, set him apart from other repealers — he is the one notable repealer to support the brewers' attacks on the 1872 Licensing Bill. In general, there is a striking consistency of voting behaviour between temperance and repeal: in the early 1870s both movements unsuccessfully put forward hopeless bills; repealers constituted between 53.5 per cent and 48 per cent of the temperance vote between 1870 and 1875; regulationists contributed between 64.5 per cent and 67.3 per cent of the drink vote.[95] After the 1880 election, the local option resolution was carried in 1880, 1881 and 1883, and again repealers were strongly for it — they were 45.7 per cent of the temperance vote in 1880, rising to 58 per cent in 1883.[96]

It was the example of vigorous organisation which made temperance important to the repeal movement — the UKA was the standard by which an agitation's energy, though not necessarily its effectiveness, was judged. In style so similar, in aim the repeal movement had a clearer task — and an easier one in that it did not have to face a formidable vested interest. In one sense though the drink interest did affect repeal. Josephine Butler recognised that the publicans had reason to fear the influence of women, and she saw their strength as a warning — in the subjected towns publicans often acted as brothel keepers which made her fear 'an equally formidable political power in the form of brothel keepers who would carry men into Parliament triumphantly, and *then* Prostitutes' petitions will be received with the utmost respect and their advice followed'.[97]

Feminism, anti-militarism, dislike of the state and of medical arrogance, admiration for the temperance movement — these are the clearest connections between the repeal movement and the network of reforming agitations. This list is, of course, far from exhaustive. The Liberation Society was as impressive as the UKA, and even more central to the political nonconformity, which was, as we have seen, a prominent force in repeal.[98] It too was moving towards the Liberal party, a fact which it recognised and welcomed. In parliament, repealers comprised about half the political nonconformity vote and, with the exception of Osborne Morgan, all its leaders — Miall, Dixon, Richard, Candlish — were repealers.[99]

What of the gamut of humanitarian and radical 'fads' which so bored the average MP in the 1870s and 1880s? Causes such as the attacks on the opium traffic (which, after the repeal of the CD Acts, became H.J. Wilson's speciality) or on the game laws; attempts to abolish capital punishment or to permit marriage with a deceased wife's sister? Evidence from an analysis of parliamentary divisions on these and other issues confirms the impression already given. MPs who voted for repeal constituted at least 40 per cent of the votes for other causes, often after 1880 considerably more. Regulationists went into the lobbies to defeat all manner of 'crotchets', and the picture on their side clouds after 1880, only because they were a smaller group given the low turnout in 1883 (it has to be remembered that repeal was one of the few successful agitations).

Opponents recognised the existence of a type of reformer who supported a range of fads promiscuously: Lucy quotes a peer parodying the all-purpose radical: 'I am a member of the National Liberal Club, a teetotaller and a passive resister. I have recently married my deceased wife's sister, and none of my children have been vaccinated.'[100] Similarly Matthew Arnold's Mr Bottles displayed an earlier range;[101] there was nothing original about making fun of reformers; indeed in so far as not all wits manifested Arnold's concern for the quality of life, such jokes become tedious and vulgar. However they do attest to the general recognition of a particular sort of reform linkage. Opponents of reform were happy to tar reformers with guilt by association: Osborne Morgan attacking the Women's Disabilities Bill in 1872 said that the only women who desired the vote were ones 'brooding over real or imaginary wrongs . . . such were the women who originated and sustained the miserable agitation for the repeal of the Contagious Diseases Acts',[102] and after suspension in 1883, Wemyss sardonically suggested that the triumphant repealers should concede local option on the Acts to the inhabitants of the subjected towns 'since they were so fond of it in the matter of drink'.[103]

The repeal movement joined together a remarkable number of agitations within this constellation of reform activity: it appealed (as did most of them) to the individualist, it was strongly moral in tone, humanitarian by instinct (despite all the problems about palliatives, there was a basic concern for the unfortunate women subjected to the Acts), and unlike most movements it attracted feminist support and gave it expression through the LNA, a particularly independent women's organisation. It was not the most important agitation by any means: the NEL had caused more of a stir, the UKA and Liberation Society were far larger, and in the heat of activity repealers often failed to put their movement in true perspective.[104] Yet it succeeded! Why did it escape the unhappy fate of its exemplars? We must now review its arguments and confront the riddle of its eventual triumph.

Notes

1. H. Ausubel, *In Hard Times: Reformers Among the Late Victorians* (New York, 1960), p. 131.

2. *Shield*, 14 Dec. 1872, pp. 1185–6.

3. FLB 5098: Josephine Butler to Mrs Ford, 30 Nov. 1872; see *Shield*, 20 June 1885, p. 89, for a half-hearted leader suggesting to the incoming Conservative government that it should repeal the Acts and leave the odium entirely with the Liberals.

4. *Shield*, 25 May 1878, p. 144.

5. J.F. Glaser, 'Nonconformity and Liberalism, 1868–1885. A Study in English Party History' (unpublished PhD thesis, Harvard University, 1948), pp. 486–7.

6. *Shield*, 1 May 1883, p. 138.

7. A.C.F. Beales, *The History of Peace* (1931), p. 78.

8. FLW Box 79 letter 980: James Stuart to H.J. Wilson, 26 Dec. 1883.

9. *Shield*, 1 May 1883, pp. 137–8.

10. Sheffield University Library (Wilson MSS) Box 5, enveolope 3: H.J. Wilson to Robert Leader, 13 Dec. 1882 (not sent).

11. See chapter 5 above; for further comments on methods generally found in reform movements see John Vincent, *The Formation of the British Liberal Party, 1857–1868* (1966), p. 75; Glaser, 'Nonconformity and Liberalism', pp. 328–37; Ausubel, *In Hard Times*, pp. 131–3.

12. NA EC Minutes, 25 Feb. 1878.

13. On interrelating memberships in general see Brian Harrison, 'The British Prohibitionists, 1853–1872' *International Review of Social History*, 15 (1970), pp. 375–465; Elizabeth Isichei, *Victorian Quakers* (Oxford, 1970), pp. 213–21; T.W. Heyck, 'British Radicals and Radicalism, 1874–1895: A Social Analysis' in R.J. Bezucha (ed.), *Modern European Social History* (1972), pp. 38–45.

14. *DNB Supplement*, p. 1064.

15. Isichei, *Victorian Quakers*, p. 221. See also D.A. Hamer, *The Politics of Electoral Pressure: A Study in the History of Victorian Reform Agitations* (1977), p. 57.

16. W.S. Jevons, *Methods of Social Reform* (1885), p. 247.

17. FWL Box 79 letter 940: Joseph Edmondson to H.J. Wilson, 13 Oct. 1883.

18. R.T. Shannon, *Gladstone and the Bulgarian Agitation* (1963), p. 142; James Stuart, *The New Abolitionists: A Narrative of a Year's Work* (1876). On antislavery see Howard Temperley, *British Antislavery 1833–1870* (1972),and for a splendid tribute to the movement, G. Kitson Clark, *The Making of Victorian England* (1962), pp. 20–1.

19. *Shield*, 11 Apr. 1870, p. 47; Ausubel, *In Hard Times*, p. 69; Josephine Butler, *Recollections of George Butler* (Bristol, *c.* 1893), p. 213; see above, chapter 6 for the influence of abolitionism on the LNA.

20. FLB 3409: James Stuart to Mrs H.J. Wilson, 18 May 1875.

21. FLB 3935: W.S. Caine to anon., 27 Aug. (1882?); Brian Harrison, 'Philanthropy and the Victorians' *Victorian Studies*, 9 (1966), p. 364.

22. *Herald of Peace*, June 1873, cited in A.C.F. Beales, *The History of Peace* (1931), p. 144.

23. FLB 3700: E. Backhouse to H.J. Wilson, 22 July 1875.

24. Sheffield University Library (Mundella-Leader correspondence) 13 May 1869; Brian Harrison, *Drink and the Victorians* (1971), p. 261.

25. See A.B. Cooke and J. Vincent, *The Governing Passion: Cabinet Government and Party Politics in Britain 1885–86* (Hassocks, 1974), pp. 21–2,

165; H.W. Lucy is the best reflection of this obsession with parliamentary behaviour – see his *Men and Manner in Parliament* (1874), *Sixty Years in the Wilderness* (1909) and a series of collected articles on successive parliaments.

26. Sheffield University Library (Mundella-Leader correspondence) *c.* 29 June–2 July 1876; see also David Roberts, *Victorian Origins of the British Welfare State* (New Haven, 1960), ch. 8.

27. William White, *The Inner Life of the House of Commons*, I (1897), pp. 18–22.

28. D.W.R. Bahlman (ed.), *The Diary of Sir Edward Hamilton* (Oxford, 1972), II, p. 737 (entry for 20 Nov. 1884).

29. FWL Box 78 letter 594: Ellis to H.J. Wilson, 18 Feb. 1883; letter 854: Ellis to H.J. Wilson, 1 Aug. 1883.

30. I.G. Sieveking, *Memoirs and Letters of F.W. Newman* (1909), pp. 7, 26.

31. FLB 3060: Josephine Butler to George Butler, July 1871.

32. Paul Smith, *Disraelian Conservatism and Social Reform* (1967), p. 190.

33. Roy M. MacLeod, 'Law, Medicine and Public Opinion: The Resistance to Compulsory Health Legislation' *Public Law* (1967), p. 126.

34. See Ausubel, *In Hard Times*, pp. 72–8.

35. FLW Box 78 letter 479: H.J. Wilson to R.F. Martineau (draft) 8 Dec. 1872.

36. FLW Box 78 letter 841: J.E. Ellis to H.J. Wilson, 19 July 1883.

37. *Review of Reviews*, 15 June 1895, p. 516.

38. See Jo Manton, *Elizabeth Garrett Anderson* (1965), pp. 250–1.

39. Sheffield Central Library, MD 2615: H.J. Wilson to Helen Wilson, 5 May 1892.

40. *Shield*, 1 May 1870, p. 74; *Shield*, 11 Dec. 1880, p. 159, Ashton Dilke MP arguing that the Acts would soon go if women had the vote.

41. FLB 3283: Josephine Butler to H.J. Wilson, 14 June 1883.

42. FLB 3975: address by Josephine Butler, *c.* 1882.

43. *Shield*, 5 Jan. 1884, p. 8, Norwood LNA on repeal and suffrage; 1 Mar. 1884, pp. 43–4; 15 Mar. 1884, pp. 50–1, the article was by the secretary of the same LNA branch.

44. See division lists for second readings of women's disabilities Bill on 4 May 1870 (DL 6) and 26 Apr. 1876 (DL 86), and for Mason's resolution on 6 July 1883 (DL 181).

45. Quoted in *Shield*, 11 July 1870, p. 162.

46. Ibid., pp. 158–62.

47. *National League Journal*, 1 Sept. 1875, p. 13.

48. FLB 3202: Mundella to H.J. Wilson, 23 Nov. 1872; on criticism of a celibate army, see Josephine Butler, *Personal Reminiscences of a Great Crusade* (1896), pp. 21, 64; *Shield*, 22 Apr. 1876, p. 131 (Lydia Becker speaking to the Lancs. and Yorks. International Arbitration Society).

49. *Shield*, 28 Jan. 1871, p. 371, Mr John Ashworth speaking at Bradford; the chairman of the meeting felt obliged to say something complimentary about military men in parliament to soften this extreme statement; *Shield*, 4 Sept. 1876, p. 268, estimated 'war members' strength to be 240 compared with 142 'commercial members'. This estimate must have been based on a generous definition of 'war member' – J.A. Thomas, *The House of Commons 1832–1901. A Study of its Economic and Functional Character* (Cardiff, 1939) estimates the gradually declining military strength to be: 1868 – 117; 1874 – 109; 1880 – 94; 1885 – 71.

50. FLB 3200: Mundella to H.J. Wilson, 20 Nov. 1872.

51. FLB 3913: Josephine Butler to 'Friends of Peace' in Bristol, 18 May (1974/75?) introducing a speaker; NCL, *6th Report for 1879 and 1880*.

52. See division lists on Mundella's opposition to army estimates, 23 Mar.
1871 (DL 31); Richard's arbitration motion, 8 July 1873 (DL 8); Lawson's
motion on size of land forces on 9 Mar. 1875 (DL 18) and 6 Mar. 1876 (DL 20);
Rylands's motion against annexation of the Transvaal, 21 Jan. 1881 (DL 8);
Richard's motion against treaties lacking parliamentary consent, 29 Apr. 1881
(DL 188); Labouchere's opposition to Lord Alcester's annuity, 19 Apr. 1883
(DL 65).

53. See, for example, Ashton Dilke's speech at Newcastle, 12 Nov. 1880,
reported *Shield*, 11 Dec. 1880, p. 159 — every attack on the aristocracy greeted
with applause.

54. FLB 3925: Josephine Butler to George Butler, 4 May 1882.

55. FLB 3958: Josephine Butler to Mrs Tanner, 4 Nov. 1882.

56. FLB 3378: address to working men signed by Edmund Jones, 1875.

57. See *Shield*, 27 Sept. 1873, pp. 314–16; 20 July 1878, pp. 204–5.

58. FLW Box 5 letter 452: Josephine Butler to repealers, 24 Aug. 1878
(circular letter).

59. *Shield*, 29 Mar. 1873, pp. 97–8, leader: 'The tendency of recent social
legislation'.

60. *Shield*, 3 May 1873, pp. 137–8, leader: 'Closed courts and sharp
practice'; 22 Oct. 1870, pp. 267–8; for justifications of state intervention see
Brian Harrison, 'State Intervention and Moral Reform in Nineteenth-century
England' in P. Hollis (ed.), *Pressure from Without* (1974), pp. 298–304.

61. *Shield*, 1 Aug. 1874, p. 164; 25 Aug. 1877, pp. 225–56; see also VA,
Annual Report for 1878, p. 6.

62. Smith, *Disraeli Conservatism*, p. 145; Tory regulationists such as Pakington,
Elphinstone and Wheelhouse supported Plimsoll.

63. I.G. Sieveking, *Memoirs and Letters of F.W. Newman* (1909), p. 295.

64. For the VA see Harrison, 'State Intervention', p. 316; Edward Bristow,
'The Liberty and Property Defence League and Individualism' *Historical Journal*,
18 (1975), pp. 772–4.

65. See VA, *Annual Report for 1872*, pp. 4, 6–10.

66. *Shield*, 1 Oct. 1874, pp. 181–3; FLW Box 2 letter 524: H.J. Wilson to
NCL EC, 14 Feb. 1876.

67. *Shield*, 15 Nov. 1884, pp. 173–5; FLW Box 78 letter 633: J.E. Ellis to
H.J. Wilson, 2 Mar. 1883.

68. *Shield*, 8 Nov. 1873, pp. 360–1, leader: 'The Police and the Public'; see Brian
Harrison, 'Animals and the State in Nineteenth-century England', *English
Historical Review*, 88 (1973), p. 811 for the RSPCA's wholly different relation-
ship with the police.

69. See *Shield*, 1 June 1874, p. 136–7, a Liverpool policeman falsely
accusing a woman of soliciting; 6 Apr. 1878, pp. 84–8, Leeds Police illegally
examining a woman.

70. VA, *Annual Report for 1878*, pp. 3–4.

71. DL 165, 3 July 1876, regulationists constituted 71 per cent of the
government's whipped majority.

72. FLW Box 5 letter 485: George Butler to H.J. Wilson and Joseph
Edmondson, 8 Oct. 1879.

73. VA, *Annual Report for 1881*, p. 25; see also Jeanne L. Brand, *Doctors and
the State: The British Medical Profession and Government Action in Public
Health, 1870–1912* (Baltimore, 1965), pp. 46–50.

74. Ibid., pp. 232–5; see also Kitson Clark, *Victorian England*, pp. 100–7,
261 and for the cheese paring attitude of the Treasury towards public health in
this period, Roy M. MacLeod, 'The Frustration of State Medicine, 1880–1899',
Medical History, 11 (1967), pp. 15–40.

75. For the Vaccination Acts see Roy M. MacLeod, 'Law, Medicine and Public Opinion: the Resistance to Compulsory Health Legislation' *Public Law* (1967), pp. 210–11.

76. See Dr Elizabeth Garrett, *An Enquiry into the Character of the Contagious Diseases Acts of 1866–69* (1870), pp. 3–5.

77. *Times*, 19 Feb. 1872, p. 12; FLB 3321: Josephine Butler to Dr W. Carter, 21 Feb. 1872.

78. *Shield*, 1 Feb. 1876, p. 33; FLB 3134: Josephine Butler to repealers, 12 Mar. 1872.

79. *Shield*, 9 Sept. 1871, pp. 647–8, Bell Taylor alleging that he had been refused permission to read a repeal paper to the BMA conference; see also LNA, *Annual Report for 1883*, p. 43, reporting that the BMA conference slipped a pro-Acts motion quietly through.

80. For Hastings and the Association see Brian Rodgers, 'The Social Science Association, 1857–1886' *The Manchester School*, 20 (1952), pp. 283–310. Hastings also obstructed discussion of the Permissive Bill in the 1860s, see Harrison, *Drink and the Victorians*, p. 238.

81. NA, *Annual Report for 1874–75*, pp. 16–17, describes the work associated with the Glasgow SSC of 1874 – 70,000 leaflets were distributed and the whole city canvassed.

82. *Pall Mall Gazette*, 21 Apr. 1883.

83. NA EC Minutes, 18 and 25 Feb. 1878; VA, *Annual Report for 1883*, p. 5, but see Birmingham Reference Library, *Minutes of the Birmingham Trades Council*, 6 (6 Jan. 1883), the council agreeing to support compulsory notification as in the interests of public health and to the advantage of the working class, by 23:3.

84. Stansfeld MSS (in family hands): Frances Power Cobbe to anon., 6 May (*c.* 1895).

85. *Shield*, 25 May 1872, pp. 951–2, denying an alleged link with anti-vaccination though without expressing any disapproval of the movement; NA EC Minutes, 30 Oct. and 6 Nov. 1882, not taking up offer of free copies of a tract by F.W. Newman because of explicit link between the two movements.

86. MacLeod, 'Law, Medicine and Public Opinion', pp. 189–211.

87. DL 95 (3 Apr. 1878); DL 4 (9 Feb. 1882).

88. *Times*, 15 Feb. 1872, p. 9 – when referring to Bruce's Bill.

89. For Stansfeld on temperance, see *Review of Reviews*, 15 June 1895, p. 521; *Morning Advertiser*, 18 Feb. 1898, 'he cannot be said to have been in touch with the trade on questions affecting its interest'.

90. FLW Box 5 letter 452: Josephine Butler to repealers, 24 Aug. 1878.

91. FLB 3160: Josephine Butler to Hudson Clark, 6 July 1872, praising Raper; FLW Box 2 letter 761: H.J. Wilson's list of temperance organisations which received NCL literature – principally the CETS, BTL, UKA, Lancs. and Yorks. Temperance Association, Yorks. Band of Hope Union.

92. See *Shield*, 17 Apr. 1880, pp. 59–60 for Josephine Butler's address to the Good Templars; *Protest*, 17 Apr. 1879, pp. 46–7, for the support of the order's head; see also *Shield*, 1 Dec. 1877, p. 296, for the support of the United Temperance Association.

93. W.S. Jevons, 'On the United Kingdom Alliance and Its Prospects of Success', *Methods of Social Reform* (1885), pp. 236–52; NA EC Minutes, 23 Feb. 1880; on Alliance methods generally, see Harrison, *Drink and the Victorians*, ch. 10, esp. pp. 226–38.

94. Welcomed by Jevons, see 'On the UK Alliance', pp. 253–76, 'Experimental Legislation and the Drink Traffic'.

95. See division lists on the Permissive Bill: DL 171 (13 July 1870); DL 63

(7 May 1873); DL 138 (16 June 1875).

96. See division lists on the local option resolution: DL 25 (18 June 1880); DL 249 (14 June 1881); DL 74 (27 Apr. 1888).

97. FLB 3255: Josephine Butler to H.J. Wilson, *c.* May 1873.

98. For the Liberation Society in this period see Glaser, 'Nonconformity and Liberalism', pp. 299–315; D.A. Hamer, *The Politics of Electoral Pressure*, ch. 8.

99. For suitable divisions illustrating the identification of the two causes, see for instance DL 277 (16 May 1873) (Miall's disestablishment motion) where repealers were 54 per cent of his minority, regulationists 64.5 per cent of the majority, or DL 193 (22 July 1873) (Dixon's amendment against clause 25 of the Education Bill), repealers 66 per cent of his minority, regulationists 58.8 per cent of the majority.

100. H.W. Lucy, *Sixty Years in the Wilderness* (1909), p. 251.

101. Quoted in Asa Briggs, *The Age of Improvement* (1959), p. 478).

102. *Hansard*, 3rd series (1 May 1872), 211 Col.56.

103. *Hansard*, 3rd series (12 June 1873), 289 Col.336; the *Shield* was furious about this intervention by the leader of the LPDL, see 16 June 1883, pp. 177–8. It illustrates the tensions between the two wings of the individualist movement touched on in Bristow, 'The Liberty and Property Reference League', pp. 773–4.

·104. See Sheffield Central Library (Wilson MSS), MD 5890: J. Chamberlain to H.J. Wilson, 10 Apr. 1876, reminding him that other causes (education, disestablishment, land reform, drink) are more important.

10 CONCLUSION

Inevitably in a study of the repeal campaign, little attention has been paid to the operation of the Acts themselves. This reflects the tendency amongst repealers to dismiss this sort of evidence as irrelevant to their moral attack. However, not all held this view, and during the 16-year course of the agitation their handling of the 'hygienic' case became sophisticated and effective.[1] But in any case, it would be careless to to take their argument at face value. Sooner or later, even the non-medical historian must face the question — did the Acts work?

Occasionally repealers were willing to concede the possibility that they did, but this was usually a tactical concession to sustain the point that 'risk-free opportunities' for vice could result only in profligacy on a grand scale.[2] Since they believed that it was wrong to protect men from the penalties of vice, it was more common for repealers to argue that the Acts provided only an illusory diminution in the incidence of venereal disease. They supported this by waging war on the reliability of official statistics which, the *Protest* joked in 1879, could be used to prove anything — even that the Rescue Society was in business to produce harlots.[3] There was much justifi-cation for this attack as the military departments were not above rigging the statistics to boost their case, and repealers had to be vigilant to prevent this. As an example, Nevins in 1884 discovered the Admiralty republishing figures which he had already forced them to acknowledge as incorrectly based. On this occasion they withdrew the figures rather gracelessly, and the *Shield* did some breast-beating about the uselessness of official statistics.[4] However, if repealers suspected the statistics for political reasons, we should suspect their veracity for medical ones. Diagnosis by means of the speculum was clearly inadequate, but the only means available, since effective scientific diagnosis of gonorrhoea was only possible after 1879 and the Wasserman blood test for syphilis was not introduced until 1906; furthermore, medical knowledge (despite the confidence of most doctors in their abilities — a confidence which is shaken by a reading of the sometimes ludicrous evidence given to Skey's committee) was inadequate. Doctors muddled the relationship between primary and secondary syphilis; and between syphilis and gonorrhoea; the causal organism of syphilis was not discovered until 1905, and Salvarsan was not available for its treatment until 1909.[5] Doubtless the figures were the best available in the state of medical knowledge in the 1870s and 1880s, but that still leaves them falling far short of the sort of reliability possible in the twentieth century. Indeed diagnoses may have been so erratic that the figures may be quite worthless; but they are all we have to go on.[6]

In the 1860s, advocates of the Acts committed two errors: they assumed that the incidence of venereal disease was increasing, and they convinced themselves (and three committees of enquiry) that an inspection system would set matters to rights. The evidence of official doctors such as W.H. Sloggett and J.C. Barr is full of confidence in the capacity of the Acts to conquer the scourge of venereal disease.[7] The first assumption appears to be incorrect. Official evidence produced before the 1879—82 select committee indicates that the incidence of venereal disease in the armed forces was steadily diminishing from 1860 onwards.[8] After 1866 this diminution merely continued in the subjected districts, that is there was no alteration in an established trend. Moreover, the confidence of the doctors appears to have been misplaced; if rates were falling all round, there was an undoubted improvement in the health of the forces, but Stansfeld was able to demonstrate, using official statistics, that very little of this was positively due to the intervention of the Acts. He conceded a small reduction in primary syphilis, but it was clear that gonorrhoea and secondary syphilis were largely unaffected.[9] Furthermore, Dr Lawson had to admit that different regiments in the same camp (Aldershot) displayed vastly different ratios of disease, which suggested that factors wholly unrelated to the Acts, such as emphasis on prophylaxis or differences in moral standards, could not be ignored.[10]

It would be foolish to suggest that the Acts effected no improvement — Stansfeld never attempted to do so — but the improvement never measured up to the claims of the Acts' promoters, and when related to the cost of the Acts was dearly bought. The minority report of the 1879—82 committee estimated (using Lawson's figures) that as a direct result of the Acts the average daily saving (from a period in hospital) was only 258 out of the 50,000 men stationed in the subjected districts; the expense of each man saved was £116 each year.[11] One may also question whether the examination system itself was wholly responsible for this improvement, for it brought with it a number of associated measures, each of which probably helped to lower VD rates.

The rigour with which the system was operated gave the subjected districts an advantage; only there were soldiers and sailors regularly examined upon entry or return from furlough, thus diminishing the risk of importation; while the attentions of police and doctors resulted in the decanting of diseased women into surrounding districts — improving the health of the subjected towns, but harming that of their neighbours (and in one case, Newport, Isle of Wight, leading to a request for the Acts as a measure of self-protection).[12] The provision of decent hospital facilities in the subjected districts was important in improving the general health of the women; and of course their incarceration for periods of up to nine months kept on removing from the market women who might otherwise infect soldiers and sailors. There is abundant evidence to show that the police were diligent in their duties, so diseased women found themselves in hospital very quickly, while juvenile and casual prostitution almost certainly diminished under this relentless scrutiny. It may be argued that it was as much the by-products of the system as the examination itself which were responsible for such improvements as were realised.[13]

On the whole the Acts, for all the efforts put into them by committed doctors and a determined police, were of marginal effect. One is struck by the bewildering variety of statistical bases and groups of stations selected for comparison by regulationists; all chosen to bolster their case, and all destroyed by Stansfeld between 1879 and 1882. They were faced with three problems which ultimately defeated their system: examining women periodically while leaving men alone was, in one sense, logically defensible (the women were selling their services, the state therefore regulated the transaction without troubling the purchaser) but hygienically absurd. Secondly, the universally agreed impossibility of extending the system meant that the rest of the country offered safe refuge for women likely to be trapped by the Acts, and served as a breeding ground for the importation of disease. Thirdly, the inadequacies of medicine meant that diagnoses could be faulty and treatment ineffective — harsh facts which doctors simply ignored. Clearly the Acts did not save the forces from VD (and nor did more thoroughgoing systems work any better in European armies); at best they had some effect in keeping it down, but the unreliability of statistics makes this difficult to prove. The disease was possibly diminishing after 1860 of its own accord, the CD Acts did little to affect this one way or the other.

The aftermath of repeal supports this view of the Acts as a medical irrelevance. Venereal disease in the armed forces continued to diminish in incidence much as did tuberculosis and other diseases; moreover, this improvement paralleled that in the civil population.[14] By 1900 the forces' infection rate had declined to 93 per 1000.[15] The military departments lost their enthusiasm for regulation in the face of this improvement, and as Florence Nightingale had always wished, were soon throwing their weight behind schemes to improve conditions for enlisted men. The Navy actively supported Agnes Weston's philanthropic efforts, and by 1894, both services were urging local commanding officers to cooperate with the efforts of the civil authorities to *repress* prostitution.[16] The official mind had turned decisively against regulation, a policy which it recognised as ineffective and likely to provoke embarrassing opposition. Indeed, during the Great War, the military departments once more resorted to misleading interpretations of statistics; but this time their aim was to minimise the increase in wartime venereal disease and so avoid being forced (by Dominion and colonial pressure) into reintroducing regulation. They had learnt the lesson that regulation was not worth the struggle involved.[17]

Nor was this the only victory over officialdom. The libertarian achievements of repeal should not be neglected. When the Acts were suspended in 1883, so too went the Metropolitan Police who enforced them. Over the years, this special force had been careless of the rights of the women for whom it was responsible, and adept at informally increasing its powers without legislative sanction. Unchecked by local control, its authoritarian tendencies were ineffectively curbed by the often distant authority of the responsible Assistant Commissioner. It is difficult to regret its departure, for as a result a dangerously autonomous 'national' force, however small, was removed,[18] and the possibility of a slide into the corruption which usually hangs over 'morals police' was averted.[19]

The defeat of the medical establishment anticipated its later defeat over vaccination and is another aspect of what has been termed 'a general characteristic of late Victorian society — a deeply flowing, often slumbering, philosophical belief in the importance of maintaining, at all costs, the "freedom of the individual" '.[20] Libertarianism on the march could combine with feminists, moralists and doctor-haters to overwhelm a profession which had been on shaky ground with regulation. Perhaps rashly, doctors had tried to compensate by advancing their orthodoxy with undue stridency. Their exaggerations served to further outrage individualists and may actually have saved repealers from some unfortunate consequences of their own extremism.[21] Individualism, for instance, led some repealers (most notably Josephine

Butler) to oppose any government involvement in the provision of hospital facilities. Separate Lock Hospitals were particularly loathed and individual, localist philanthropy thought sufficient.[22] There were repealers who accepted the case for separate Lock provision, and were even willing to see the state intervening as long as this was in the direction of higher moral standards,[23] but this potentially embarrassing division hardly mattered, given the medical profession's better exposed failings.

However, individualism did not have things all its own way. The libertarian approach of repealers, such as Josephine Butler herself, who were also members of the Vigilance Association (later the Personal Rights Association) was increasingly at odds with a phenomenon which was otherwise a great boon to their cause: the late nineteenth-century wave of moral revivalism, the creation of a 'respectable sexual ideology'.[24] The advantage of this was that it created a climate of opinion in which the CD Acts stood out as reflecting a male, libertine view of sexual behaviour. The disadvantage was that the Social Purity campaigners, organised after 1885 into the similarly named National Vigilance Association, were prepared to countenance repressive methods far from the original libertarian ethos of the repeal movement.

In the early 1880s the problem scarcely arose. The campaign against the white slave traffic assisted repeal inasmuch as it demonstrated the corruption and complicity of a 'morals police'. Alfred Dyer's part in the exposure of the traffic made it very much a repeal *cause célèbre*; it was part of the turning tide of middle-class concern, and provided ammunition for those in parliament who sought to raise the age of consent — again a prime concern for many repealers.[25]

Yet beneath the surface of these associated issues was a repressionist tendency typified by Dyer and his fellow WMNL stalwart, W.A. Coote. This willingness to use coercion to achieve morality was perhaps more representative of the rank and file repealer than has usually been admitted.[26] It is easy to see how, once the Acts had been suspended in 1883, repeal activists might be attracted to a more strident, though still related, agitation. The authoritarian beliefs of men such as Joseph Edmondson and Henry Wilson, whose 1875 scheme to outlaw fornication had been vigorously resisted by Mrs Butler, were much more in tune with the mood of the early 1880s.[27]

W.T. Stead's sensational revelations in 1885, with which Josephine Butler was closely associated, made Social Purity a national issue. In the ensuing scramble to be seen to be doing something, scruples and caution went to the wall. A libertarian like C.H. Hopwood was prepared to continue resisting interventionist measures for the protection of young girls (very bitterly too, revealing a suspicion, commonly found amongst repealers, of Stead and his followers) but most repealers were swept along by the agitation.[28] The LNA was prominent in the great Purity Demonstration in Hyde Park in August 1885, and the Wesleyan repealer, Dr William Arthur, pointedly contrasted the glare of righteous publicity in which the Criminal Law Amendment Bill was discussed with the secrecy which had surrounded the CD Acts twenty years before.[29]

Stead's agitation shows the way the wind was blowing. The House of Commons deferring to public opinion, raised the age of consent and granted the police wide powers of enforcement; the National Vigilance Association with the remorseless Coote as its Secretary was set up to guard public morals — repealers flocked to join.[30] Under the new regime, it was impossible for public figures such as Dilke and Parnell to escape censure for private behaviour perhaps once condonable. Purity campaigners demonstrated a new confidence in their assaults on 'indecency' in the arts and entertainment. In one sense individualism did remain, for the NVA believed in inflicting its collective conscience upon society through independent prosecutions, but to argue thus is to traduce the integrity of the true individualism of the earlier phases of the repeal movement which had openly and bravely achieved its moral victory over the Acts.

Despite her role in the Stead controversy, Josphine Butler did not sympathise with these developments. Virtually alone amongst repeal organisations, the LNA remained in existence to continue the work of raising and equalising moral standards — its aim had always been broader than simple repeal.[31] But most moralist activity was henceforth devoted towards repressing the outward signs of vice. By the 1890s the NVA's zealotry was tending towards hysterical kill-joyism, and Mrs Butler's patrician temperament reacted against the threat of conventional middle-class morality:

> I have *never* heartily sympathised with the work of the Vigilance Society, and yet undoubtedly they have done much good, many good things. But there is a constant tendency towards *external* pressure, and inside that a tendency to let the pressure fall almost exclusively on women because it is more difficult, they say to get at men. It is dangerous work, in reference to personal liberty, but few people care for liberty or personal rights now. Our *only* hope is in a higher standard.[32]

The impact of the repeal campaign on the women's movement has to be judged in the context of the studied moderation of the pioneering feminists. In their cautious manner, gradually eroding male resistance, they were extending opportunities for women's higher education, expanding employment prospects, using philanthropic activity as a means of liberating middle-class women from the home, and, of course, attempting to secure the parliamentary vote. This awakening was encouraged by the *Englishwoman's Journal* founded in 1858; its appearance has been said to mark the beginning of the organised women's movement, but it still remained dependent on friendly male support. The early feminists were careful not to press their claims too strongly.[33] The suffrage movement was as cautious as any; The National Society for Women's Suffrage had been founded in 1867 in the aftermath of John Stuart Mill's female suffrage amendment.[34] In its early years, public meetings and debates were rare, the petition and the private drawing room meeting were more discreet weapons and preferred for that reason. The redoubtable Mrs Fawcett made her first public speech only in July 1869 (at a meeting chaired by Mrs P.A. Taylor) and described herself as 'terrified' before it, even though she was supported on the platform by a strong group of male sympathisers. Henry Fawcett and P.A. Taylor were later criticised in parliament for allowing their wives to behave in so 'advanced' and 'unsexing' a fashion.[35]

Then in 1870 the Ladies' Protest against the CD Acts delivered a frontal attack on male assumptions and shattered the careful, possibly even timid, strategy pursued by earlier feminists. Here was a disreputable subject, connected with immorality, lust, prostitution being championed by women whose object was to force the matter out into the open. Hitherto, the thrust of the women's campaign had been towards enlisting male assistance and cooperation, now the LNA proclaimed its aggressive independence, and Josephine Butler courageously stood up to the abuse of the *Saturday Review* and its cohorts.

Was this spectacular development one which potentially might have united feminists? It was a principled agitation — a clear case which could be argued both in terms of morality, and of the discrimination against women to support male lust. Unlike other feminist activities, it saw middle-class women disinterestedly rising to the defence of their working-class sisters because of the slight to their sex (though this class gulf had a practical advantage in so far as the LNA had no 'constituency' urging it towards compromise so as to improve conditions). The LNA got off to an excellent start — an impressive range of prominent women signed the protest, publicity came easily, and there were male repealers to shelter its members from the worst taunts of the anti-feminists. Yet, despite all this, the leaders of the feminist movement held aloof, as did many of their followers. They were gradualists, committed to cautious advance, fearful of jeopardising hard-won gains, and temperamentally out of sympathy with Mrs Butler's crusading spirit. Emily Davies, leader of the educationalists had already shied away from the suffrage movement as being too advanced; the pioneer woman doctor, Elizabeth Garrett Anderson, followed medical orthodoxy and approved of the Acts.[36]

The suffrage movement split over the issue. The majority led by Mrs Fawcett feared confusing an already unpopular question with a new, much more controversial one. The minority, which included Mrs Butler and Miss Lydia Becker, thought it possible to work for both causes. Indeed Mrs Butler, while giving more time to the cause of equal morality than to that of equal suffrage, was aware that keeping the vote from women perpetuated injustice and immorality; in 1873 she wrote, 'I feel more keenly than I ever did the great importance of our having votes *as a means* of self-preservation.'[37] Mrs Fawcett was privately sympathetic but 'deliberately and after careful consideration, she stood aside from it [repeal], and though this decision cost her a great effort, she believed to the end of her life that it had been right'.[38] The majority were determined to err on the side of caution and took it to such extremes that in 1874 they considered dismissing their parliamentary representative, Jacob Bright, because he supported repeal.

Caution initially appeared justified. For every MP like J.W. Henley whose horror of the Acts brought him to look favourably on women's suffrage for the first time,[39] there was one like Hanbury whose support for it

> had been destroyed by the course which had been adopted by those ladies who, acting, doubtless, from very high motives, had taken part in an agitation on a subject to which he would not further allude, but which was one which he believed women ought never to touch in public.[40]

Opponents of the suffrage happily incorporated the LNA's activities into their armoury as Mrs Fawcett feared they would. We have already encountered Osborne Morgan doing so; the LNA, he said, 'flooded gentlemen's breakfast tables with abominable literature — not

addressed to themselves only, but also to their wives and daughters'.[41]
Not for the first or last time were the nation's breakfast tables under
siege![42]

The panic was exaggerated; despite its sensational concern with
prostitution, repeal was an essentially moral cause and the coarse
rebukes of men like Cavendish-Bentinck served only to elicit firm
declarations of support for women repealers from their male
colleagues. Then again, repeal was broader than any of the women's
rights issues and enlisted the support of those not primarily concerned
with feminist objectives, but with moral or constitutional ones. This
too served to protect LNA members who were part of a wide campaign
with abundant male support. Indeed Henry Fawcett pointed out how
religious and working-class involvement in the repeal campaign made
it stronger than the suffrage campaign.[43] The division fostered by his
wife failed to protect suffragists, while those who supported both
movements weathered the storm to see the LNA become a wholly
respectable organisation.[44]

The place of Josephine Butler and the LNA in the history of
women's rights is assured today, but is it accurate? The official historian
of the suffrage movement deals sketchily with its career, but then
compensates by conceding that the LNA:

> changed the whole basis of sex morality and swept away a
> multitude of shams. When Mrs. Butler came forward in the cause,
> a double moral standard was not only tolerated but widely upheld;
> before she had been working a year that comfortable illusion was
> upset. Not that there were not still innumerable men and women
> to support it, not that it does not to this day influence and bias
> the judgement of society, but its hold on thoughtful and
> serious people was destroyed.[45]

Generous though this is, it surely reflects a desire to incorporate a
certain view of Josephine Butler into the suffragist pantheon. Was the
LNA really this successful? One has to guard against taking the
assumptions of committed historians at face value; it did, after all, take
16 years and a great deal of male help to 'sweep away' a single
manifestation of the double standard.[46] In 1870, Mrs Butler and her
supporters succeeded not so much in weakening it, as in forcing it out
into the open and involving women themselves in the fight. Unequal
moral standards persist to this day, and the repeal movement,
though important in attacking a particularly provocative example, was

but an attack on a single front. Indeed it is arguable that the birth control movement, though quite unrelated to official feminism, was more responsible for equalising moral standards, and that Annie Besant's front was more important in the long term than Josephine Butler's.[47] Writing in the 1920s, Ray Strachey was prepared to rank Mrs Butler amongst feminism's heroines while ignoring Annie Besant; the situation has not much changed today.[48]

Since the LNA is so highly esteemed, it is curious that judgements seldom extend to pointing out how important a precedent organising and conducting an independent women's pressure group was. The LNA showed that women could run a campaign without male interference, and while its lack of political experience made it initially over-optimistic,[49] it persevered, forced its moral attitudes upon male repealers, and eventually triumphed. As the *Echo* put it, 'the despised "shrieking sisterhood" stands avenged'.[50] This victory assisted feminism in another respect: the participation of women in the repeal campaign had been controversial; their success legitimised many other less controversial but then untried activities. If women could campaign for equal moral standards, most other demands assumed a moderation they had not possessed before. Mrs Fawcett nobly recognised this when she reviewed her life's work: 'Mrs. Butler's victory was an immense encouragement to us; for her task had been immeasurably more difficult than ours, and her triumph helped us to believe that all things were possible.'[51] Hesitations were quickly forgotten once success was attained. Indeed the LNA's vigour positively recommended it to suffragettes. Mrs Pethick-Lawrence wrote:

> Mrs. Josephine Butler and her friends were the first in England to discover the effectiveness of the militant by-election policy . . . the story . . . offers many parallels to the history of the militant campaign of women for the vote.[52]

Whether Mrs Butler would have welcomed this tribute is doubtful; in old age she dismissed the militants' claim to be modernisers of the LNA tradition — far from it: 'The suffrage women are going mad. I am disgusted.'[53]

We must now turn to the question of repeal's success. How was it that the despised cranks of 1870 were able to defeat the forces of official medicine by 1886? Two factors have already been turned up: the failure of the Acts to achieve what had been claimed for them, and the change in society's attitude to morality. Something more positive is needed though, and for this we should look to the movement itself. By the 1880s it had assembled an extremely strong coalition of support, which James Stuart enumerated to the 1884 LNA Annual Meeting:

> We have on our side, *without any exception whatever*, the whole of the Nonconformist bodies in the U.K. in their corporate capacity . . . We have the National Liberal Federation which has passed a resolution that the time for repealing the Acts has come; and we have the representative body of the working classes of this country — the Trades' Union Congress which . . . whilst thanking the Government for what it has up to this moment done, called upon it to repeal these Acts and finish its work.[54]

No Liberal government could afford to ignore a coalition so precisely attuned to major sources of Liberal support, and it was this advantage which provincial repealers successfully exploited after 1880. Indeed in looking at the evolution of the strategy pursued by H.J. Wilson and his associates, one is observing the growth of political awareness of a provincial radical élite which by the end of the campaign was itself moving into parliament, having lost much of its old loathing for Westminster.

The paradox of the repeal campaign is the conversion of the Londoners from a moderate parliament-orientated position in the early 1870s to an erratic militancy in the 1880s, while provincials moved the other way, eventually becoming the realists, the practical politicians. One explanation of this may be that the Londoners had been directing the agitation since its inception. They were accustomed to controlling it, prided themselves on the excellence of their organisation, and resorted to militancy only to prove their continued ability to lead. But essentially they had become a bureaucratised clique which, as Josephine Butler had predicted, had perfected its machinery at the expense of individual initiative, 'substituting stereotyped office work for the vitality of missionary work'.[55] If the NA persisted in its belief that the force of argument had a bipartisan appeal, the provincials were much more alive to party politics. In the 1870s they believed they could storm the political system and bludgeon the Liberal party into acquiescence. By the 1880s their strategy was adjusted towards infiltrating repeal into the Liberal programme.

Persistence is another important feature of the agitation. The

campaign kept going however black its prospects: its militant strategy
in the early 1870s collapsed disastrously, and there was no cheer
during the Disraeli government. This may be put down to firmness
of principle, holiness of character, or whatever pleases the reader. The
point is that the agitation plainly would not go away, and after 1880,
Liberal politicians had to reckon with this: disappoint the repealers
and they would be around for ever. Furthermore, persistence paid off
in terms of propaganda; public opinion was moulded to the repeal
view, for instance, the Lord Advocate flatteringly conceded to an
SNA deputation in 1882:

> There seemed to be a very growing feeling of repugnance through-
> out the country towards the Acts . . . Many persons who at one
> time were so strongly impressed with the great evils that existed in
> garrison towns that they were prepared to make a large sacrifice of
> considerations which were usually paramount, now thought that,
> both on sanitary and moral grounds, that the Acts ought to be
> repealed. That, he thought, was the growing feeling in the country,
> he thought it would be very dispassionately and very carefully
> considered by the Legislature.[56]

Repealers succeeded in establishing themselves in areas sensitive for any
Liberal government: while their failure in dockyard and military towns
was embarrassing, it was not politically harmful — the Liberal party's
hopes did not rest on success in military-dominated towns in the south
of England. They did, however, rest on success in the urban areas of
the midlands and north (Scotland and Wales too, of course, but for this
purpose we are looking for areas of repeal strength) and here repeal
embedded itself firmly. The NCL was the most successful repeal body
in enlisting the support of MPs and in petitioning. The MCEU, with
the midland shires as part of its area, illustrated this urban bias
supremely well: its 1882 annual meeting was told that only five
county members supported repeal while 39 were regulationists, whereas
borough members divided 32:14 against the Acts.[57]

Success in parliament was of course partly a function of success
within the Liberal party, but two other factors help to explain the
surprising ease with which the Commons carried repeal votes in 1883
and 1886. The first concerns the government's attitude. Only once,
in 1875, had a government ever whipped the majority against repeal;
more usually, governments stuck by the Acts but scarcely treated them
as matters of confidence. The 1880—5 government was very obviously

divided on the issue, with the service ministers remaining strong for the
Acts, while others, notably Childers, Chamberlain and Dilke were
only too aware of the restraint being shown by repealers (as well as
other reformers) and were eager to offer some satisfaction.[58] Under
these circumstances, not only did government resistance collapse
easily in 1883, but once a majority of the House had condemned the
Acts, it hastened to suspend their most obnoxious provisions in the
hope that calm would return. Stansfeld held his forces in check thereafter, conscious that the government's aim was to find a solution
which would avoid alienating its many followers who supported repeal.
Politically speaking, the only one which would fit the bill was total
repeal, and early in 1886, Stansfeld was able to capitalise on
Gladstone's desire to seize hold of radicalism for the coming crisis,
and slip repeal through with government assistance.

The second factor has often been touched upon: parliament's
dislike of the whole subject and its preference for discretion. Stansfeld
explained this to his electors in 1871: 'it was not that the House was
not cognizant of them, but that there was a general feeling . . . that
on a subject of this character it would be better to legislate without
much public speaking'.[59] Perseverance here was vital for success.
However much they hated doing so, repeal MPs had to bring their
question up each year in order to show the majority of MPs that
there was no escape. They did so in the mid-1870s when the subject
had gone stale; they did so all the more in 1882 and 1883 when they
scented success. Stansfeld also led his followers along the same
parliamentary path used by the enemy ten years before. Just as the
select committees of 1868 and 1869 had produced results their sponsors
desired (common enough in the nineteenth century) so he determined
to use the 1879–82 committee to blow open the regulationist case;
and though his was a minority report, it was an exceptionally cogent
one. By 1883 the message to the majority of MPs must have been
clear; the Acts had not brought about the promised transformation in
military health, and their opponents would not go away. The
abstainers got Stansfeld's resolution through.

This helps to solve a final problem. Why did repealers succeed when
their richer, better organised and more powerful exemplars, the UKA
and the Liberation Society were frustrated? The answer surely lies
with the strength of the opposition to be overcome. Despite over-
drawn estimates of medical influence, the doctors were not much of
a force in the House of Commons; they lost on vaccination and were
forced to accept restrictions on vivisection. The military interest was

stronger, but its preoccupations were considerably wider — especially in periods of Gladstonian retrenchment. Regulationists had lost command of the House (indeed had they ever really enjoyed it, since the Acts had been carried by stealth?), they had abandoned ideas of extension as long ago as 1873, and their failure to reinstate examination in any form after 1883 suggests that most MPs found their zeal for the Acts as much a nuisance as repealers' determination to overthrow them had always been. Compared to this, the UKA faced the drink trade, and more significantly, challenged the social reflexes of the majority of the male population; while the Liberation Society threatened a national institution which the Tory party was pledged to defend, and which again could probably enlist an enormous amount of passive support. Their failure underlines something which few repealers were prepared to acknowledge; fidelity of principle, strength of purpose, excellence of organisation, militancy of behaviour, though all splendid characteristics, in themselves guaranteed nothing.

In the harsh world of politics, the morality of a cause was debatably a necessary condition of success; it certainly was not sufficient in itself. Repealers were zealous, earnest, principled, but so were their counterparts in other agitations. Judged in terms of commitment, most Victorian reformers deserved to win. Repealers could triumph because theirs was basically a winnable cause, not a true 'forlorn hope' and their leadership was able to exploit this indispensable touch of luck. Yet final victory came just in time. Within a few months the Home Rule split in the Liberal party had destroyed the strategic basis of this success. So, at the very end of the struggle, Gladstone rather curiously justified Josephine Butler's earlier confidence in him; by giving the repeal bill government backing, he ensured that it got through in a much preoccupied session. It was a now forgotten narrow squeak, but the Acts were well and truly buried before the Conservatives returned.

That parliamentary tactics should have been so crucial in the 1880s may incline the reader to dismiss the high-minded idealism of most repealers as foolish or unworldly. This would be a bleak judgement, for, if principles alone could not win the day, their absence would have consigned the movement to the historical oblivion of the compromisers and time-servers. It should not be forgotten that, especially for women, holding repeal principles did require courage in the early years. Ridicule, hostility even violence had all to be faced. The remarkable tenacity with which the movement held to its simple demand for 'total, immediate and unconditional repeal' at least ensured that compromises such as Bruce's Bill would never succeed: it was the Acts or nothing, and eventually the repealers were rewarded with complete success. It need not have been so — and this study has attempted to redress the balance away from the view that success was morally inevitable — but who is to deny that the repealers deserved their triumph? Their efforts resulted in the dismantling of a threatening system of police control over the individual, the abandonment of a medically ineffective attempt to regulate public health by compulsion, and the recognition that the law should not be used to underpin a double standard of sexual morality.

These achievements were not won without cost. On the face of it, Mrs Butler appears a self-possessed, resilient leader and her reputation rests on her forcefulness as a prominent late-Victorian woman. But behind this facade, we know that she was plagued by illness and actually made ill by the nature of her work; her commitments obliged her to spend long periods separated from her family; she must surely have known that her activism had wrecked her husband's career in the church,[60] and both of them were ostracised by many of his friends and colleagues because of her repeal work.[61] Stansfeld's sacrifice is the better known: he took up repeal fully aware of the risk to his career,[62] and the fact that he remained ambitious and was hurt by his exclusion in 1880, serves only to emphasise what he had thereby lost. His return for a mere three months in 1886 was a bittersweet reward — a tantalising glimpse of the satisfactions of office, yet inadequate recompense. In 1892, despite service on the front bench during the Salisbury government, he was again passed over, this time on grounds of age.

Let us turn to Mrs Fawcett for the last word. For all her hesitation in the early years, she was always generous in making amends, and she appreciated the wider significance of repeal for the movement of which she was the head. In 1886 on the day after Stansfeld carried his resolution, she congratulated him movingly:

Your long years of noble and persevering effort are crowned with success, and you and all who have laboured with you have placed women of England under a debt of gratitude that they can never hope to repay.[63]

Notes

1. Yet even a medically qualified repealer, Dr Cameron, MP, felt obliged to apologise for arguing at his opponents' level when offering a rigorous 'cost-benefit analysis' of the Acts at the 1884 Exeter Hall Meeting; see *Shield*, 16 Feb. 1884, pp. 25–31.

2. See for instance, FLB 3460: circular letter from Northern Counties League in support of repeal bill, 18 June 1875.

3. *Protest*, 17 Apr. 1879, p. 39.

4. *Shield*, 5 Apr. 1884, pp. 52–4.

5. R.S. Morton, *Venereal Diseases* (Harmondsworth, 1966), pp. 21, 28.

6. F.B. Smith, 'Ethics and Disease in the Later Nineteenth Century', *Historical Studies* (University of Melbourne), 15 (1971), pp. 130–2, discusses the statistics informatively and argues that 'the figures are a mare's nest'.

7. *PP*, 1868–69 (306), vii QQ55–6, 104 (Dr Sloggett); QQ673, 713 (Dr Barr).

8. See for instance, *PP* 1881 (351), viii Appendix A; between 1860 and 1866 the figures for primary venereal sores per 1,000 men fell from 146 to 87 in stations which were later subjected to the Acts, and from 132 to 84 in stations never under the Acts. See also the illuminating discussion of hospital treatment and VD rates in J.R. Walkowitz, ' "We are not beasts of the field": Prostitution and the Campaign Against the Contagious Diseases Acts, 1869–1886' (unpublished PhD thesis, Rochester University, 1974), ch. 8, esp. pp. 294–5.

9. James Stansfeld, *On the Failure of the Contagious Diseases Acts as Proved by the Official Evidence* (1881), pp. 8–9.

10. *PP*, 1878–79 (323), viii Q409: Dr Lawson (Inspector General of the Army Medical Department) noting that in two comparable regiments the ratio of 'primary sores' found was 23 per 1,000 in one, 146 per 1,000 in the other.

11. *PP*, 1882 (340), ix, minority report, paragraph 6; *Shield*, 8 Mar. 1879, pp. 33–5, implementing the Acts cost £32,413 in 1878–9.

12. FLB 3353a: Joseph Edmondson in a letter to the *British Medical Journal*, 2 Mar. 1875.

13. See Smith, 'Ethics and Disease', pp. 126–7. For the professionalisation of prostitution under the impact of the Acts, see Walkowitz, ' "We are not beasts of the field" ', pp. 266–7.

14. A. Ramsay Skelley, *The Victorian Army at Home* (1977), pp. 25, 53–8.

15. Morton, *Venereal Diseases*, p. 30.

16. Agnes Weston, *My Life Among the Bluejackets* (1909); Edward J. Bristow, *Vice and Vigilance: Purity Movements in Britain since 1700* (Dublin, 1978), p. 160.

17. Suzann Buckley, 'The Failure to Resolve the Problem of Venereal Disease Among the Troops in Britain During World War One', in B. Bond and I. Roy (eds.), *War and Society*, 2 (1977), pp. 66, 73.

18. R.J. Evans, 'Prostitution, State and Society in Imperial Germany', *Past and Present*, 70 (1976), pp. 110, 126, notes the autonomy of German police forces and their ability, albeit unrestrained by legislation, to widen their powers.

19. For the tendency towards corruption, see Bristow, *Vice and Vigilance*, p. 180; and C.H. Rolph, *Times Literary Supplement*, 12 May 1978, p. 522.

20. Roy M. MacLeod, 'Law, Medicine and Public Opinion', *Public Law* (Summer–Autumn, 1967), p. 211.

21. See H.R.E. Ware, *The Recruitment, Regulation and Role of Prostitution in Britain from the Middle of the Nineteenth Century to the Present Day* (unpublished PhD thesis, London University, 1969), pp. 219–27.

22. *Shield*, 22 Mar. 1875, pp. 93–4; 1 Aug. 1875, pp. 237–9; 5 Apr. 1879,

pp. 49–50.

23. The Bristol branch of the LNA actively supported a Voluntary Lock Hospital, see *Shield*, 18 Mar. 1871, p. 425; 6 Mar. 1880, p. 37.

24. For which see Peter T. Cominos, 'Late Victorian Sexual Respectability and the Social System', *International Review of Social History*, 8 (1963).

25. See above p. 193; for Dyer as a 'working-class radical puritan' see Bristow, *Vice and Vigilance*, p. 87; for a particularly good analysis of the white slave agitation, see Deborah Gorham, 'The Maiden-Tribute of Modern Babylon Re-examined: Child Prostitution and the Idea of Childhood in Late Victorian England', *Victorian Studies*, 21 (1978), pp. 357–62.

26. See above pp. 146–47; Bristow, *Vice and Vigilance*, pp. 77, 155.

27. J.W. Walkowitz, ' "We are not beasts of the field" ', pp. 355–6.

28. *Shield*, 18 July 1885, pp. 105–6, 108–10; 1 Aug. 1885, pp. 123–4; 5 sept. 1885, pp. 133–5, 138–9; Gorham, 'The Maiden-Tribute', pp. 366–8 discusses the pressures on libertarians.

29. Dr William Arthur, *Hush or Speak Out?* (1885).

30. Bristow, *Vice and Vigilance*, pp. 117–121; Walkowitz, ' "We are not beasts of the field" ', pp. 369–72; F.B. Smith, 'Labouchere's amendment to the Criminal Law Amendment Bill', *Historical Studies*, 17 (1976), pp. 165–73 demonstrates the extent to which decency and restraint were lost sight of in 1885.

31. FLB 4075: Josephine Butler to Miss Priestman, May 1886; LNA, *Annual Report for 1886*, p. 43.

32. FLB Box 2E: Josephine Butler to Anon. 5 Nov. (1896?); see above pp. 18–19 for Mrs Butler's temperament; R.J. Evans, *The Feminists* (1977), p. 67 for the NVA; G. Stedman Jones, 'Working-Class Culture and Working-Class Politics in London, 1870–1900', *Journal of Social History*, 7 (1974), pp. 495–6 for its activities.

33. See Jo Manton, *Elizabeth Garrett Anderson* (1965), p. 44; Kathleen E. McCrone, 'The Assertion of Women's Rights in Mid-Victorian England', *Historical Papers (Canadian Historical Association)*, 1972, p. 39 stresses the importance to the mid-Victorian feminist of 'social standing' and 'personal reputation'.

34. C. Rover, *Women's Suffrage and Party Politics in Britain, 1866–1914* (1967), pp. 5–6, 53–5.

35. R. Strachey, *The Cause, a Short History of the Women's Movement in Great Britain* (1928), pp. 118–21; R. Strachey, *Millicent Garrett Fawcett* (1931), pp. 45–6.

36. Strachey, *The Cause*, pp. 197–8; Jo Manton, *Elizabeth Garrett Anderson* (1865), pp. 178–80.

37. FLB 3313: Josephine Butler to Mrs H.J. Wilson, 12 Nov. 1873.

38. R. Strachey, *Millicent Garrett Fawcett* (1931), pp. 52–3.

39. *Hansard*, 3rd Series (21 May 1873), 216 Cols.263–4.

40. Ibid., (6 June 1877), 231 Cols.1363–4.

41. Ibid., (1 May 1872), 211 Cols.56.

42. See J.A. and O. Banks, 'The Bradlaugh-Besant Trial and the English Newspapers', *Population Studies*, 8–9 (1954–6), pp. 22–35 for later examples of this onslaught; see above p. 58 for an earlier one.

43. FLB 3312: James Stuart to H.J. Wilson, Saturday (n.d., possibly 1873) quoting Fawcett.

44. Strachey, *The Cause*, pp. 196–9, 266–9, discusses the division from the suffrage point of view; Rover, *Women's Suffrage*, pp. 53–5 places it in the context of the suffrage movement's tendency to divide (this schism lasted seven years: 1871–1878); J.A. and O. Banks, *Feminism and Family Planning in Victorian England* (Liverpool 1964), pp. 94–6, discuss it from the morality aspect.

45. Strachey, *The Cause*, p. 204.

46. J.A. and O. Banks, 'Feminism and Social Change', in G.K. Zollschan and W. Hirsch (eds.), *Explorations in Social Change* (1st edn, 1964) provide a valuable note of caution. See also Brian Harrison, *Separate Spheres: The Opposition to Women's Suffrage in Britain* (1978), p. 73, for a controversial assessment of the *willingness* of male parliaments to respond to female demands.

47. J.A. and O. Banks, *Feminism and Family Planning*, pp. 9–10, ch. 7; the work of Angus McLaren, e.g. 'Women's Work and Regulation of Family Size: The Question of Abortion in the Nineteenth Century', *History Workshop Journal*, 4 (1977), pp. 70–81, seriously modifies the feminist and malthusian aspects of birth control.

48. See Constance Rover, *Love, Morals and the Feminists* (1970), p. 2.

49. A fault the suffragists shared. Because 80 MPs voted with Mill in 1867, they believed they would win within a year or two; see Strachey, *The Cause*, p. 109.

50. *Echo*, 21 Apr. 1883.

51. Millicent Garrett Fawcett, *What I Remember* (1924), p. 128.

52. *Votes for Women*, 28 May 1909, pp. 720–21. I owe this reference to Dr Brian Harrison.

53. Liverpool University Library (Butler MSS) undated fragment, c. 1903–4.

54. LNA, *Annual Report for 1884*, p. 15.

55. FLB 3899: Josephine Butler to British, Continental and General Federation EC, 11 Jan. 1879.

56. *Shield*, 11 Feb. 1882, p. 27.

57. Ibid., 11 Feb. 1882, p. 20; see also above p. 236 for borough strength.

58. See D.A. Hamer, *Liberal Politics in the Age of Gladstone and Rosebery* (1972), ch. 4.

59. *Shield*, 18 Mar. 1871, p. 423.

60. Sir Edward Hamilton's diary confirms this, see D.W.R. Bahlman (ed.), *The Diary of Sir Edward Hamilton*, I, pp. 281–2 (2 June 1882), p. 376 (17 Dec. 1882), II, pp. 612–13 (8 May 1884).

61. Liverpool University Library (Butler MSS) MS 8.4(2): Josephine Butler to Rhoda Butler, no date (1890s), she describes how, at the Harrow speeches, all but one of George Butler's friends literally turned their backs on her; 'It made him unhappy for weeks'.

62. E. Moberly Bell, *Josephine Butler, Flame of Fire* (1962), p. 114.

63. Stansfeld MSS (in family hands): Mrs M.G. Fawcett to James Stansfeld, 17 Mar. 1886.

APPENDIX A: THE PRINCIPAL REPEAL ASSOCIATIONS AS AT 1 JUNE 1880

National Association (1869–86)
2, Westminster Chambers, London, SW
    William Shaen, MA, Chairman
    William T. Malleson, BA, Vice-Chairman
    Frederick Charles Banks, Secretary
Ladies National Association (1869–1915)
348, Park Road, Liverpool, and 2 Westminster Chambers, London, SW
    Josephine E. Butler, Hon. Secretary
    Margaret Tanner, Treasurer
National Medical Association (1874–86)
    J. Birkbeck Nevins, MD, President
    William Carter, MD
    Thomas Carson, MRCSI, Hon. Secretaries
Midland Counties Electoral Union (1872–86)
20 Paradise Street, Birmingham
    Robert Francis Martineau, Chairman of Committee
    John Edward Baker, Treasurer
    Arthur J. Naish
    Thomas Worth, MRCS, Hon. Secretaries
    William Wastell, Secretary
Northern Counties League (1872–86)
255, Pitsmoor, Sheffield
    Henry J. Wilson, Hon. Secretary
    Joseph Edmondson, Treasurer
Scottish National Association (1873–86)
5, St Andrew's Square, Edinburgh
    David McLaren, Chairman
    Professor H. Calderwood
    Rev. W.D. Moffat, Hon. Secretaries
Wesleyan Society (1874–84)
    Percy Bunting, MA
    Rev. Hugh Price Hughes, BA
    Rev. Allan Rees, Hon. Secretaries

Friends' Association (1873–?)
1 & 2, The Poultry, London EC
   William Fowler, MP, President
   Frederic Wheeler, Chairman of Committee
   Samuel Gurney, Treasurer
Congregational Committee (1875–86)
   Rev. J.P. Gledstone, Hon. Secretary
   Edward Crossley, Treasurer
British Continental and General Federation for the Abolition of State-
Regulated Prostitution (1873–present)
2, Westminster Chambers, London, SW and 348 Park Road, Liverpool
   James Stuart, MA, LLD, Professor of Mechanism in the University
      of Cambridge, Financial Secretary
   Josephine E. Butler, Hon. Secretary
City of London Committee (1877–86)
   Samuel Morley, MP, Chairman
   William McArthur, MP, Vice-Chairman
   R.C.L. Bevan, Treasurer
   Benjamin Scott, FRAS
   James B. Porter, Hon. Secretaries
Working Men's National League (1875–86)
1 & 2, The Poultry, London, EC
   Edmund Jones, President
   Joesph Joyce, Secretary
   Sidney Goult, Organising Secretary

Source: *National League Journal*, 1 June 1880, p. 4.

APPENDIX B: INCOME AND EXPENDITURE FIGURES

Table B.1
(See above, chapter 3, p. 88, for some comparable figures for other agitations.)

	National Association			Ladies' National Association		
	Income	Subscriptions + donations	Expenditure	Income	Subscriptions + donations	Expenditure
1870–1	2778. 2 1	1091.11. 6	2609. 2. 0	1079.16. 8	992.16. 1	975.18. 9
1871–2	2520.12. 2	1738.10. 0	2454. 0. 5	1321.15. 0½	990.18. 9½	896. 6. 1
1872–3	2728.19. 7	2029.17. 1	2617. 8. 9	2064.13. 3	1633.13. 4½	1906. 9. 1½
1873–4	3513. 1. 0		3330.14. 2	1441.16. 5½	982.13. 6	1183.11. 0
1874–5	3797. 6. 6	3147. 6. 7	3409. 8. 8	1229. 0. 2	914. 1. 3	1198. 1. 5
1875–6	3494.17. 0		3396. 5. 3	1133. 2. 0	1032. 3. 3	1074. 8. 7½
1876–7				1238. 3. 1½	1160. 9. 9	1097.13. 1½
1877–8				1090. 7. 5	942.16. 3	1090. 7. 5
1878–9				916. 5. 6		891.18. 7
1879–80	2238. 8. 9	1812.17. 5	2710.15. 5	697. 5.11	672.19. 0	345.18.10
1880–1	2523. 4. 2	2162. 8. 0	2689.15. 7	1113.10. 9	750. 3. 8	897.15. 5
1881–2	2605.15. 9	2287. 9. 2	2520.15.11	992.13. 8	776.18. 4	792.11. 2½
1882–3	2680. 7.10	2336. 5.10	2596.17. 4	1117.18. 4	854.10. 4	1084.12. 0
1883–4	1973.15. 2	1761.18. 0	2164. 2. 8	842. 4. 7	635 16. 6	371. 8. 8
1884–5	2316.10.10	2119. 9. 2	2227.14.10	1004. 6. 5	523.19. 6	474. 0. 4

Source: *Annual Reports* (where available).

Table B.2

	British Continental and General Federation		Wesleyan Society		
1877–8	1020. 0.10		198. 1. 9	165.11. 9	278.10. 1
1878–9	967.18. 8	881.13. 9	127. 1. 7	120.15. 0	291. 1.11
1879–80	991.18. 3	1075.15.10	567.10. 9	76. 5. 2	438. 4.11

Source: *Protest*, 18 June 1879, p. 69; 19 June 1889, p. 69.

Source: *Protest*, 16 Oct. 1878, p. 90; 17 Oct. 1879, p. 88; 20 Nov. 1880, p. 101.

Table B.3

Working Men's National League

	Income	Subscription + donations	Expenditure
1875–6	276.18.11		357.11.11
1877–8	314.14. 9	314.14. 9	339.14. 3
1878–9	254. 6. 9	243. 5. 5	254. 6. 9

Source: *National League Journal*, 1 August 1876; 1 January 1879; 1 April 1880.

Table B.4

	National Medical Association		
	Income	Subscriptions + donations	Expenditure
1876–7	964.14. 2½		976.14. 6
1878–9	466. 7. 6		886.19. 1½

Source: *Methodist Protest*, 16 April 1877, pp. 47–8.

Table B.5

	Friends' Association		
1878–9	808. 5. 0		766. 0. 5
1883–4	1160. 4.10		1235. 5. 3
1884–5	634. 5. 7		642.15.10

Source: *Shield*, 8 March 1879, pp. 39–40; Friends' Association, *Annual Reports* (where available).

Table B.6

	City of London Committee		
1877–8	114.11. 0		96. 7.11
1878–9	114. 7. 5		116. 4. 1
1879–80	109. 9. 6	96. 1. 6	102.13. 4
1880–1	138. 2. 0	103. 8.10	124.19. 8
1881–2	125. 7. 9	105.13. 0	110. 8. 4

Source: *Protest*, 16 March 1878, p. 33; 17 March 1879, p. 30; 25 March 1881, p. 58; 26 March 1882, p. 55; 30 March 1883, p. 18.

APPENDIX C: SOME EMPLOYEES OF REPEAL ASSOCIATIONS AND SALARIES

(Salaries, if known, expressed per annum.)

National Association

Secretary	F.C. Banks	1870–6	Nov. 1872: £250, Jan. 1874: £400
Asst. Secretary	Miss E. Harrison		Oct. 1876: £80
Asst. Secretary	Mrs F.C. Banks		Oct. 1876: £80
Male Clerk	Mr Burfoot	1876–9	Oct. 1876: £80, Mar. 1877: £105 dismissed Aug. 1879 for 'irregularities' in the office.
Editor of *Shield*	Mme Venturi	1870–86	Nov. 1876: £150
Agents	John Marshall (Plymouth)		Nov. 1876: £90, probably raised later.
	S. MacDonald	1872–3	£150
	W. Charles	1872–3	£100
	Rev. W. Knox	Feb.– May 73	£150
	J. Coutts	1873–5	£200 then became agent of the SNA.
	J. Johnson	1873–4	£150 dismissed in disgrace.
	Rev. J.H. Lynn	1874–6	£150
	Rev. J.H. Lynn	1879–86	initially helping in office at 4 guineas per week.
	W.T. Swan	1877–81	£250

Northern Counties League

A clerk was always employed at the office (Wilson's home) to do routine work.

Agents	J. Hardy	1872–3	£143
	W.T. Swan	1873–7	£200
	W. Burgess	1873–4	£250 (jointly with LNA)

Agents	J. Elliott	1873–	part-time
	J.P.Gledstone	1875–7	
	E. Barton	1878–9	
	C. Payne	1879–80	

when the NCL advertised for an agent in 1877, it offered £150–£300 according to experience.

Ladies' National Association

Mrs Butler employed a secretary at her Liverpool home/office.

Agents	W. Burgess	1873–7	£250 (jointly with NCL 1873–4).
	S. Fothergill	1872–7	
	H. Bligh	1873–6	
	Mrs Goulder	1877–9	£100 rising to £150 in Apr. 1878.
	Mrs Campbell	1880–3	
	Miss J. Craigen	1880–3	

Others

In 1876 the Midland Counties Electoral Union employed an Organising Secretary, S.J. Ainge; a Travelling Secretary and Lecturer, Rev. W. Wastell and an Asst. Secretary, John Craig. By 1878, Wastell had replaced Ainge and was described as Secretary.

The Working Men's National League paid its President and employed a Secretary. The Scottish National Association employed a Secretary and sometimes an agent. The Bristol Gentlemen's Association employed a Secretary, Rev. E.S. Bayliffe, from 1879–83, after which he was employed by its successor the South Western Counties Union.

This bibliography is arranged as follows:

Primary Sources

Manuscript Sources
Printed Sources
- (a) Official Publications
- (b) Works of Reference
- (c) Reports
- (d) Newspapers and periodicals
- (e) Contemporary tracts and pamphlets
- (f) Contemporary biographies and autobiographies
- (g) Other contemporary printed sources

Secondary Sources

Unpublished Theses
Books
Articles

Unless otherwise stated, place of publication is London.

Primary Sources

Manuscript Sources

Birmingham Reference Library
   Minutes of the Birmingham Trades Council, 1–6, 1870–84
Birmingham University Library
   Harriet Martineau Papers
British Museum
   Gladstone Papers
   Florence Nightingale Papers
   Ripon Papers
   T.G. Balfour Papers
Fawcett Library
   Josephine Butler Papers (FLB)
   H.J. Wilson Papers (FLW)

Minute Books of the National Association, 1871–86
Minute Books of the Ladies' National Association, 1875–84
Letter Book of the National Association, 1883–6
Friends' Library
   Minute Books of the Friends' Association, 1873–86
Liverpool University Library
   Josephine Butler Papers
Public Record Office
   Home Office Papers
Sheffield Central Library
   H.J. Wilson Papers
Sheffield University Library
   H.J. Wilson Papers
   Mundella-Leader Correspondence
In the possession of W.J. Stansfeld Esq.
   James Stansfeld Papers

Printed Sources

(a) Official Publications

*Report of the Committee appointed to enquire into the pathology
   and treatment of Venereal Disease with the view to diminish its
   injurious effects on the men of the Army and Navy*, PP 1867–68
   (4031), xxxvii, 425
*Report from the Select Committee of the House of Lords on the
   Contagious Diseases Act, 1866*, session 1867–68 (46)
Report from the Select Committee on the Contagious Diseases Act,
   PP 1868–69 (306), vii, 1
*Royal Commission upon the administration and operation of the
   Contagious Diseases Acts*, PP 1871 (c. 408 + 408–1), xix
*Reports from the Select Committee on the Contagious Diseases
   Acts (1866–69)*, PP 1878–79 (323), viii, 397; PP 1880 (114), viii,
   283; PP 1880 (308), viii, 361; PP 1881 (351), viii, 193; PP 1882
   (340), ix, 1
House of Commons Division Lists, sessions 1867–68 to 1886

(b) Works of Reference

Annual Monitor
Boase, F., *Modern English Biography* (Truro, 1892–1921)
Cook, C. and B. Keith (eds.), *British Historical Facts, 1830–1900*
   (1975)

Dictionary of National Biography
Dictionary of Quaker Biography (at Friends' Library)
Dod's Parliamentary Companion
Hansard's Parliamentary Debates, 3rd series

(c) Reports

National Association (NA), *Annual Reports*, 1870–5, 1880–6
Ladies' National Association (LNA), *Annual Reports*, 1870–1915
Northern Counties League (NCL), *Annual Reports*, 1873–85
Friends' Association (FA), *Annual Reports*, 1879–81, 1884–8
Vigilance Association (VA), *Annual Reports*, 1871–84
Association for promoting the extension of the Contagious Diseases Acts (EA), *Reports on the Operation of the CD Acts*, 1870–5
Harveian Medical Society of London, *Report of the Committee for the Prevention of Venereal Diseases* (1867)
Rescue Society, *15th Annual Report for 1868, 16th Annual Report for 1869*
Birmingham branch of the National Association for promoting the extension of the Contagious Diseases Act, *Report of the Committee for 1868*
Birmingham Association for procuring the repeal of the Contagious Diseases Acts, *Report for 1870*
Minutes of the Wesleyan Methodist Conference, 1870–86
Minutes of the Primitive Methodist Conference, 1870–85
Minutes of the United Methodist Free Churches Annual Assembly, 1870–86
Minutes of the Methodist New Connexion Conference, 1870–86

(d) Newspapers and Journals

The Times
Westminster Review
Pall Mall Gazette
Daily Telegraph
Liverpool Daily Courier
Birmingham Post
Devonport Independent
Saturday Review
Daily News
Echo
Manchester Examiner
Liverpool Daily Post
Northern Echo
Western Morning News

Shield
Methodist Protest (later *Protest*)
Medical Enquirer
National League Journal
Occasional Paper
Journal (of the VA)
Sentinel (social purity journal published by Dyer Brothers)

(e) Contemporary Tracts and Pamphlets

Arthur, Dr William, *Hush or Speak Out* (1885)

Blackwell, Dr Elizabeth, *Rescue Work in Relation to Prostitution and Disease* (1881)

Butler, Josephine, *Paper on the Moral Reclaimability of Prostitutes* (1870)

—— *The Constitution Violated* (1871)

—— *Address Delivered in Craigie Hall, Edinburgh, 24 February 1871* (Manchester, 1871)

—— *Address delivered at Croydon, 3 July 1871* (1871)

—— *Sursum Corda; Annual Address to the LNA* (Liverpool, 1871)

—— *Some Thoughts on the Present Aspect of the Crusade Against the State Regulation of Vice* (Liverpool, 1874)

—— *Government by Police* (1879)

Birmingham Anti-Contagious Diseases Acts Association, *Report of the Deputation to Plymouth* (Birmingham, 1870)

Circular letter from the joint secretaries of the Extensionist Association, May 1873

Garrett, Dr Elizabeth, *An Enquiry into the Character of the Contagious Diseases Acts of 1866–69* (1870)

Gledstone, Rev. J.P., *Observations on the Recent Select Committee of the House of Commons* (1882)

Nevins, J. Birkbeck, *Statement on the Grounds Upon Which the Contagious Diseases Acts are Opposed, Addressed to the Rt. Hon. R.A. Cross, MP* (Liverpool, 1874)

Newman, F.W., *The Political Side of the Vaccination System* (1874)

—— *The Coming Revolution* (1882)

Shaen, William, *Suggestions on the Limits of Legitimate Legislation on the Subject of Prostitution* (delivered at the Geneva Congress, 1877)

—— *The Common Law in Its Relation to Personal Liberty and the State-Regulation of Vice* (delivered at the Geneva Congress, 1880)

Stansfeld, James, *On the Failure of the Contagious Diseases Acts as proved by the Official Evidence* (1881)

—— *Speech on the Contagious Diseases Acts* (1874)

Stuart, James, *The New Abolitionists: A Narrative of a Year's Work* (1876)

(f) Contemporary Biographies and Autobiographies

Butler, Josephine, *Recollections of George Butler* (Bristol, *c.* 1893)

—— *Personal Reminiscences of a Great Crusade* (1896)

Dyer, G.H., *Edmund Jones* (1879)
—— *Sir Wilfrid Lawson* (1878)
—— *Benjamin Lucraft* (1879)   all penny biographies
—— *William Lloyd Garrison* (1878)
Heath, H.J.B., *Margaret Bright Lucas. The Life Story of a 'British Woman'* (1890)
Stead, W.T. (?), 'Sir James Stansfeld: A Character Sketch', *Review of Reviews* (15 June 1895), pp. 504–21.
Stuart, James, *Reminiscenses* (1911)

(g) Other Contemporary Printed Sources

Acton, William, *Prostitution, Considered in its Moral, Social and Sanitary Aspects in London and Other Large Cities and garrison towns: With Proposals for the Mitigation and Prevention of Its Attendant Evils* (2nd edn 1870). Republished in Fitzroy edn, introduction by Peter Fryer (ed.) (1968).
Amos, Sheldon, *Laws for the Regulation of Vice* (1877)
Gregory, M., *The Crowning Crime of Christendom: with a Short History of the Society of Friends for its Abolition* (1896)
——*A Short Summary of the Parliamentary History of State Regulated Vice in the United Kingdom* (1900)
Jevons, W.S., *Methods of Social Reform* (1885)
Lecky, W.E.H., *History of European Morals from Augustus to Charlemagne* (1869), 10th edn (1892)
Scott, Benjamin, *A State Iniquity: Its Rise, Extension and Overthrow* (1890)
Wilson, H.J., *A Rough Record of Events and Incidents Connected the Repeal of the Contagious Diseases Acts* (Sheffield, 1907)

Secondary Sources

Unpublished Theses

Glaser, J.F., 'Nonconformity and Liberalism, 1868–1885. A Study in English Party History (unpublished PhD thesis, Harvard University, 1948)
Walkowitz, J.R., ' "We are not beasts of the Field": Prostitution and the Campaign Against the Contagious Diseases Acts, 1869–1886' (unpublished PhD thesis, Rochester University, 1974)
Ware, H.R.E., 'The Recruitment, Regulation and Role of Prostitution in Britain from the Middle of the Nineteenth Century to the Present Day' (unpublished PhD thesis, London University, 1969)

Books

Anderson, Mosa, *H.J. Wilson, Fighter for Freedom* (1953)

Armytage, W.H.G., *A.J. Mundella, 1825–1897, The Liberal Background to the Labour Movement* (1951)

Ausubel, H., *In Hard Times: Reformers among the Late Victorians* (New York, 1960)

Bahlman, D.W.R. (ed.), *The Diary of Sir Edward Hamilton* (Oxford, 1972)

Bamford, T.W., *The Rise of the Public Schools* (1967)

Banks, J.A. and O., *Feminism and Family Planning in Victorian England* (Liverpool, 1964)

Banks, J.A., *Prosperity and Parenthood* (1954)

Bassett, A. Tilney, *The Life of the Rt. Hon. John Edward Ellis, MP* (1914)

Beales, A.C.F., *The History of Peace* (1931)

Beales, Derek, *England and Italy, 1859–1860* (1961)

Bell, E. Moberly, *Josephine Butler, Flame of Fire* (1962)

Best, G., *Mid-Victorian Britain, 1851–1875* (1971)

Bevington, M.M., *The Saturday Review 1855–1865* (New York, 1941)

Bowen, D., *The Idea of the Victorian Church* (Montreal, 1968)

Branca, Patricia, *Women in Europe Since 1750* (1978)

Brand, Jeanne L., *Doctors and the State: The British Medical Profession and Government Action in Public Health, 1870–1912* (Baltimore, 1965)

Briggs, Asa, *The Age of Improvement* (1959)

Bristow, Edward J., *Vice and Vigilance: Purity Movements in Britain since 1700* (Dublin, 1978)

Burn, W.L., *The Age of Equipoise, A Study of the Mid-Victorian Generation* (1964)

Butler, A.S.G., *Portrait of Josephine Butler* (1954)

Chesney, Kellow, *The Victorian Underworld* (1970)

Cooke, A.B. and J. Vincent, *The Governing Passion: Cabinet Government and Party Politics in Britain, 1885–86* (Hassocks, 1974)

Cunningham, Hugh, *The Volunteer Force* (1975)

Davidson, J.M., *Eminent Radicals in and out of Parliament* (1880)

Evans, Richard J., *The Feminists* (1978)

Fawcett, Millicent Garrett, *What I Remember* (1924)

Fawcett, M.G. and E.M. Turner, *Josephine Butler: Her Work, Principles, and their meaning for the Twentieth Century* (1927)

Fowler, W.S., *A Study in Radicalism and Dissent: The Life and Times of Henry Joseph Wilson, 1833–1914* (1961)

French, R.D., *Antivivisection and Medical Science in Victorian Society* (Princeton, 1975)

Grisewood, H., *Ideas and beliefs of the Victorians* (1949)

Grosskurth, Phyllis, *John Addington Symonds* (1964)

Hamer, D.A., *Liberal Politics in the Age of Gladstone and Rosebery* (Oxford, 1972)

Hamer, D.A., *The Politics of Electoral Pressure: A Study in the History of Victorian Reform Agitations* (Hassocks, 1977)

Hammond, J.L., *Gladstone and the Irish Nation* (2nd edn, 1964)

Hammond, J.L. and B., *James Stansfeld: A Victorian Champion of Sex Equality* (1932)

Hanham, H.J., *Elections and Party Management: Politics in the Times of Disraeli and Gladstone* (1959)

Harries-Jenkins, G., *The Army in Victorian Society* (1977)

Harrison, Brian, *Drink and the Victorians: The Temperance Question in England, 1815–1872* (1971)

—— *Separate Spheres: The Opposition to Women's Suffrage in Britain* (1978)

Harrison, Royden, *Before the Socialists: Studies in Labour and Politics, 1861–1881* (1965)

Heyck, T.W., *The Dimensions of British Radicalism: The Case of Ireland 1874–1895* (Urbana, 1974)

Houghton, Walter, *The Victorian Frame of Mind, 1830–1870* (New Haven, 1957)

Humphrey, A.W., *Robert Applegarth: Trade Unionist, Educationalist, Reformer* (1913)

Isichei, Elizabeth, *Victorian Quakers* (Oxford, 1970)

Johnson, G.W. and L.A., *Josephine E. Butler: An Autobiographical Memoir* (Bristol, 1909)

Jones, Andrew, *The Politics of Reform: 1884* (Cambridge, 1972)

Kelly, C.H., *Memoirs* (1910)

Kamm, Josephine, *Rapiers and Battleaxes: The Women's Movement and Its Aftermath* (1966)

Kitson Clark, G., *The Making of Victorian England* (1962)

Koss, Stephen, *Nonconformity in Modern British Politics* (1975)

Lambert, Royston, *Sir John Simon, 1816–1904, and English Social Administration* (1963)

Lovell Cocks, H., *The Nonconformist Conscience* (1943)

Lloyd, C. and J.L.S. Coulter, *Medicine and the Navy, 1200–1900:*

Volume 4, 1815–1900 (Edinburgh and London, 1963)

Lloyd, T., *The General Election of 1880* (Oxford, 1968)

Lucy, Henry W., *Men and Manner in Parliament* (1919, 1st edn, 1874)

—— *A Diary of Two Parliaments. The Disraeli Parliament, 1874–1880* (1885)

—— *Sixty Years in the Wilderness* (1909)

Manton, Jo, *Elizabeth Garrett Anderson* (1965)

Marcus, Steven, *The Other Victorians* (New York, 1966)

Morton, R.S., *Venereal Diseases* (Harmondsworth, 1966)

Nield, Keith (ed.), *Prostitution in the Victorian Age* (1973)

Pearl, Cyril, *The Girl with the Swansdown Seat* (1955)

Pearsall, Ronald, *The Worm in the Bud* (1969)

Pelling, Henry, *Social Geography of British Elections* (London, 1967)

—— *Popular Politics and Society in Late-Victorian Britain* (1968)

Perkin, Harold, *The Origins of Modern English Society* (1969)

Petrie, Glen, *A Singular Iniquity: The Campaigns of Josephine Butler* (1971)

Remelson, Marion, *The Petticoat Rebellion* (1967)

Rasor, Eugene L., *Reform in the Royal Navy: A Society History of the Lower Deck 1850–1880* (Hamden, Conn, 1976)

Roberts, David, *Victorian Origins of the British Welfare State* (New Haven, 1960)

Rover, Constance, *Women's Suffrage and Party Politics in Britain, 1866–1914* (1967)

—— *Love, Morals and the Feminists* (1970

Rowbotham, Sheila, *Hidden from History: 300 Years of Women's Oppression and the Fight Against It* (1973)

Salter, F.R., *Dissenters and Public Affairs in Mid-Victorian England* (1967)

Shaen, M.J., *William Shaen: A Brief Sketch Edited by His Daughter* (1912)

Shannon, R.T., *Gladstone and the Bulgarian Agitation, 1876* (1963)

Sieveking, I.G., *Memoir and Letters of F.W. Newman* (1909)

Simey, Margaret, *Charitable Effort in Liverpool in the Nineteenth Century* (Liverpool, 1951)

Skelley, A. Ramsay, *The Victorian Army at Home: The Recruitment and Terms and Conditions of the British Regular, 1859–1899* (1977)

Smith, Paul, *Disraelian Conservatism and Social Reform* (1967)

Spender, J.A., *Life of Sir Henry Campbell-Bannerman G.C.B.* (1923)

Stocks, Mary, *Josephine Butler and the Moral Standards of Today* (1967)

Strachey, Ray, *The Cause: A Short History of the Women's Movement in Great Britain* (1928)

—— *Millicent Garrett Fawcett* (1931)

Temperley, Howard, *British Anti-Slavery, 1833–1870* (1972)

Thomas, J.A., *The House of Commons, 1832–1901. A Study of its Economical and Functional Character* (Cardiff, 1939)

Vincent, John, *The Formation of the British Liberal Party, 1857–1868* (1966)

Watkins, Owen Spencer, *Soldiers and Preachers Too* (1906)

Wainwright, D., *Liverpool Gentlemen* (1960)

Webb, R.K., *Harriet Martineau, a Radical Victorian* (1960)

Weston, Agnes, *My Life among the Bluejackets* (1909)

White, William, *The Inner Life of the House of Commons* (1897) 2 vols.

Woodham-Smith, C., *Florence Nightingale* (1950)

Zeldin, Theodore, *France 1848–1945*, vol. 1 (Oxford, 1973)

Articles

Annan, Noel, 'The Intellectual Aristocracy' in J.H. Plumb (ed.), *Studies in Social History* (1955)

Banks, J.A. and O., 'The Bradlaugh-Besant trial and the English Newspapers', *Population Studies* 8–9 (1954–6)

—— 'Feminism and Social Change' in G.K. Zollschan and W. Hirsch (eds.), *Explorations in Social Change* (1st edn, 1964)

Beales, H.L. and Edward Glover, 'Victorian Ideas of Sex' in H. Grisewood (ed.), *Ideas and Beliefs of the Victorians* (1949)

Beck, Ann F., 'Issues in the Anti-Vaccination Movement in England', *Medical History* 4 (1960)

Berrington, Hugh, 'Partisanship and Dissidence in the Nineteenth-Century House of Commons', *Parliamentary Affairs* 21 (1967–8)

Blanco, R.L., 'Attempted Control of Venereal Disease in the Army of Mid-Victorian England', *Journal of the Society for Army Historical Research* 45 (1967)

Bristow, Edward, 'The Liberty and Property Defence League and Individualism', *Historical Journal*, 18 (1975)

Cromwell, Valerie, 'Interpretations of Nineteenth-Century Administration: An Analysis', *Victorian Studies*, 9 (1966)

Buckley, Suzann, 'The Failure to Resolve the Problem of Venereal Disease Among the Troops in Britain During World War One' in B. Bond and I. Roy (eds.), *War and Society*, 2 (1977)

Cominos, Peter T., 'Late Victorian Sexual Respectability and the

Social System', *International Review of Social History*, 8 (1963)

Drus, Ethel (ed.), 'A Journal of Events During the Gladstone Ministry, 1868–1874, by John, first Earl of Kimberley', *Camden Miscellany*, 21 (1958)

Ellegard, Alvar, 'The Readership of the Periodical Press in Mid-Victorian Britain', *Goteborgs Universitets Arsskrift*, 63 (1957)

Evans, Richard J., 'Prostitution, State and Society in Imperial Germany', *Past and Present*, 70 (1976)

Glaser, John F., 'English Nonconformity and the Decline of Liberalism', *American Historical Review*, 63 (1958)

Gorham, Deborah, 'The Maiden-Tribute of Modern Babylon Re-examined; Child Prostituion and the Idea of Childhood in Late-Victorian England', *Victorian Studies*, 21 (1978)

Hanham, H.J., 'Religion and Nationality in the Mid-Victorian Army', in M.R.D. Foot (ed.), *War and Society* (1973)

Harrison, Brian, 'The Sunday Trading Riots of 1855', *Historical Journal*, 8 (1965)

—— 'Philanthropy and the Victorians', *Victorian Studies*, 9 (1966)

—— 'Underneath the Victorians', *Victorian Studies*, 10 (1966–7)

—— 'Religion and Recreation in Nineteenth-Century England', *Past and Present*, 38 (1967)

—— 'The British Prohibitionists' 1853–1872', *International Review of Social History*, 15 (1970)

—— 'Animals and the State in Nineteenth-Century England', *English Historical Review*, 88 (1973)

—— 'Josephine Butler' in J.F.C. Harrison, B. Taylor and I. Armstrong (eds.), *Eminently Victorian* (1974)

—— 'State Intervention and Moral Reform in Nineteenth-Century England' in P. Hollis (ed.), *Pressure from Without* (1974)

Harrison, B.H. and A.E. Dingle, 'Cardinal Manning as Temperance Reformer', *Historical Journal*, 12 (1969)

Heyck, T.W., 'British Radicals and Radicalism, 1874–1895: A Social Analysis' in R.J. Bezucha (ed.), *Modern European Social History* (1972)

Ingham, S.M., 'The Disestablishment Movement in England, 1868–1874', *Journal of Religious History*, 3 (1964)

Inglis, K.S., 'English Nonconformity and Social Reform, 1800–1900', *Past and Present*, 13 (1958)

Kent, John, 'Hugh Price Hughes and the Nonconformist Conscience' in G.V. Bennett and J.D. Walsh (eds.), *Essays in Modern Church History* (1966)

Lowell, A.L., 'The Influence of Party upon Legislation in England and America', *Annual Report of the American Historical Association 1901*, Part 2 (Washington 1902)

L'Esperance, Jean, 'The Work of the Ladies' National Association for the Repeal of the Contagious Diseases Acts', *Bulletin of the Society for the Study of Labour History*, 26 (1973)

—— 'Doctors and Women in Nineteenth-Century Society: Sexuality and Role' in J. Woodward and D. Richards (Eds.), *Health Care and Popular Medicine in Nineteenth-Century England* (1977)

McCrone, Kathleen E., 'The Assertion of Women's Rights in Mid-Victorian England', *HIstorical Papers (Canadian Historical Association)* (1972)

McLaren, Angus, 'Women's Work and Regulation of Family Size: The Question of Abortion in the Nineteenth Century', *History Workshop Journal*, 4 (1977)

MacLeod, Roy M., 'Medico-Legal Issues in Victorian Medical Care', *Medical History*, 10 (1966)

—— 'The Frustration of State Medicine, 1880–1899', *Medical History*, 11 (1967)

—— 'Law, Medicine and Public Opinion: The Resistance to Compulsory Health Legislation, 1870–1907', *Public Law* (Summer-Autumn 1967)

Neilans, Alison, 'Changes in Sex Morality' in R. Strachey (ed.), *Our Freedom and Its Results* (1936)

Post, J.B., 'A Foreign Office Survey of Venereal Disease and Prostitution Control, 1869–70', *Medical History*, 22 (1978)

Ramelson, Marion, 'The Fight Against the Contagious Diseases Acts', *Marxism Today* (June 1964)

Rodgers, Brian, 'The Social Science Association, 1857–1886', *The Manchester School of Economic and Social Studies*, 20 (1952)

Shiman, Lillian L., 'The Band of Hope Movement: Respectable Recreation for Working-Class Children', *Victorian Studies*, 17 (1973–4)

Sigsworth, E.M. and T.J. Wyke, 'A Study of Victorian Prostitution and Venereal Disease' in M. Vicinus (ed.), *Suffer and Be Still* (Bloomington, 1972)

Smith, F.B., 'Ethics and Disease in the later-Nineteenth Century: The Contagious Diseases Acts', *Historical Studies* (University of Melbourne), 15 (1971)

—— 'Sexuality in Britain, 1800–1900', *University of Newcastle (NSW) Historical Journal*, 2 (1974)

Smith, F.B., 'Labouchere's Amendment to the Criminal Law Amendment Bill', *Historical Studies*, 17 (1976)

Stedman Jones, Gareth, 'Working-Class Culture and Working-Class Politics in London 1870–1900: Notes on the Remaking of the Working-Class', *Journal of Social History*, 7 (1974)

Thomas, Keith, 'The Double Standard', *Journal of the History of Ideas*, 20 (1959)

Thompson, David, 'The Liberation Society, 1844–1868' in P. Hollis (ed.), *Pressure from Without* (1974)

Walkowitz, J.R. and D.J. ' "We are not beasts of the field". Prostitution and the Poor in Plymouth and Southampton under the Contagious Diseases Acts', *Feminist Studies* (1974)

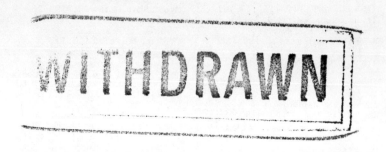